International Best Practices for Evaluation in the Health Professions

Edited by
WILLIAM C. MCGAGHIE, PHD
Jacob R. Suker, MD, Professor of Medical Education,
Professor of Preventive Medicine, Center for Education in Medicine,
Northwestern University Feinberg School of Medicine, Chicago, IL

Editorial Assistance by
MADELINE M. HINKAMP

Foreword by
RONALD M. HARDEN

Radcliffe Publishing
London • New York

Radcliffe Publishing Ltd
33–41 Dallington Street
London
EC1V 0BB
United Kingdom

www.radcliffehealth.com

British Library Cataloguing in Publication Data

A catalogue record for this book is available from the British Library.

ISBN-13: 978 184619 515 0

Typeset by Darkriver Design, Auckland, New Zealand
Printed and bound by Cadmus Communications, USA

Contents

Contents

Foreword by Ronald M. Harden

THIS IS A BOOK ABOUT ASSESSMENT OF STUDENTS AND PRACTITIONERS in the health professions: it looks at assessment from a number of perspectives. Without doubt, the assessment of competence is one of the most important responsibilities for all engaged in health professions education. It provides a clear statement as to what we value and care about, it defines what is regarded as important, and it exerts a powerful influence on students' behavior and styles of learning. Carried out inappropriately, assessment can have a negative effect and can even undermine rather than underpin the process of learning. If carried out effectively, however, assessment can exert a major influence on the curriculum and can reassure the public that the practitioner responsible for their management has the necessary knowledge, skills, and attitudes.

In curriculum planning, attention is often focused on the expected learning outcomes and the prescribed content, the educational strategies to be promoted, and the teaching and learning methods to be adopted, including the use of the new learning technologies. Assessment, unfortunately, is sometimes an afterthought and fails to receive the necessary attention, with the almost inevitable result that it is done badly or at least not as well as it should be. The fact that assessment can drive both the curriculum and the concept of assessment-led innovation is not sufficiently well recognized. Moreover, assessment is a complex subject and decisions relating to assessment represent some of the most difficult challenges facing medical education. Teachers, educationists, psychometricians, content experts, and technologists all have a contribution to make. This book synthesizes from these different viewpoints answers to common assessment challenges. It reviews traditional practices and new approaches and highlights the major developments in the field over recent decades.

In June 1985, an international conference organized by Ian Hart and Ronald Harden on the topic of assessment of clinical competence was held in Ottawa, Canada, to facilitate the sharing of views and experiences from different countries. Recognizing the importance of assessment for health care delivery, Jake Epp, then minister of National Health and Welfare of Canada, in opening the ceremony, said, "It is my hope that this meeting will encourage the development of international standards of medical education which will lead to further improvements in health care and health care delivery around the world." [A paraphrase of this statement was published later.[1]] Since then, on alternate years, conferences with this aim have been held in major cities around the world. These have provided updates and reviews of established techniques in assessment and have explored exciting new developments and methodologies. The fourteenth Ottawa conference, held in Miami in 2010, examined what was considered to be good practice for assessment in the health professions. Working groups produced position papers that served as a basis for discussion and debate at the conference. Six chapters in this book highlight some of the key recommendations that resulted from the process. Other chapters address important topics on today's agenda such as assessment of teamwork, assessment of leadership skills, and assessment in continuing education and recertification. Bill McGaghie is to be congratulated on putting together in one volume what must be the most definitive guide available today on the assessment of competence in the health professions.

Six key questions are addressed across the chapters in the context of a testing and assessment scene that is changing rapidly. *What should be assessed? How should it be assessed? Why should it be assessed? When should it be assessed? Who should carry out the assessment? Where should assessment take place?* A consideration of the answers to these questions will without doubt improve the standard of assessment practice and medical education.

Key to any discussion about assessment is a consideration of *what should be assessed*. It has been asserted that the most important development in medical education in the past 4 decades has been the move to outcome- or competency-based education, where the product or learning outcomes are viewed as more important than the process or method of getting there. Implicit in outcome-based education is that there is a system of assessment in place that guarantees that learners have achieved the expected learning outcomes and that the practicing doctor has the necessary competencies. Frameworks for looking at assessment in terms of what is assessed, including Miller's pyramid, Kirkpatrick's four-level scheme, and the T1–T3 model, are presented eloquently in different chapters of this book.

Few would disagree that too much attention has been paid in the past to the bottom level of Miller's pyramid and to assessment of the acquisition and recall of knowledge, often using multiple-choice questions (MCQs). The ability to answer correctly a set of MCQs, however, does not necessarily guarantee a good doctor. The outcome-based education movement has focused attention on the assessment of a wider range of competencies including clinical and communication skills, professionalism, teamwork, and leadership skills. Some of these competencies are the focus of specific chapters in this book. The discussion on the assessment of professionalism in Chapter 8 recognizes that there is, at present, no unified consensus as to what signifies professionalism, given the different ways in which the phenomenon is understood. Professionalism may vary across cultures and consequently the assessment will vary. While it is not in dispute that the professional behavior of students and practitioners should be assessed, we have still to establish the elements that constitute appropriate professional behavior and how these elements should be assessed. There is also a need for a consensus model that describes the teamwork competencies to be acquired and assessed at the different stages in the curriculum. Teamwork is critical to safe and effective health care delivery, and competence in this area must be assessed. Teamwork assessment, as described in Chapter 9, may be somewhat messy, requiring the assessment of knowledge, skills, and abilities that underlie effective cooperation.

In addressing the question *"How should it be assessed?"* the chapters in this book highlight that there is no single magic bullet. One assessment methodology does not fit all purposes and is likely to be more effective at assessing some learning outcomes than others. The authors in the different chapters argue for a more authentic approach to assessment with greater use made of tools such as the objective structured clinical examination (OSCE), the mini-clinical evaluation exercise, case-based discussion, the objective structured long case examination record, and the use of portfolios for assessment purposes. As discussed in Chapters 3 and 13, the application of technologies to assessment can broaden the competencies to be assessed and have far-reaching consequences for assessment. With appropriate technology, patient outcome data can be linked to the assessment of practical performance.

Much of the work on assessment in the United Kingdom in the 1970s was around the use of the OSCE, which, as described in Chapter 6, became the gold standard for performance assessment. Issues such as the psychometrics and reliability of the examination have, to a much greater extent, determined the choice of assessment approach in North America, with MCQs dominating the assessment scene. Despite the recent emphasis on performance assessment, MCQs still have a role to play and can contribute to the overall assessment of competency, as described in Chapter 7.

Just as important as the method selected from the examiner's tool kit is how the approach is introduced in practice. Is the method implemented fairly with individuals evaluated accurately, and the scoring rules applied consistently? Is the method practical and cost-effective? Does it yield sufficiently precise measures of achievement? Will it allow the examiner to make justifiable inferences concerning the learning outcomes that are being assessed? These key issues and questions are addressed in Chapter 2 and the principles proposed for good assessment can be applied to whatever method of assessment is adopted.

Various chapters in this book provide answers to the question, "*Why should we assess the learner?*" The traditional aim for assessment, passing or failing a student or determining whether a doctor has the necessary competence to practice, remains a key function and is in line with the demand for greater transparency and accountability in medical education. Issues relating to the recertification of the physician are considered in Chapter 13, with a description of what is described as "best practice" around the world involving both a legislatively led top-down and a professionally led bottom-up approach. Illustrated in Chapter 12 and throughout the book are the other important purposes that assessment can serve. Among these is the provision of feedback to the learner. It is suggested that a major flaw with traditional assessment is its narrow focus on a test without equal attention being paid to formative assessment to improve learning. We see today a move from thinking of assessment as "assessment of learning" to "assessment for learning" and "assessment as learning," where assessment is incorporated as a powerful tool in the learning process.

The question "*When should students be assessed?*" also merits consideration. As highlighted in Chapter 9, the right frequency of assessment and the specific timing depends on issues such as the purpose and method of assessment. Students can be assessed at the beginning of, during, and at the end of a course of study. Frequent assessment is required for the purposes of feedback. A key challenge is the assessment of students before their admission to medical studies. Developments in this area are reviewed in Chapter 5, including a move from reliance on estimates of academic achievement. The importance of considering other abilities and attitudes is now recognized, and instruments such as the multiple mini-interview, a modified OSCE approach, have been adopted.

Important issues need to be addressed in relation to *who should carry out the assessment*. Should a central national organization, such as the National Board of Medical Examiners in the United States, be charged with the responsibility, or should it be left to individual schools supervised by a national accrediting body, such as the General Medical Council in the United Kingdom? The need to assess student competence in a range of learning outcomes over time using direct measures of their performance inevitably places more responsibility on the school where the student is studying and the teachers in the school rather than on a central national body. Within a school, the use of peer assessment is attracting increasing interest, and some areas such as assessment of professionalism can offer insights not readily obtained from other methods. Self-assessment, while notoriously unreliable, also has an important role to play, with self-assessment skills recognized as an important learning outcome. This is reflected in the definition of a professional as someone who is an enquirer into his or her own competence.

The question *"Where should assessment take place?"* has been the subject of much recent interest. Assessment in the workplace rather than in the classroom, as described in Chapter 12, can apply not just to the practicing doctor but also to students. It implies direct observation of performance conducted in the workplace. This may be important because doctors are known to perform differently in the controlled setting of a clinical performance examination than in a real work setting. The variety of performance that is likely to be observed in the context of the workplace is likely to be different than in the classroom or simulated setting.

Given current thinking and developments in the field of assessment, to what extent do we need to reshape our current practices? This book will help to provide some of the answers. The contributors highlight that assessment has to be an integral part of medical education: it does not exist in isolation and it must be closely aligned with the curriculum, the learning outcomes, and the learning experience. This book paints a broad picture of assessment in terms of the abilities expected of a doctor rather than presenting a more traditional approach where the emphasis is on measures of academic achievement. For these reasons alone this book merits close study. Other strong messages include the importance of quality control and the recognition that bad examiners can be as serious a problem as bad examinations. Too often in the past, for the examinee, the examination may have been like playing a game of tennis blindfolded, with the opponent, the examiner, also being the umpire and the only person who knows the rules, and changing the rules every game. Hopefully things are different today and poor assessment practice, due to a culture of ignorance in those responsible, to insufficient allocation of resources, or to a lack of attention to detail in implementation, will become a thing of the past. This book should encourage all those engaged with medical education to attach to assessment in their schools or organizations the importance required. This book offers an insight into what is now regarded as good practice in the area. It addresses the factors governing the choice of the appropriate tool in different contexts to assess different outcomes and provides ground rules as to how the tools are best employed. This book provides good examples of how assessment can be used to take into account new goals for the curriculum such as professionalism, teamwork, and leadership skills and to drive the curriculum in the desired direction.

This book, with its international contributors, recognizes that assessment practices may differ around the world and in different contexts. The terms "assessment" and "evaluation," for example, are used differently on the two sides of the Atlantic. In the United Kingdom, emphasis has been placed on validity and on the assessment of clinical skills; in the United States, there is an emphasis on psychometrics and written assessment. Some of the cross-cultural differences with regard to assessment around the world are described in Chapter 11.

As highlighted by Bill McGaghie in the first chapter, assessment practice in the health care profession has come a long way in the last century. This book is written in the belief that a better understanding of these developments and of assessment principles and concepts and tools and technologies can help medical education to respond to the challenges of the next century. This book is important because it can help set the agenda for future developments in assessment, not only of students and doctors but also, as described in Chapters 14 and 15, of the educational program as a whole. The challenge for assessment will be to meet the needs of different stakeholders: on the one hand, the legitimate demands of government and the public for improved standards and accountability and for assessment that encapsulates the range of learning outcomes and competencies expected of the doctor at various stages in their training; on the other hand, the demands from teachers and students for assessment to be integrated as part of the curriculum and as part of the learning process.

Reference

1. Epp J. Achieving health for all: a framework for health promotion. *Health Promot Int.* 1986; **1**(4): 419–28.

Ronald M. Harden
AMEE General Secretary
Editor of *Medical Teacher*
Emeritus Professor of Medical Education
University of Dundee, UK
Professor of Medical Education
Al-Imam University, Riyadh, Kingdom of Saudi Arabia
September 2012

Preface

THIS IS A BOOK FOR EDUCATORS IN THE HEALTH PROFESSIONS, WORLD-wide. Health professions educators are individuals, teams, and administrative champions who are responsible for teaching others to deliver health care to persons in need. Evaluation is a key feature of health professions education. Evaluation informs educators about the readiness of learners to receive instruction, gauges learner progress toward educational goals, and judges whether learners have achieved competency outcome standards. Health professions educators need rigorous evaluation to be effective. This book addresses current evaluation *best practices* in the health professions to identify today's evaluation benchmarks, reveal evaluation limits, address improvement pathways, and map a research agenda to boost future evaluation practices.

The audience for *International Best Practices for Evaluation in the Health Professions* is both broad and deep. The professions and occupational groups who provide health care services around the world—human medicine, nursing, dentistry, midwifery, physiotherapy, clinical psychology, veterinary medicine, and many others—shape audience breadth. The duration and quality of experience that defines the status quo of professional practice—today's competency criteria and expectations for individuals and teams, codes of professional conduct, interdisciplinary rules, and ethical standards—govern audience depth. The audience is also formed by variation in country and culture, because methods of health professions practice and education are not uniform worldwide. The contributors to this book know that cultural differences are real and present but also that these differences can be bridged. *International Best Practices for Evaluation in the Health Professions* aims to provide such a span.

This book is unique because it presents a comprehensive narrative about why and how we need to evaluate health professions students for practice in the twenty-first century. Advancements in information and communication technology, bioscience and behavioral research, and worldwide travel are dissolving barriers that have separated professions, countries, and cultures for centuries. *International Best Practices for Evaluation in the Health Professions* both celebrates these achievements and recognizes next steps temperately. This book recognizes the huge improvements that have been made in evaluation practices within the health professions over the past 40 years but also asks for more. It calls for added reform as the international health professions community studies and better understands current practice from different social, cultural, and educational perspectives; values cross-professional programs that span boundaries; and acknowledges the authority of the future rather than historical baggage.

This book originates in part from the fourteenth Ottawa Conference on Evaluation in the Health Professions, held in Miami, Florida, in the United States during May 2010. Planning for that conference involved the formation of six consensus groups of international experts. The international consensus groups were challenged to write state-of-the-art summary reports about evaluation best practices in the health professions. The 2010 Ottawa Conference consensus group reports addressed the following topics:

- Criteria for a good assessment (Chairperson: John Norcini, United States)
- Technology-based assessment (Chairperson: Zubair Amin, Singapore)
- Performance assessment (Chairperson: Katharine Boursicot, United Kingdom)
- Assessment of professionalism (Chairperson: Brian Hodges, Canada)
- Assessment for selection for the health care professions and specialty training (Chairperson: David Prideaux, Australia)
- Research in assessment (Chairperson: Lambert Schuwirth, the Netherlands).

The 2010 Ottawa Conference consensus group reports were published as six journal articles during 2011 in *Medical Teacher* (Vol. 33, Nos. 3 and 5). Three of these journal articles are reprinted verbatim as chapters in this book with permission from the copyright holder, Informa Healthcare. The reprinted materials are Technology-Enabled Assessment of Health Professions Education (Chapter 3), Assessment for Selection for the Health Care Professions and Specialty Training (Chapter 5), and Clinical Competence Assessment (formerly Performance in Assessment) (Chapter 6).

Several of the 2010 Ottawa Conference consensus group reports inspired preparation of new and different manuscripts that are presented as chapters in this book. These chapters are Criteria for a Good Assessment (Chapter 2), Research on Assessment Practices (Chapter 4), and Assessment of Professionalism (Chapter 8).

This book is organized to tell the story of *International Best Practices for Evaluation in the Health Professions* as a straightforward, compelling narrative. It begins with a short statement about the history and current practice in the field and proceeds with state-of-the-art scholarly chapters on assessment criteria, technology-enabled assessment, and research on assessment practices. Scholarship and professional practice are united in the next four chapters covering assessment for selection and specialty training, clinical competence assessment, evaluation of knowledge acquisition, and assessment of professionalism. The book continues by breaking new ground in scholarship and practice from chapters that address measuring health care team performance; evaluating outcomes in continuing education and training; culture, medical education, and assessment; and workplace-based assessment. International policy and organizational issues shaped by evaluation are covered by chapters on recertification and revalidation of physicians, evaluation of health professions leadership and management, and evaluation for program and school accreditation. This book concludes with a visionary look to the future.

The authors and the editor of this book wish to acknowledge key contributors to the volume whose names do not appear on the masthead. They include the biannual Ottawa Conference and its sponsors; the Michael S. Gordon Center for Research in Medical Education at the University of Miami Miller School of Medicine; the Jacob R. Suker, MD, professorship in medical education at the Northwestern University Feinberg School of Medicine; and the Ottawa Conference's Founders, Ian Hart and Ronald Harden. Each of these contributors provided professional resources that enabled production of this volume.

Finally, I am indebted to Madeline M. Hinkamp who provided editorial assistance in the later stages of book production.

William C. McGaghie, PhD
Chicago, IL
September 2012

About the Editor

Dr. McGaghie is the Jacob R. Suker, MD, Professor of Medical Education and Professor of Preventive Medicine at the Northwestern University Feinberg School of Medicine in Chicago, Illinois, where he has served since 1992. Dr. McGaghie's research and writing in medical education and preventive medicine ranges widely, including such topics as personnel and program evaluation, research methodology, medical simulations, attitude measurement, medical student selection, concept mapping, curriculum development, faculty development, standardized patients, and geriatrics. Dr. McGaghie has authored or edited eight books and has published more than 250 journal articles, textbook chapters, and book reviews in health professions education, simulation-based education, preventive medicine, and related fields.

List of Contributors

Zubair Amin, MBBS, MHPE, Associate Professor, Department of Paediatrics, Yong Loo Lin School of Medicine, National University of Singapore and Senior Consultant, Department of Neonatology, National University Hospital, Singapore

Barbara Barzansky, PhD, MHPE, Co-Secretary, Liaison Committee on Medical Education, American Medical Association, Chicago, IL, USA

Taylor E. Berens, BS, Graduate Assistant, Department of Psychology, University of Maryland Baltimore County, Baltimore, MD, USA

John R. Boulet, PhD, Associate Vice President, Research and Data Resources, Foundation for Advancement of International Medical Education and Research, Philadelphia, PA, USA

Katharine Boursicot, BSc, MBBS, MRCOG, MAHPE, FHEA, Reader in Medical Education and Head of Assessment, Division of Population Health Sciences and Education, St. George's, University of London, London, UK

Vanessa Burch, MBBCh, MMed, PhD, FCP, FRCP, Professor and Chair of Clinical Medicine, Department of Medicine, Faculty of Health Sciences, University of Cape Town and Groote Schuur Hospital, Cape Town, South Africa

Nick Busing, MD, President, Association of Faculties of Medicine of Canada, Ottawa, ON, Canada

Francisco Eduardo de Campos, MD, MPH, PhD, Professor of Public Health, Federal University of Minas Gerais, Belo Horizonte, Brazil; Board Member of the Global Health Workforce Alliance, Geneva, Switzerland; Executive Secretary to the Open University of Brazil's Unique National Health System (UNASUS), Brasilia, Brazil

Henry de Holanda Campos, MD, MSc, PhD, Professor of Internal Medicine, Vice-Rector, Federal University of Ceará, Fortaleza, Brazil; Director, FAIMER Brazil Regional Institute of Education for the Health Professions, Fortaleza, Brazil

Angel Centeno, MD, PhD, Professor and Director, Department of Biomedical Education, Faculty of Biomedical Sciences, Austral University, Buenos Aires, Argentina

Jerry Colliver, PhD, Professor, Statistics and Research Consulting, Southern Illinois University School of Medicine, Springfield, IL, USA

David A. Cook, MD, MHPE, Professor of Medicine, Professor of Medical Education, and Director, Office of Education Research, College of Medicine, Mayo Clinic, Rochester, MN, USA

W. Dale Dauphinee, MD, FRCPC, FCAHS, Senior Scientist and Senior Mentor, Foundation for the Advancement of International Medical Education and Research, Philadelphia PA, USA; Adjunct Professor, Division of Clinical Epidemiology, Department of Medicine, McGill University, Montreal, QC, Canada

David A. Davis, MD, CCFP, FCFP, FRCPC (Hon), Senior Director, Continuing Education and Performance Improvement, Association of American Medical Colleges, Washington, DC, USA; Adjunct Professor, Family and Community Medicine, and Health Policy, Management and Evaluation, University of Toronto, Toronto, ON, Canada

Rachel Ellaway, PhD, Assistant Dean Curriculum and Planning, Associate Professor, Northern Ontario School of Medicine, Sudbury, ON, Canada

Luci Etheridge, MBChB, MRCPaeds, Clinical Academic Teaching Fellow, University College London, London, UK

Kevin Eva, PhD, Senior Scientist, Centre for Health Education Scholarship, Associate Professor and Director, Educational Research and Scholarship, Department of Medicine, University of British Columbia, Vancouver, BC, Canada

Ahmad Fahal, MBBS, FRCS, Professor of Surgery, University of Khartoum, Sudan

Moshe Feldman, PhD, Assistant Professor, Office of Assessment and Evaluation, Virginia Commonwealth University School of Medicine, Richmond, VA, USA

Stacey Friedman, PhD, Associate Director for Evaluation and Planning, Foundation for Advancement of International Medical Education and Research, Philadelphia, PA, USA

Shiphra Ginsburg, MD, MEd, Associate Professor of Medicine and Scientist, Wilson Centre for Research in Education, Faculty of Medicine, University of Toronto, Toronto, ON, Canada

Larry Gruppen, PhD, Josiah Macy Jr. Professor of Medical Education, Chair, Department of Medical Education, University of Michigan Medical School, Ann Arbor, MI, USA

Ana Estela Haddad, DDS, MSc, PhD, Professor, Faculty of Dentistry,

University of São Paulo, São Paulo, Brazil; Program Director, Secretariat of Labor Management and Health Education, Ministry of Health, Brasilia, Brazil

Ronald M. Harden, AMEE General Secretary, Editor of *Medical Teacher*, Emeritus Professor of Medical Education, University of Dundee, UK and Professor of Medical Education at Al-Imam University, Riyadh, Kingdom of Saudi Arabia

Madeline M. Hinkamp, BA, Feinberg Academy of Medical Educators Research Fellow, Center for Education in Medicine, Northwestern University Feinberg School of Medicine, Chicago, IL, USA

Brian David Hodges, MD, PhD, FRCPC, Vice President, University Health Network, Richard and Elizabeth Currie Chair in Health Professions Education Research, Professor of Psychiatry, Faculty of Medicine, and Scientist, Wilson Centre for Research in Education, University of Toronto, Toronto, ON, Canada

Dan Hunt, MD, MBA, Co-Secretary, Liaison Committee on Medical Education, Association of American Medical Colleges, Washington, DC, USA

S. Barry Issenberg, MD, FACP, Michael S. Gordon Professor of Medicine and Director; Associate Dean, Research in Medical Education, Michael S. Gordon Center for Research in Medical Education, University of Miami Miller School of Medicine, Miami, FL, USA

Dorthea Juul, PhD, Vice President, Research and Development, American Board of Psychiatry and Neurology, Inc., Buffalo Grove, IL, USA

Jean Ker, MRCGP, Director of Clinical Skills Center, University of Dundee, Dundee, Scotland, UK

Roger Kneebone, PhD, FRCS, FRCSEd, FRCGP, Professor of Surgical Education, Department of Surgery and Cancer, Imperial College, London, UK

Clarence Kreiter, PhD, Professor, Office of Consultation and Research in Medical Education and Department of Family Medicine, University of Iowa Carver College of Medicine, Iowa City, IA, USA

Enoch Kwizera, MB ChB, MSc, PhD, ACCP, Professor and Head of Department of Pharmacology, Faculty of Health Sciences, Walter Sisulu University, Mthatha, South Africa

Moira Maley, PhD, Associate Professor of Medical Education (Technology), Rural Clinical School of Western Australia (Albany), Faculty of Medicine, Dentistry and Health Science, The University of Western Australia, Perth, Western Australia, Australia

Paul E. Mazmanian, PhD, Associate Dean, Assessment and Evaluation Studies, School of Medicine, Virginia Commonwealth University (VCU) and Director of Evaluation, VCU Center for Clinical and Translational Research, Richmond, VA, USA

Peter McCrorie, PhD, Professor of Medical Education, St. George's, University of London, London, UK

William C. McGaghie, PhD, Jacob R. Suker, MD, Professor of Medical Education, Professor of Preventive Medicine, Center for Education in Medicine, Northwestern University Feinberg School of Medicine, Chicago, IL, USA

Danette W. McKinley, PhD, Director, Research and Data Resources, Foundation for Advancement of International Medical Education and Research, Philadelphia, PA, USA

Chris McManus, FMedSci, Professor of Psychology and Medical Education, Research Department of Clinical, Educational and Health Psychology, University College of London, London, UK

Stewart Mennin, PhD, Professor Emeritus, Department of Cell Biology and Physiology, Assistant Dean Emeritus, Educational Development and Research, University of New Mexico School of Medicine, Albuquerque, NM, USA (current residence: São Paulo, Brazil)

Page S. Morahan, PhD, Professor, Drexel University College of Medicine, Co-Director, Foundation for Advancement of International Medical Education and Research, Philadelphia, PA, USA

John J. Norcini, PhD, President and CEO, Foundation for Advancement of International Medical Education and Research (FAIMER), Philadelphia, PA, USA

Hirotaka Onishi, MD, MHPE, International Research Center for Medical Education, University of Tokyo, Tokyo, Japan

Doris Østergaard, MD, DMSc, MHPE, Associate Professor, Danish Institute for Medical Simulation, Herlev Hospital, Capital Region of Denmark and Copenhagen University, Copenhagen, Denmark

Louis Pangaro, MD, MACP, Professor and Chair, Department of Medicine, F. Edward Hebert School of Medicine, Uniformed Services University of the Health Sciences, Bethesda, MD, USA

Fiona Patterson, PhD, Professor of Psychology, University of Cambridge and Work Psychology Group, Cambridge, UK

Gominda Ponnamperuma, PhD, Senior Lecturer in Medical Education, Centre for Medical Education Development and Research Centre, Faculty of Medicine, University of Colombo, Colombo, Sri Lanka

David Powis, PhD, Conjoint Professor in the School of Psychology, University of Newcastle, Newcastle, New South Wales, Australia

David Prideaux, PhD, Emeritus Professor of Medical Education, Health Professional Education, School of Medicine, Flinders University, Adelaide, South Australia, Australia

Charlotte Ringsted, MD, MHPE, PhD, Professor of Medical Education and Director, Centre for Clinical Education, University of Copenhagen and Capital Region, Copenhagen, Denmark

Chris Roberts, MBBS, PhD, Associate Professor and Director of Community Engaged Learning and Teaching, Office of the Deputy Vice Chancellor (Education), University of Sydney, Sydney, New South Wales, Australia

Michael A. Rosen, PhD, Assistant Professor, Armstrong Institute for Patient Safety and Quality, Department of Anesthesiology and Critical Care Medicine, The Johns Hopkins University School of Medicine, Baltimore, MD, USA

Eduardo Salas, PhD, Pegasus and Trustee Chair Professor, Department of Psychology, Institute for Simulation and Training, University of Central Florida, Orlando, FL, USA

Elango Sambandam, FACS, Associate Director, Center for Medical Education, International Medical University, Kuala Lumpur, Malaysia

Lambert Schuwirth, MD, PhD, Professor of Medical Education, Flinders Innovation in Clinical Education, Flinders University, Adelaide, Australia and Professor for Innovative Assessment, Department of Educational Development and Research, Faculty of Health, Medicine, and Life Sciences, Maastricht, the Netherlands

Zeryab Setna, MRCOG, Clinical Academic Teaching Fellow, University College London, London, UK

Tejinder Singh, MD, MSc HPE, Program Director, CMCL-FAIMER Regional Institute, Professor of Paediatrics and Vice Principal, Christian Medical College, Ludhiana, India

Sydney Smee, PhD, Medical Council of Canada, Ottawa, ON, Canada

Rita Sood, MBBS, MD, MMEd, FRCP, Professor, Department of Medicine, All India Institute of Medical Sciences, New Delhi, India

Alison Sturrock, MRCP, Senior Lecturer, University College London, London, UK

David Swanson, PhD, Vice President for Program Development and Special Projects, National Board of Medical Examiners, Philadelphia, PA, USA

Ara Tekian, PhD, MHPE, Associate Professor of Medical Education, Department of Medical Education, and Associate Dean of International Affairs, University of Illinois at Chicago College of Medicine, Chicago, IL, USA

Luiz E. A. Troncon, MD, PhD, Full Professor of Internal Medicine, Ribeirão Preto Faculty of Medicine, University of São Paulo, São Paulo, Brazil

Cees van der Vleuten, PhD, Professor of Education, Director, School of Health Professions Education, Chair, Department of Educational Development and Research, Faculty of Health, Medicine and Life Sciences, Maastricht University, Maastricht, the Netherlands

Michaela Wagner, Mag. Dr., Medical University of Vienna, Department of Medical Education, Vienna, Austria

Andy Wearn, MMedSc, MRCGP, Associate Professor and Director, Clinical Skills Centre, Faculty of Medical and Health Sciences, The University of Auckland, Auckland, New Zealand

Sallie J. Weaver, PhD, Assistant Professor, Armstrong Institute for Patient Safety and Quality, Department of Anesthesiology and Critical Care Medicine, The Johns Hopkins University School of Medicine, Baltimore, MD, USA

Angela P. Wetzel, PhD, Director of Assessment, Department of Foundations of Education, Virginia Commonwealth University School of Education, Richmond, VA, USA

David Wilkinson, MD, PhD, Dean of Medicine, School of Medicine, University of Queensland, Brisbane, Queensland, Australia

Amitai Ziv, MD, MHA, Clinical Associate Professor and Chairman, Medical Education Department, Sackler Medical School, Tel-Aviv University, Israel; Deputy Director, Chaim Sheba Medical Center and Director, Department of Patient Safety and Risk Management; Director, Israel Center for Medical Simulation (MSR), Chaim Sheba Medical Center, Tel Hashomer, Israel

This book is dedicated to the memory of four
pioneers in the field of health professions
education: Howard S. Barrows, Miriam Friedman,
Christine H. McGuire, and George E. Miller.

We stand on the shoulders of giants.

Evaluation in the Health Professions

History and Current Practice

William C. McGaghie

THE IDEA THAT PROFESSIONALS SHOULD BE EVALUATED BEFORE starting practice and throughout their careers is not new. The historical record teaches that ancient Chinese civil service examinations were established during the Han dynasty (206 BCE–220 CE) to recruit and empower men on grounds of merit rather than on the basis of family or political connections.[1] Ability and virtue, grounded in Confucian philosophy, were valued and assessed. This examination system was later credited as an important means of holding the country together and has been called "one of the most successful political devices ever invented by man."[2] The Chinese civil service examination system was prescient. It set the ideological stage for professional evaluation practices for centuries.

Recent scholars have noted:

> As far as we know, the oldest application of testing for licensure in the Western World was in the field of medicine. In the early 700s, following a physician error that had resulted in the death of a member of the Court, the Caliph of Baghdad decreed that physicians practicing in his Court be examined regularly. In the mid 900s King Roger of Sicily instituted a similar practice, and from there the requirement spread slowly through Europe for physicians attending powerful people.[3]

The Western medical profession advanced slowly through the Middle Ages from Alexandria in Egypt to European hubs in Padua, Vienna, Berlin, Paris, London, Amsterdam, and elsewhere.[4] Evaluation of physicians about their fitness for professional practice also advanced slowly, chiefly through a system of European guilds that controlled professional access, prestige, and compensation. Assessment of doctors' readiness for professional practice became more systematic as technology and ideas about social accountability evolved from the Enlightenment. Competence evaluation for the medical profession has historical precedent. The by-laws of the Royal College of Physicians (1693) state:

> Before anyone be admitted either into the Order of the Fellows or Candidates, let him be examined thrice in lawful Meetings, whether greater or lesser, according to the pleasure of the President and Censors...
>
> Let the form of the examination be after this manner.
>
> First, let him be examined in the Physiologic part, and the very rudiments of Medicine...
>
> Secondly, let him be examined in the Pathologic part, or concerning the causes, differences, symptoms, and signs of diseases, which physicians make use of to know the essence of diseases...
>
> Thirdly, let him be examined concerning the use and exercise of medicine, or the reason of healing.[5]

This sequential, three-part format is identical to the approach endorsed by the National Board of Medical Examiners in 1919 after an international exchange of scholars from the United States, England, Scotland, and France.

> As a result of this international exchange, Dr. Stewart Rodman proposed an examination following the pattern of the established procedures of the Triple Qualifying Board of Scotland and the Conjoint Examining Board of England. ... Part I was usually taken by students at the end of the second year of medical school and Part II toward the end of the fourth year. A year of internship was required for admission to Part III. Thus, as the student proceeded through his years of formal education and acquired an M.D. degree, he had the opportunity to qualify for a state license by taking and passing the three-part series of extramural examinations.[6]

The three-part structure remains in use to evaluate the fitness of US candidates for medical licensure in 2012.[7] Today, the tests are named United States Medical

Licensing Examination (USMLE): Step 1, basic sciences; Step 2, clinical knowledge and clinical skills; and Step 3, general medical practice. As noted in prior writing:

> The titles are different but the purposes are the same. For more than three centuries, students of Western medicine have submitted to knowledge assessments of basic science, clinical science and clinical practice, respectively. The examination content has evolved due to scientific and technical advances. The examination format, by contrast, appears immutable.[8]

Medical education reflects the general cultural level and the structure of medicine in a given society. Medical historian Kenneth Ludmerer[9,10] has written that the period of the late nineteenth and early twentieth centuries was a watershed for advancement of medical thought, technology, and education. Scientific advancements in fields such as bacteriology (e.g., Louis Pasteur's germ theory),[11,12] improvements in public health knowledge and research, and technological progression from the Industrial Revolution—with its emphasis on efficiency, mass production, fast communication, and improved transportation—coalesced to provide the medical profession new opportunities for patient care and social service. Medical education reforms, especially acknowledging the importance of grounding medical training in a university setting with a graded curriculum focused on both bioscience and clinical care, and rigorous trainee selection and assessment, gradually became the norm.[9,10]

Sir William Osler addressed the New York Academy of Medicine in 1903 on the topic of "The Hospital as a College."[13] Osler spoke about the newborn Johns Hopkins medical curriculum based on the German model, featuring a 2-year foundation of course and laboratory work in the basic medical sciences later amplified by 2 years of supervised clinical work on hospital wards and outpatient services. Osler's passion was educating superb clinicians grounded in biomedical science and refined habits of thought. His concern was to train competent medical doctors as scientist-practitioners and to embed their preparation in patient care experiences. Osler asked:

> How can we make the work of the student in the third and fourth years as practical as it is in the first and second? Osler responded ... take him from the lecture-room, take him from the amphitheatre—put him in the outpatient department—put him in the wards. ... Ask any physician of twenty years' standing how he has become proficient in his art, and he will reply, by

constant contact with disease; and he will add that the medicine he learned in the schools was totally different from the medicine he learned at the bedside.[13]

Osler concluded, "Teach him how to observe, give him plenty of facts to observe, and the lessons will come out of the facts themselves."[13] Note that Osler was silent about the role of assessment, feedback, and summative evaluation to document graded medical education achievement and overall clinical competence.

Ludmerer's historical synthesis coupled with Osler's prescription for clinical medical education in the early twentieth century set the stage for methods used to educate doctors worldwide today. The nearly universal set of US and Canadian third-year clinical clerkships and fifth-year clerkships in Europe and other world regions that cover medicine, surgery, pediatrics, obstetrics and gynecology, psychiatry, and other disciplines; subsequent selectives and sub-internships grounded in patient care experiences; and postgraduate residencies and fellowships in clinical specialties are all derived from the Osler clinical education model of 1903. Today, in 2012, we aim to educate twenty-first-century physicians using a nineteenth-century intellectual model. Chapter 16 (this volume) sets forth an educational agenda to modernize medical education training and assessment goals.

The Flexner Report, written in 1910 and titled *Medical Education in the United States and Canada*,[14] is widely credited as a watershed event for advancements in North American medical education and medical personnel evaluation for at least a century.[15] However, Ludmerer[9,10] and other medical historians teach that many of the reforms advocated in the Flexner Report (e.g., selective student admission, prior baccalaureate preparation, graded curriculum, emphasis on science and clinical practice) happened because of secular trends already underway. Abraham Flexner was one voice in a chorus whose debut started roughly with Pasteur and Sir Francis Galton. An accelerating evolution of thought and technology spurred advancements in medical education and personnel evaluation in the late nineteenth and early twentieth centuries in the Western world.

The rise of standardized testing was a key technological development coincident with advancement in late nineteenth- and early twentieth-century medical science.[16] Standardized testing among medicine and other health professions originates from the science and writing of Sir Francis Galton, cousin of Charles Darwin, in the 1880s and 1890s, through new biometric understanding about the Gaussian normal curve, and the emergence of psychometric science. One of the earliest introductions of psychometric science as an agent of public policy was the creation and use of Army Alpha and Army Beta, classification tests used to sort US military recruits during World War I. This led to development of early mental (i.e., intelligence) tests by Alfred Binet and Théodore Simon. Psychometric science and educational measurement became legitimate academic disciplines in the early twentieth century and established a platform for applied projects in personnel evaluation for the health professions for future decades.[16]

One of the most important, and lasting, applications of psychometric science in Western medical education was the creation and subsequent evolution of the Medical College Admission Test (MCAT).[17] The MCAT was launched in 1928 by the Association of American Medical Colleges in response to the high attrition rate (5%–50%) of students admitted to medical school at that time. The MCAT has undergone five revisions since its inception, which demonstrates that "the definition of aptitude for medical education reflects the professional and social mores and values of the time."[17] A sixth revision of the MCAT is now underway at the time of writing (June, 2012). In the United States, the MCAT has been a huge success as a medical school screening device because the medical school attrition rate for all reasons is now 1.4%.[18] This means that the decision to admit an individual to medical school is equivalent (within measurement error) to granting that person a license to practice medicine.

Similar advancements in student selection for health professions education using sophisticated psychometric technologies have been implemented in many countries and cultures around the world. Scholarly writing about fixed-quota student selection for high-stakes careers in the health professions uniformly points out the tension between reliance on grades and test scores as indicators of educational readiness for professional education versus measures of personal qualities, ethnic fit, gender equity, or cultural justice as student selection metrics (*see* especially Chapter 5 of this volume by Prideaux and colleagues).[19,20] These controversies will not go away. Student selection problems will vex health professions educators until an acceptable calculus can be reached that places academic measures and personal qualities in proper balance.

The post-World War II expansion of the medical profession into a health care industry was a source of great growth in national and international bioscience, advancements in clinical practice, public health attention and interventions, and improved medical education. Post-war introduction and widespread use of antibiotics, rapid growth of the National Institutes of Health in the United States, creation and use of the Salk and Sabin vaccines for polio prevention, growth in the number of medical schools worldwide, and the nascent development of medical and health professions education as legitimate academic disciplines took shape in the 1950s and 1960s.[21]

George Miller and the so-called "Buffalo Group"—including Stephen

Abrahamson, Hilliard Jason, Ira S. Cohen, Harold P. Graser, Robert S. Harnack, Edwin F. Rosinski, and Adelle Land—were early pioneers in the US medical education movement in the mid-twentieth century. Working at the State University of New York at Buffalo, this group of physicians and educators broke new ground in medical curriculum development, learner assessment and evaluation, and faculty development that laid a solid foundation for today's work in these fields. This fledgling group sought to (a) systematically study medical education processes, (b) engineer and manage better approaches to educating doctors, and (c) evaluate medical education outcomes rigorously. Scholarship by the Buffalo Group is captured in the volume *Teaching and Learning in Medical School*,[22] edited by George Miller and published in 1961. Many of the book's ideas and educational prescriptions are as timely today as when they were pronounced over 50 years ago.

Seminal work in medical education by the Buffalo Group later seeded colonies of medical education excellence at several US and Canadian university sites. George Miller and his protégés established centers of medical education research and development at several North American medical universities, including the State University of New York at Buffalo (Hilliard Jason), the University of Illinois at Chicago (George Miller, Christine McGuire), the University of Southern California (Stephen Abrahamson), the University of Washington at Seattle (Charles Dohner), Michigan State University (Lee Shulman, Arthur Elstein), and McMaster University in Hamilton, Ontario, Canada (Howard Barrows). George Miller was also a catalyst for formation of the Regional Teacher Training Centers under auspices of the World Health Organization in the 1970s. These organizational achievements and the financial commitments they received cemented medical and health professions education in the university community worldwide and set the stage for today's program development and scholarship.

North American advancements in medical education born from the 1950s through the 1970s spread quickly across the globe thanks to at least 10 coincident reasons: (1) new communication technologies; (2) international collaboration; (3) scholarship in psychological science about human learning, retention, and transfer by individuals and teams; (4) integrated curricula and integrated assessments; (5) improved methods to evaluate readiness for medical practice and medical education; (6) a broad view of professionalism in health professions education, especially as a field of scholarship and professional expression; (7) greater emphasis on outcomes assessment; (8) technology-enhanced assessment; (9) new knowledge about implementation science; and (10) the psychometric integration of reliability and validity as indexes of data quality and interpretive accuracy.

New communication technologies have revolutionized health professions education and professional practice in ways that were unknown 30 years ago. A small sample of illustrations include formation of the internet, personal computing, mushrooming software development, exponential growth in data processing capacity, miniaturization of devices, and the shrinking scale of technological costs. These and many other technological innovations simultaneously simplify and make more efficient the delivery of educational curricula and formation of educational networks among students, faculty, and other stakeholders worldwide. New communication technologies compress the world, boost information transfer efficiency, and link health professions learners and faculty across countries and cultures. Technological advancement will accelerate continually and will affect health professions education in ways that cannot be fully anticipated today.

International collaboration spurred by technological advancement is now a hallmark of health professions education. Growth in prominence and attendance at the biennial Ottawa Conference on Evaluation in Health Professions Education, the annual conferences of the Association for Medical Education in Europe, the Association of American Medical Colleges, and the International Association of Medical Science Educators, national and regional professional meetings in China, Southeast Asia, Latin America, Africa, and many other locations clearly show that attention to health professions education is now a global enterprise. International professional meetings and conferences act as principal outlets for dialogue and educational research reporting. Sharing ideas, innovations, learner and program evaluation practices, and research data worldwide will become easier, more efficient, and more widespread in the future.

Scholarship in psychological science and about human learning, retention, and transfer of training has become increasingly sophisticated and has direct applications to the education of health professionals as individuals and teams. Pertinent examples include the work of learning psychologist Richard E. Mayer on applying the science of learning to medical education in general[23] and neurosurgery in particular.[24] Research and writing by K. Anders Ericsson about the deliberate practice construct has had a major impact on health professions education.[25,26] This is especially evident in medical education research that demonstrates the power of deliberate practice in combination with mastery learning to achieve robust skill acquisition outcomes among learners that transfer directly to better patient care practices and improved patient outcomes.[27] Five excellent chapters that address human learning are also available in the *International Handbook of Research in Medical Education*, published in 2002.[28]

Psychologist Eduardo Salas and his colleagues have published seminal work about the formation, education, and maintenance of expert medical teams in a variety of disciplines (*see* especially Chapter 9 of this volume by Salas et al).[29] A key message from this science is that with rare exceptions, no one works alone anymore. The best clinical and scientific work is now done by teams, rather than by individual clinicians or scholars laboring in isolation. Steps toward optimizing individual and team performance in health care will continue to move ahead through psychological science progress.

European medical educators were the first to recognize and address the disconnect between the objectives of medical education and the methods used to evaluate medical education outcomes. Writing in 1968, Charles University (Czechoslovakia) medical professor Josef Charvat and colleagues[30] pointed out the gap between competent practice of clinical medicine and the procedures then in use to judge the readiness of students and other trainees for such work. In the late 1960s, medical clinical competence was evaluated chiefly by multiple-choice tests, oral examinations (viva voce), or long case clinical assessments. The reliability, validity, and clinical realism of these outcome measurement methods were doubtful. By contrast, Charvat and colleagues[30] advocated a "process approach" to the evaluation of clinical competence. The process approach would integrate medical education and medical assessment and would

> require the student to make a judgment of the type he would have to make as a physician, about clinical data presented in a realistic form: *Certain findings are made. What lesion could account for them and what are their practical consequences?* The student records his decisions in a fashion that permits both objective and reliable assessment of their accuracy.

The Charvat et al.[30] "process approach" sought to integrate medical education and medical personnel evaluation. It argued for moving learner evaluation close to the clinic and bedside, rather than relying on detached measures of acquired knowledge. A decade later, Harden and Gleeson[31] observed, "in the U.S.A. the tendency has been to move away from examinations at the bedside and towards [written] patient management problems." This became a point of departure for competency-based, objective measurement of clinical fitness that is the foundation of current evaluation practice.

Improved methods to evaluate competence for professional practice and readiness for health professions education have been developed and taken hold since the 1970s.

A major advancement in clinical competence evaluation was the introduction of the objective structured clinical examination (OSCE) in the United Kingdom by Harden and Gleeson[31] and Harden et al.[32] in 1975. In contrast with written (multiple-choice) tests of acquired knowledge and oral examinations (viva voce) to presumably assess judgment and reasoning, OSCEs were specifically designed "to assess clinical competence at the bedside."[31]

> [S]tudents rotate round a series of stations in the hospital ward. At one station they are asked to carry out a procedure, such as take a history, undertake one aspect of physical examination, or interpret laboratory investigations in light of a patient's problem, and at the next station they have to answer questions on the findings at the previous station and their interpretation.[32]

OSCE results are typically combined across a series of test stations to provide a clinical competence profile for each examinee. Decisions about candidate advancement in the curriculum or need for remedial education experiences are shaped by reliable OSCE data.

The straightforward, practical approach to medical competence evaluation captured by OSCEs has received acceptance throughout the medical education community worldwide. OSCEs are now used for formative and summative assessment of health professions learners in rich and poor nations and across many cultures. This approach to learner assessment, and its many variations, combines the best of rigorous (reliable) clinical education measurement and evaluations focused on clinical skills that matter (validity) to care for patients and their families.

Historically, readiness for health professions education—especially medicine, dentistry, and veterinary medicine—has been assessed chiefly using measures of academic aptitude, secondary school or college grades, and narrative endorsements from teachers or other influential people.[20] A candidate's fund of knowledge and academic aptitude were weighted most heavily. One's personal qualities and interpersonal skills—both key features of professional practice—received less emphasis.

Introduction of the multiple mini-interview (MMI) measurement procedure at McMaster University in Canada in the early 2000s was intended to change the face of selective admissions to health professions education programs. The MMI is an admissions OSCE.[33] Its rationale and utility are based on evidence that shows traditional selective admission interviews are not standardized, yield unreliable data, and do not contribute to accurate health professions student selection decisions. After selection goals are set,

> the MMI is intended to consist of a large number of short stations, each with a different examiner. The MMI is not, however, objective. Nor is it clinical. Research [...] has shown that subjective ratings can be reliable and valid estimates of an individual's abilities.[33]

MMI stations focus on such general attributes as communication skills under pressure, critical thinking, ethical decision making, and knowledge of the health care system. A connected series of experiments at McMaster University showed the MMI produced reliable data and that measurement context reduces the validity of traditional admissions interviews.[33]

Subsequent research studies about the MMI measurement procedure present data that reinforce its utility for selective admission decisions. "Both candidates [86% international medical graduates] and interviewers agreed that the MMI format was reliable, fair, and asked appropriate, easy-to-understand questions" in a UK regional pediatric training program.[34] A qualitative evaluation study in Australia amplifies a "quantitative evaluation [that] has demonstrated robustness of the MMI including its reliability, aspects of validity and acceptability to candidates and interviewers in undergraduate and postgraduate settings."[35] The qualitative investigators identified key MMI measurement themes and concluded, "We gained a deeper understanding of participants' experiences of a high-stakes, decision-making process for selection into a graduate-entry medical school."[35] An Israeli variation on the MMI (MOR, a Hebrew acronym for "selection for medicine") measured medical school candidates' personal and interpersonal attributes: interpersonal communication, ability to handle stress, initiative and responsibility, self-awareness. The Israeli scientists conclude, "MOR is a reliable tool for measuring non-cognitive attributes in medical school candidates [...] its implementation conveys the importance of maintaining humanist characteristics in the medical profession to students and faculty staff."[36]

Important conceptual progress has also been made about health professional personnel evaluation. The US Accreditation Council for Graduate Medical Education has published and promulgated a set of six core competencies to shape postgraduate medical education and resident evaluation in the United States.[37] The six core competencies are (1) patient care, (2) medical knowledge, (3) practice-based learning and improvement, (4) interpersonal and communication skills, (5) professionalism, and (6) systems-based practice. Residency program directors use the core competencies as a framework to design educational activities and prepare resident evaluation exercises. A similar set of European competency expectations is embodied in the *Scottish Doctors* report that endorses medical student achievement in 12 domains as the foundation for competent medical practice in Scotland.[38] The domains are (1) clinical skills; (2) practical procedures; (3) patient investigations; (4) patient management; (5) communication; (6) health promotion and disease prevention; (7) medical informatics; (8) basic, social, and clinical sciences and underlying principles; (9) attitudes, ethical understanding, and legal responsibilities; (10) decision-making skills, and clinical reasoning and judgment; (11) role of the doctor within the health service; and (12) professional development. The *Scottish Doctors* competencies differ from those of the Accreditation Council for Graduate Medical Education because they focus on undergraduate medical students and are more granular.[38] The two lists are similar because they give focus to medical education curricula and outcome evaluation among learners.

The dedication and hard work of George Miller and many other mid-twentieth-century pioneers in health professions education has created a new sense of professionalism in the field. For many years the post-World War II educational agenda was the stepchild of Western academic medical centers, where basic and clinical biomedical research and clinical patient care were the topmost priorities. The educational agenda took a backseat. However, evidence is now growing from several sources that health professions education and its improvement are growing in importance at health science centers globally. For example, faculty promotion policies in most health professions educational institutions have been changed to give greater weight to teaching in many forms: curriculum and test development, student advising and mentoring, educational research, community service, and other educational expressions. Such policies were unheard of at most academic health science centers 30–40 years ago. Another sign of growing professionalism is the rapid proliferation of master's degree programs in health professions education worldwide.[39] In 1996, there were only seven such programs in health professions education. Today there are 76 health professions education master's degree programs in Europe, North America, Asia, Latin America, the Middle East, Australia, and Africa.[39] The growth of professionalism in the field is evident from these data.

The number and quality of outlets for scholarship in health professions education has grown at a fast pace. These journals range from publications that address single professions (e.g., *Medical Teacher, Journal of Nursing Research, Medical Education, Academic Medicine, Journal of Veterinary Medical Education*), to publications that span professional boundaries (e.g., *Advances in Health Sciences Education, Journal of Allied Health, Qualitative Health Research, Simulation in Healthcare*). Many specialty journals, including *BMJ, Chest,* and *JAMA,* are now receptive to high-quality manuscript submissions about educational issues. The message is that the rise of professionalism in health professions education is growing and is no longer in doubt.

Increased emphasis on outcomes assessment is another advancement that has taken hold in health professions education and is being implemented worldwide. Outcome assessment by educational programs acknowledges that such *measured educational results* as gains in knowledge, clinical skill, professionalism, and teamwork are the *raison d'être* for program operation. This underscores the maxim, "we value what we measure and we measure what we value." Measured educational outcomes demonstrate that curricula are effective, satisfy accreditation requirements, certify learner competence, and fulfill public expectations that health professions graduates are safe and effective.

Outcome assessment among health professions learners and programs originates from the competency-based medical education movement first articulated in the late 1970s.[40] Recent scholarly writings about this approach to education are available in Association for Medical Education in Europe Guide No. 14, *Outcome-Based Education*, published in 1999[41] and in a thematic issue of *Medical Teacher* (Vol. 32, No. 8) on competency-based medical education published in August 2010. One article in that issue specifically addresses the theory and practice of competency-based medical education.[42]

It is important to point out that educational outcome assessment is conceptualized not just as an educational endpoint measured at the classroom, clinic, or simulation laboratory exit door. These results, of course, are very important. However, educational outcomes that really matter are better patient care practices and improved patient and public health linked directly to educational interventions. Such educational outcomes reveal what health professionals *do* as a consequence of education and the benefits their competent behavior yields. Useful taxonomies to classify hierarchical levels of educational outcomes are found in the Miller pyramid,[43] Kirkpatrick's four-level scheme for evaluating training programs,[44] and a recent mechanism that views downstream results (i.e., patient care practices, patient improvement) derived from educational interventions as "translational science."[27,45]

Technology-enhanced assessment is discussed in detail in Chapter 3 of this volume, authored by Zubair Amin and his colleagues. These scholars argue that the uptake of information and communication technologies (ICTs) in health professions education can have far reaching consequences on assessment. The medical education community needs to develop a deeper understanding of how technology can underpin and extend assessment practices. ICTs are constantly changing in assessment settings. In addition, users need to recognize the importance of aligning technology-enabled assessment with local context and needs, the need for better evidence to support use of technologies in health professions education assessment, and a number of challenges, particularly validity threats, that need to be addressed while incorporating technology in assessment.

No matter what ICTs are used, users must adhere to principles of good assessment[46] (*see* Chapter 2, this volume), the need to develop coherent institutional assessment policy, using technologies to broaden the competencies to be assessed, linking patient outcome data to assessment of practitioner performance, and capitalizing on technologies for management of the entire life cycle of assessment.

Implementation science (IS) is producing a growing influence on expansion and quality improvement in health professions education around the world. IS is a novel academic discipline and also the title of a new open-access journal, now in its seventh volume (2012). The journal states its research focus is

> the scientific study of methods to promote the systematic uptake of clinical research findings and other evidence-based practices into routine practice, and hence to improve the quality and effectiveness of healthcare. It includes the study of influences on healthcare professional and organisational behaviour. [This] is scientifically important because it identifies the behaviour of healthcare professionals and healthcare organisations as key sources of variance requiring improved empirical and theoretical understanding before effective interventions can be reliably achieved.[47]

IS studies and aims to overcome health care organizational silos and barriers, pockets of cultural inertia, professional hierarchies, educational roadblocks, and financial disincentives that reduce health care efficiency and effectiveness.

In hospitals and clinics, IS addresses the science of health care delivery. Advances in IS are no less important than new drug discoveries and surgical innovations. The impact and effectiveness of health care is diminished when its delivery is substandard.

Historically, classical test theory separated the reliability of educational measurements and the validity of measurement data including its interpretation and use.[16] Reliability then and now addresses the accuracy, consistency, and reproducibility of assessment scores—data quality revealed as precision.[48] Test validation has experienced a scholarly evolution because the idea started as a property of assessments (content validity) and their uses (concurrent and predictive validity).[16] Today, validation of educational measurement data is considered an interpretive argument where reliable, context-specific evidence is weighed and judged about its utility for informing practical decisions or scientific inferences.[49,50]

The *Standards for Educational and Psychological Testing*,[51] published jointly by the American Educational Research Association, the American Psychological Association, and the National Council on Measurement in Education, point out that a comprehensive picture of test validation (construct validity) has at least five elements that combine traditional ideas about reliability and validity: (1) content, (2) response process, (3) internal structure, (4) relationship to other variables, and (5) consequences. Each of the five elements must be supported by logic and data to advance a validity argument about the strength and utility (i.e., integrity) of an educational evaluation and its practical consequences.

Psychometrician Steven Downing[49] notes:

> Validity is always approached as hypothesis, such that the desired interpretive meaning associated with assessment data is first hypothesized and then data are collected and assembled to support or refute the validity hypothesis. In this conceptualization, *assessment data are more or less valid for some very specific purpose, meaning or interpretation, at a given point in time and only for some well-defined population* [emphasis added]. The assessment itself is never said to be "valid" or "invalid" rather one speaks of the scientifically sound evidence presented to either support or refute the proposed interpretation of assessment scores, at a particular time period in which the validity evidence was collected.

Such data-based logic was used recently to argue against the widespread US practice of using USMLE Step 1 and Step 2 scores to inform postgraduate medical specialty selection decisions.[52] USMLE Part 1 and Part 2 scores are solid measures of acquired medical knowledge. However, their failure to correlate with other variables that measure clinical skill acquisition cast doubt on their usefulness for selecting postgraduate medical residents.

Gregory Cizek[53] has recently proposed an even simpler intellectual model for defining and distinguishing validity. Cizek asserts that the essence of validation resides simply in the internal structure of measurements and the consequences of their use. Whether this view has "traction" and life will be seen as the integrated scientific validity debate plays out over time.

The overall message of this book, conveyed in its 16 chapters, is that evaluation practices in health professions education have come a long way in the last century. Evaluation practices are far more sophisticated and yield data having higher reliability than ever before. Reliable data, of course, are essential for faculty and institutional authorities to reach valid decisions on the progress or competence of learners in the health professions. This presentation of current thought and technology about *International Best Practices for Evaluation in the Health Professions* acknowledges the contributions of predecessors and sets the stage for subsequent scholarship.

References

1. Franke W. *The Reform and Abolition of the Traditional Chinese Examination System.* Cambridge, MA: Center for East Asian Studies, Harvard University [distributed by Harvard University Press]; 1960.
2. Latourette KSL. Chinese history. In: *Encyclopedia Britannica.* 14th ed., vol. 5. New York, NY: Encyclopedia Britannica; 1929. p. 535.
3. McGuire CH, Tekian A, McGaghie WC, editors. Preface to *Innovative Simulations for Assessing Professional Competence.* Chicago: Department of Medical Education, University of Illinois at Chicago; 1999. p. iv.
4. Puschmann T. *A History of Medical Education.* New York, NY: Hafner Publishing; 1966 (originally published 1891).
5. Royal College of Physicians. *By-Laws of the Royal College of Physicians* [microfilm]. London: Royal College of Physicians; 1693.
6. Hubbard JP. *Measuring Medical Education: the tests and the experience of the National Board of Medical Examiners.* 2nd ed. Philadelphia, PA: Lea & Febiger; 1978.
7. Federation of State Medical Boards of the United States and National Board of Medical Examiners (NBME). *United States Medical Licensing Examination (USMLE) Bulletin of Information.* Philadelphia, PA: NBME; 2012.
8. McGaghie WC. Evaluating competence for professional practice. In: Curry L, Wergin JF, editors. *Educating Professionals.* San Francisco, CA: Jossey-Bass; 1993. pp. 229–61.
9. Ludmerer KM. *Learning to Heal: the development of American medical education.* Baltimore, MD: The Johns Hopkins University Press; 1985.
10. Ludmerer KM. *Time to Heal: American medical education from the turn of the century to the era of managed care.* New York, NY: Oxford University Press; 1999.
11. Pasteur L. The germ theory and its application to medicine and surgery [translated by Harold C. Ernst]. In: Eliot CW, editor. *Scientific Papers* (Harvard Classics Vol. 38). New York, NY: Collier; 1910. pp. 382–9. Originally read before the French Academy of Sciences, April 29, 1878. Available at: www.bartleby.com/38/7/ (accessed January 4, 2012).
12. Pasteur L. On the extension of the germ theory to the etiology of certain common diseases [translated by Harold C. Ernst]. In: Eliot CW, editor. *Scientific Papers* (Harvard

Classics Vol. 38). New York, NY: Collier; 1910. pp. 390–402. Originally read before the French Academy of Sciences, May 3, 1880. Available at: www.bartleby. com/38/7/ (accessed January 4, 2012).

13. Osler W. The hospital as a college [1903]. In: Osler W, editor. *Aequanimitas.* Philadelphia, PA: P. Blakiston's Son; 1932. pp. 313–25.

14. Flexner A. *Medical Education in the United States and Canada.* Bulletin No. 4. New York, NY: Carnegie Foundation for the Advancement of Teaching; 1910.

15. Cooke M, Irby DM, O'Brien BC. *Educating Physicians: a call for reform of medical school and residency.* San Francisco, CA: Jossey-Bass; 2010.

16. Anastasi A. *Psychological Testing.* 5th ed. New York, NY: Macmillan; 1982.

17. McGaghie WC. Assessing readiness for medical education: evolution of the Medical College Admission Test. *JAMA.* 2002; **288**(9): 1085–90.

18. Brewer L, Grbic D. Medical students' socioeconomic background and their completion of the first two years of medical school. *AAMC Analysis in Brief.* 2010; **9**(11): 1–2.

19. Adam J, Dowell J, Greatrix R. Use of UCAT scores in student selection by U.K. medical schools, 2006–2010. *BMC Med Educ.* 2011; **11**: 98.

20. McGaghie WC. Student selection. In: Norman GR, van der Vleuten CPM, Newble DI, editors. *International Handbook of Research in Medical Education.* Part I. Dordrecht, the Netherlands: Kluwer Academic Publishers; 2002. pp. 303–35.

21. Kuper A, Albert M, Hodges BD. The origins of the field of medical education research. *Acad Med.* 2010; **85**(8): 1347–53.

22. Miller, GE, editor. *Teaching and Learning in Medical School.* Cambridge, MA: Harvard University Press for the Commonwealth Fund; 1961.

23. Mayer RE. Applying the science of learning to medical education. *Med Educ.* 2010; **44**(6): 543–9.

24. Mayer RE. What neurosurgeons should discover about the science of learning. *Clin Neurosurg.* 2009; **56**: 57–65.

25. Ericsson KA. Deliberate practice and the acquisition and maintenance of expert performance in medicine and related domains. *Acad Med.* 2004; **79**(Suppl. 10): S70–81.

26. Ericsson KA. Enhancing the development of professional performance: implications from the study of deliberate practice. In: Ericsson KA, editor. *Development of Professional Expertise: toward measurement of expert performance and design of optimal learning environments.* New York, NY: Cambridge University Press; 2009. pp. 405–31.

27. McGaghie WC, Draycott TJ, Dunn WF, et al. Evaluating the impact of simulation on translational patient outcomes. *Simul Healthc.* 2011; 6 Suppl.: S42–7.

28. Norman GR, van der Vleuten CPM, Newble DI, editors. *International Handbook of Research in Medical Education.* Parts I and II. Dordrecht, the Netherlands: Kluwer Academic Publishers; 2002.

29. Salas E, Frush K, editors. *Improving Patient Safety through Teamwork and Team Training.* New York, NY: Oxford University Press; 2012.

30. Charvat J, McGuire C, Parsons V. *A Review of the Nature and Uses of Examinations in*

Medical Education. Public Health Paper No. 36. Geneva: World Health Organization; 1968.

31. Harden RM, Gleeson FA. Assessment of clinical competence using an objective structured clinical examination (OSCE). *Med Educ.* 1979; **13**(1): 41–54.

32. Harden RM, Stevenson M, Downie WW, et al. Assessment of clinical competence using objective structured examination. *BMJ.* 1975; **1**(5955): 447–51.

33. Eva KW, Rosenfeld J, Reiter HI, et al. An admissions OSCE: the multiple mini-interview. *Med Educ.* 2004; **38**(3): 314–26.

34. Humphrey S, Dowson S, Wall D, et al. Multiple mini-interviews: opinions of candidates and interviewers. *Med Educ.* 2008; **42**(2): 207–13.

35. Kumar K, Roberts C, Rothnie I, et al. Experiences of the multiple mini-interview: a qualitative analysis. *Med Educ.* 2009; **43**(4): 360–7.

36. Ziv A, Rubin O, Moshinsky A, et al. MOR: a simulation-based assessment centre for evaluating the personal and interpersonal qualities of medical school candidates. *Med Educ.* 2008; **42**(10): 991–8.

37. Stewart MG. *Core Competencies.* Accreditation Council for Graduate Medical Education; 2001. Available at: www.acgme.org/acwebsite/RRC_280/280_corecomp.asp (accessed February 27, 2012).

38. Scottish Dean's Medical Curriculum Group. *Learning Outcomes for the Medical Undergraduate in Scotland: a foundation for competent and reflective practitioners.* 3rd ed. August 2007. Available at: www.scottishdoctor.org/resources/scottishdoctor3.doc (accessed September 27, 2012).

39. Tekian A, Harris I. Preparing health professions education leaders worldwide: a description of masters-level programs. *Med Teacher.* 2012; **34**(1): 52–8.

40. McGaghie WC, Miller GE, Sajid AW, et al. *Competency-Based Curriculum Development in Medical Education.* Public Health Paper No. 68. Geneva: World Health Organization; 1978.

41. Smith SR, Dollase R. Outcome-based education: part 2. Planning, implementing and evaluating a competency-based curriculum. AMEE Guide No. 14. *Med Teach.* 1999; **21**(1): 15–22.

42. Frank JR, Snell LS, ten Cate O, et al. Competency-based medical education: theory to practice. *Med Teach.* 2010; **32**(8): 638–45.

43. Miller GE. The assessment of clinical skills/competence/performance. *Acad Med.* 1990; **65**(Suppl. 9): S63–7.

44. Kirkpatrick DL. *Evaluating Training Programs.* 2nd ed. San Francisco, CA: Berrett-Kohler Publishers; 1998.

45. McGaghie WC. Medical education research as translational science. *Sci Transl Med.* 2010; **2**(19): 19cm8.

46. Amin Z, Seng CY, Eng KH. *Practical Guide to Medical Student Assessment.* Singapore: World Scientific Publishing; 2006.

47. About *Implementation Science.* London: Implementation Science. Available at: www.implementationscience.com/about (accessed February 27, 2012).

48. Downing SM. Reliability: on the reproducibility of assessment data. *Med Educ.* 2004; **38**(9): 1006–12.

49. Downing SM. Validity: on the meaningful interpretation of assessment data. *Med Educ*. 2003; **37**(9): 830–7.

50. Kane MT. Validation. In: Brennan RL, editor. *Educational Measurement*. 4th ed. Westport, CT: American Council on Education/Praeger Publishers; 2006. pp. 17–64.

51. American Educational Research Association, American Psychological Association, National Council on Measurement in Education. *Standards for Educational and Psychological Testing*. Washington, DC: American Educational Research Association; 1999.

52. McGaghie WC, Cohen ER, Wayne DB. Are United States Medical Licensing Exam Step 1 and Step 2 scores valid measures for postgraduate medical residency selection decisions? *Acad Med*. 2011; **86**(1): 48–52.

53. Cizek GJ. Defining and distinguishing validity: interpretations of score meaning and justifications of test use. *Psychol Methods*. 2012; **17**(1): 31–43.

Criteria for a
Good Assessment

John R. Boulet and Danette W. McKinley

THE PROPER ASSESSMENT AND EVALUATION OF HEALTH CARE WORKERS is paramount, given their role in patient care activities. Throughout their education, physicians, nurses, and other health care professionals are exposed to a wide array of assessments. These assessments can be used for formative (educational) or summative (e.g., establish competence) purposes. Regardless of how they are used, the evaluation tools must yield outcomes (e.g., scores, decisions) that are fair, meaningful, and defensible.

This chapter will focus on describing and justifying the criteria for good assessments. Examples of the use of assessments in the health care fields will be presented. In general, assessments must be practical, yield sufficiently precise measures of ability, and allow one to make justifiable inferences concerning the qualities or abilities of those being evaluated. While the specific purpose of the assessment can influence how stringently various quality criteria are applied, individuals responsible for evaluating health care workers, either as part of educational activities or for credentialing and licensing purposes, must gather evidence to support the use of their assessment results. The types of evidence collected, and their utility with respect to explaining performance, serve to define the criteria for good assessment.

Methods of Assessment
• •

In health care professions education, there are numerous assessment method-ologies, including multiple-choice items, various short-answer formats, patient management problems, computer-based case evaluations, objective structure clinical examinations (OSCEs), mannequin-based simulations, oral examina-tions, and peer assessments.[1–10] For most assessments, these methods can be broadly categorized as either selected or constructed response. For selected-response formats, examinees (candidates) choose, or match, responses based on a fixed list of options.[11] The most common selected-response format is a multiple-choice question (MCQ). Examinees read a question, which may be based on a clinical case scenario, and attempt to select the correct answer from a list that includes a number of distracters (incorrect answers). MCQs, which typically measure knowledge-based constructs, can be administered as paper-and-pencil or computer-based examinations. For computer-based assessments, the content of examination can be varied over the course of the administration to better align item characteristics (e.g., difficulty) and examinee abilities. This is known as adaptive testing.

Constructed-response formats demand that the examinee (candidate) produce something. The most common constructed-response format is an essay or short-answer question. In the health care professions, for example, an examinee may be asked to write about common and alternative therapies in the treatment of breast cancer. Often, these types of assessments are graded, either analytically or holistically, by experts.

With respect to the evaluation of health care workers, there has been a move-ment toward more authentic assessments and an associated emphasis on patient safety.[12,13] This coincides with improvements in technology and educational measurement techniques, effectively broadening the scope of the assessment domain, especially for constructed-response formats. For the evaluation of health care workers, either as part of training, or for certification and licensure decisions, some manner of practice-based assessment is often employed.[14–16] Computer-based case simulations, where examinees work through one or more patient management problems on the computer, are often administered to measure clini-cal reasoning or clinical decision-making skills.[17–19] By using the computer, the evaluator can present information (e.g., lab results) in (simulated) real time, and see how examinees interpret the information and subsequently adapt their treat-ment plan (e.g., asks for a consultation, orders medication). In the health care professions, one of the most common forms of "authentic" assessment involves the use of standardized patients (SPs), laypeople trained to portray mannerisms and complaints of "real" patients.[20] The use of SPs, often as part of an OSCE, is valuable because it allows for the assessment of what examinees can do (e.g., correctly perform a physical examination, communicate with a patient), compared with what they know. Having the necessary knowledge (typically assessed via MCQs), or the ability to know what to do when presented with a patient management problem, is not enough. From a patient safety perspective, we also need to evaluate what the candidate (physician, nurse, pharmacist, etc.) can do, either in a simulated environment or, more important, in a real patient care setting.

In developing assessment methods that tap what a candidate can do (e.g., insert a central line, interview a patient), other modalities, or even combinations of modalities, have also been used.[21,22] With the current emphasis on maintenance of competence (or maintenance of certification) in many health care professions, the use of various workplace-based assessments, including chart reviews and 360-degree evaluations, have been instituted.[23] Many of these assessments, typically used as quality improvement measures, involve peer review, evaluation of practice outcomes, and patient or client satisfaction measures.[24] More recently, the development of part-task trainers and high-fidelity mannequins provides an opportunity to measure technical and procedural skills.[12,13] By combining tools (e.g., SPs, mannequins), more authentic assessments can be built, often covering skill areas that, historically, were difficult to measure, at least with any degree of standardization.[25,26]

Although the criteria for judging the quality of an assessment should not depend on the mode of administration or the format, strategies to gather evidence to support any statements of quality may differ substantially. More important, given the introduction of new assessment modalities, often involving novel scoring and scaling methods, and different assessment cohorts (e.g., teams instead of individuals), making judgments about quality can be complicated, multifaceted, and, from a research perspective, time-consuming and expensive.[27] Thus it is important that all stakeholders, especially those directly involved with the development of assessments for health care professionals, are aware of the standards by which to evaluate the quality of assessments and, therefore, the strength of the inferences that one can make based on the assessment results.

Frameworks for Guiding the Development of Quality Indicators for Assessments
· ·

There are a number of frameworks that can help guide the identification and amalgamation of criteria that could, and should, be used to judge the quality of assessments that health professionals encounter as part of their selection, training or, where applicable, certification. These models will be briefly discussed, followed by synthesis of their combined utility to outline criteria for either constructing or judging the quality of assessments. The reader should keep in mind that assessments are used for many purposes, including ranking individuals for selection purposes (e.g., for entry into medical or nursing programs) and establishing competence or minimal proficiency. As a result, while general criteria to judge the quality of assessments can be formulated, the strictness by which they are applied can vary as a function of intended use of the assessment results.

Kirkpatrick's Four-Level Training Evaluation Model
Kirkpatrick's four-level training evaluation model provides a framework for judging the quality and effectiveness of training programs.[28] Since training or education programs often have an assessment component, Kirkpatrick's model can yield some generic criteria for the appraisal of assessment quality. The four levels of evaluation are (1) *reaction* (how the learners react to the learning process), (2) *learning* (the extent to which the learners gain knowledge and skills), (3) *behavior* (capability to perform learned skills while on the job), and (4) *results* (impact of the training program, e.g., on patient safety). The hierarchical specification of the model implies a natural order for the importance of evaluation criteria. While measuring how learners react to the learning process (training) is important, their perceptions may have little impact on their performance or skill acquisition. For example, learners (e.g., medical or nursing students) may indicate that they are comfortable performing a certain procedural skill in the simulated environment (as part of an assessment) even though they have had little opportunity to practice this skill in any setting. Those charged with evaluating the quality of an assessment often stop data gathering at level 1, simply concluding that the participants were satisfied with the conditions under which they were assessed and the perceived scope, or content coverage, of the examination. This constitutes weak evidence of quality because it is based solely on the potentially biased opinions of those who developed the assessment and those to whom it was administered. If an assessment, either formative (e.g., as part of educational activities) or summative (e.g., as part of credentialing), is to be judged effective,

evidence must be gathered to support that learning has occurred, that abilities measured translate to on-the-job performance (e.g., the content of the assessment is appropriate), and that the assessment yields positive outcomes (e.g., efficiencies, cost savings, changes in the behaviors of those being assessed).

Standards for Educational and Psychological Testing

The *Standards for Education and Psychological Testing*[29] provide detailed information on specific criteria to judge the quality of an assessment (i.e., sources of validity evidence), including evidence based on *test content* (e.g., format of the exercises, procedures for administration and scoring), evidence based on *response processes* (e.g., documentation of how individuals proceed through the assessment, application of scoring criteria by judges), evidence based on *internal structure* (e.g., do different groups of examinees with similar ability have, on average, systematically different responses to an item or a task?), evidence based on *relations to other variables* (e.g., do those individuals with more experience receive higher scores?), and evidence based on *consequences of testing* (e.g., is there any appreciable benefit associated with the assessment program such as decreased training costs and/or improvement in patient outcomes?). The *Standards* also provide a comprehensive section on the reliability, or precision, of assessment scores. The critical information on reliability includes the identification of sources of measurement error and quantifying the extent to which the scores generalize across alternate test forms, administrations, or other relevant dimensions. If scores are not reasonably precise, their utility for making any inferences concerning ability is suspect. Taken together, gathering evidence to support the validity and reliability of assessment scores, or decisions based on assessment scores, is the basis for any decision, positive or negative, regarding the quality of an assessment.

Kane's Framework

Although there is a long history of test theory,[30] and associated test score validation, the work by Kane[31,32] and Kane et al.[33] provides a useful framework for thinking about, and evaluating, the quality of assessments. The structure of Kane's view of validity rests on a series of assertions and assumptions that support the interpretation of the assessment scores. The four components of Kane's inferential chain are labeled *scoring, generalization, extrapolation,* and *interpretation/decision.* The *scoring* component includes evidence that the assessment was administered fairly (in a standardized way), individuals were evaluated accurately, and the scoring rules were applied consistently. The *generalization* component requires evidence that the observations (e.g., MCQs, simulation scenarios) were sampled adequately from the "universe" of available observations. In addition, with respect to *generalization*, it is essential to gather evidence to suggest that the sample of observations is large enough to produce scores with reasonable precision. Here, the question of interest is whether the assessment yields reliable scores and decisions. The *extrapolation* component requires evidence that the observations represented by the assessment scores are relevant to the construct of interest. This also requires evidence that the assessment scores (e.g., ratings, checklists) were not unduly influenced by sources of variance that are not related to the construct that is being measured. The *interpretation/decision* component of the argument requires evidence to be procured to establish that the theoretical framework required for score interpretation can be supported. Likewise, where decision rules are employed (e.g., pass or fail), evidence to support the proce- dure, and the utility of the resultant placement or categorization of those being assessed, should be gathered.

Synthesis of Frameworks

Although Kirkpatrick's model, the *Standards for Educational and Psychological Measurement*, and Kane's framework are not the only structures that can be used to define criteria for ascertaining the quality of an assessment,[34,35] they make it clear that both reliability (precision of scores or outcomes) and validity (the assessment's ability to measure what it was intended to measure) are key components. Of special note, if the assessment scores (or decisions based on the scores) are not sufficiently precise (reliability issue) then it does not much matter what we are measuring (validity issue). From an assessment perspective, measur- ing the wrong construct with great precision is not helpful (e.g., using a lengthy, well-constructed, multiple-choice examination to evaluate communication skills). This interplay between reliability and validity suggests that after an assessment is constructed and initial scoring rubrics are formulated, efforts should first be directed at quantifying sources of measurement error and, through this process, identifying an administrative design that will yield sufficiently precise scores. Kane's framework, as well as the *Standards*, provides a discussion of validity generalization—the degree to which evidence of validity based on assessment- criterion relations can be generalized to a new situation without further study of validity in that new situation. This is particularly important for new assessments because, referring to level 4 of Kirkpatrick's model, we frequently want to predict how an individual will perform in "real," non-assessment, conditions. Given the variations in both assessment and practice environments, some skills may generalize and others may not. Thus, the study of validity generalization, at least for some assessments, is paramount.

To develop or, more appropriately, to synthesize specific criteria for good assessment, Kane's framework is not only useful to identify issues related to the reliability (generalizability) and validity of assessment scores but also to define, in more detail, the criteria by which we can judge whether an assessment is high or low quality. In terms of identifying general criteria that define good assessments, the frameworks discussed earlier can easily be subsumed under Kane's. Following a brief review of previous work aimed at delineating criteria for good assessment, we provide a more detailed review of how Kane's framework, with appropriate examples from the health professions assessment literature, can be used to guide the collection of data to support the use of assessment scores. The choice of what data to collect, how to collect it, and, once secured, how to interpret what it means in terms of making inferences about examinee abilities is at the core of any argument that seeks to define the qualities of good assessment.

Previous Work

Before outlining how Kane's framework can be used to define the qualities of good assessment, it is important to acknowledge that much work has already been completed in this area. Most educational measurement textbooks have sections on test and item development, estimating measurement error, validity considerations, and quality assurance measures.[36] With respect to medical education, several articles have been published that describe assessment techniques and express criteria by which to judge the relevance and adequacy of the scores.[37–40] Recently, Norcini et al.[41] published a consensus statement on the qualities of good assessment. This comprehensive work, guided by a number of experts in the field, provides broad-based guidelines for judging the quality of assessments. Their recommendations, which extend beyond measurement principles, are keyed to criteria that recognize the legitimacy and incorporate the perspectives of the patients and the public. Here, in addition to psychometric rigor, the overriding principle of a good assessment is that it results in quality improvement of those being assessed. Assessment should have a catalytic effect, driving future learning forward, and improving practitioner knowledge and skills. Ultimately, albeit difficult to measure, this should help protect the public and improve patient care. Clauser et al.[42] provide a comprehensive synthesis of validity and reliability issues for assessments in medical education. While not specifically devoted to delimiting the qualities of good assessment, the authors also use Kane's framework to discuss key measurement issues and how they impact the utility of an assessment. Taken together, the existing work on assessment quality, both from psychometric and program perspectives, suggests that we need to pay specific attention to what we want to evaluate and that we need to create tools (rating scales, items, etc.) that allow collection of data that can be used to generate reasonably precise estimates of individual or group ability that, ultimately, are indicative of true proficiencies.

In the next sections of this chapter, we employ Kane's framework to discuss numerous assessment-related issues. By referencing existing studies, and discussing examples of good and poor assessment practices, practical criteria for judging the value of an assessment can be advanced.

Kane's Framework and the Quality of Good Assessments

Scoring

There have been numerous studies that have looked at the applicability of various scoring models, the accuracy of the scores, the influence of changes in assessment administration protocols on scores, and the influence of standardization and fidelity of examination conditions on examinee/candidate performance.[43-49] Unfortunately, given the plethora of scoring models, and their unique application for specific assessment modalities, these studies are far from complete. They do, however, provide a basis, often through documentation of poor assessment practices, for delineating criteria for good assessment. With reference to the scoring component of the validity argument, there are a number of questions that test developers, and even those using the tests, can ask. Some of these questions are outlined here and, where appropriate, effective and ineffective strategies for addressing them, both for selected-response and constructed-response examination formats, are provided.

For scoring, one of the major issues centers on standardization. The concept of standardized testing really refers to the conditions under which an assessment is delivered. While the level of "standardization" can vary somewhat as a function of the stakes of the evaluation, the proper interpretation of test scores demands that individuals are assessed under similar conditions. This is especially true for higher-stakes examinations such as those used for credentialing and licensure.

Here, it is important the administration conditions (e.g., lighting, time allowed for a task, screen size for computer-based examinations) are controlled. For typical multiple-choice examinations, it is fairly straightforward to standardize the administration conditions. For other types of assessments, such as those that employ raters or SPs, the task is far more difficult. For simulations, subtle variations in the fidelity of the simulation (e.g., SP portrayal of a specific scenario) or the reaction of the simulator to any management interventions (e.g., administering a drug to a mannequin) may cause those who are being assessed to alter their data collection or management strategies. To the extent that the scores are linked to the performance, and the performance conditions vary from one person to the next, the assessment results may have little meaning. For example, although the term "standardized patient" is widely used, it is very difficult to truly standardize patient actors. Unlike two actors in a play, the conversation between an SP and doctor (or nurse, or pharmacist) is semi-structured, and potentially impacted by a host of factors related to conversational dynamics. Likewise, subtle variations in the portrayal by an SP (e.g., level of depression) may lead candidates (examinees) on different management pathways, potentially leading to different diagnoses. In this case, if diagnosis was part of the scoring rubric, and the two examinees are not similarly exposed to the same testing conditions, differences in their performance may not be interpretable. That is, even though one person's score is higher than another's, it may not mean that his or her ability on the construct of interest is greater.

Even when the assessment conditions can be reasonably standardized, one needs to have appropriate, meaningful, scoring tools. At the heart of this issue is the alignment of the scores with the construct, or constructs, being measured. The scores could reflect the process (e.g., checklists for capturing data-gathering skills on an SP assessment) or outcomes (e.g., correct diagnosis on a patient management problem, correct answer on a multiple-choice item). For some assessments (e.g., selection tests such as multiple-choice examinations of knowledge), the scoring domains (e.g., knowledge of anatomy) and scoring processes are well developed. Years of work have yielded numerous scoring models ranging from the very simple (sum correct responses and divide by total number of test items) to the complex (e.g., item response theory).[46] For other types of assessments (e.g., constructed-response formats), the choice of scoring tools, and associated scoring models is not as clear. This is especially true for performance-based assessments, where those being assessed may employ divergent strategies in completing a task or exercise. Likewise, test developers, even with the help of content experts, may not achieve consensus about the host of potential correct responses.[50] For example, SP-based assessments commonly use checklists for assessing data-gathering skills. For a given simulated scenario (e.g., middle-aged male patient presenting with left side chest pain), and a defined target skill level of those being assessed, there may be no consensus on what checklist items (e.g., history taking, physical examination maneuvers) should be scored. Furthermore, the dynamic nature of health care, especially patient management strategies, suggests that the scoring criteria used today may be different sometime in the future. Finally, if the candidates know they are being assessed with checklists, and there is no mechanism to take into account irrelevant questions or inappropriate physical examination maneuvers, then individuals who "shotgun" questions and do as many maneuvers as possible within the time frame will score well. This score, at least as a measure of ability to interview and assess the patient appropriately, will necessarily be flawed.

For other types of performance assessments, the development of suitable scoring algorithms can be even more challenging. For example, some health care professional assessments employ mannequins to measure critical care skills. Given the nature of these events, the straight use of checklists is problematic because timing (e.g., quickly establishing an airway) and sequencing can be extremely important. If these facets are not captured in the scoring rubric, the interpretability of any ability measures could be faulty. Finally, test developers need to pay attention to how scores are aggregated. Often, scores from dissimilar constructs are added together to form a global measure of ability. If examinees can compensate for deficiencies in one area with better performance in others, the total score may not be appropriate for making inferences about some specific abilities.

Given that the assessment conditions are reasonably standardized, and the scoring rubrics make sense, one still needs to be certain that the scoring rules are consistently applied. For selected-response examinations (e.g., MCQs), often administered on a computer, it is reasonably straightforward to collect accurate data (responses to the items) and apply consistent scoring rules (e.g., calculate some form of ability measure through aggregation of responses). Likewise, rules governing the treatment of missing responses, weighting specific components, or the elimination of certain items based on post-administration analyses (e.g., key validation), can be applied consistently. For performance-based assessments, the application of consistent scoring rules is often more difficult. Where examiners (raters) are employed, they may have different levels of training, and they may not fully understand the scoring rubrics or, if employed over time, they may exhibit some drift in their performance expectations, potentially affecting how they apply the scoring criteria.[51–53] As a result, without adjustment to the ratings (e.g., equating scores) some examinees may have an advantage over others, regardless of their ability. Historically, this has been a problem with oral examinations where an examinee's ability estimate may be more a function of the choice of rater than the choice of task, or tasks. Regardless of the type of assessment employed, quality assurance measures are necessary to ensure that the scoring rules are employed consistently and that the scores are accurate.[54,55] For selected-response formats, this may entail scoring the examination on different computer systems or post hoc review of item responses. For constructed response assessments, especially those that employ raters, double-scoring select performances combined with analyses of rating patterns can help ensure that the scoring rules have been applied in a fair and consistent manner.

A final, but arguably less important, scoring issue concerns the application of appropriate security procedures. For all assessments, whether formative or summative, high or low stakes, or selected response or constructed response, prior exposure to the test material may provide some advantage to some examinees. Clearly, if examinees have previous access to specific test content on an MCQ examination, and correct answers to some or all of the items, their scores will be higher and may not necessarily reflect their ability. Similarly, even though it may have little impact unless the specific scoring rubrics are exposed, examinees who have prior information about the content of a performance-based assessment would be expected to obtain higher scores. In both of these situations, examinee ability estimates will likely be wrong, compromising any attempts to make meaningful interpretations of the scores. To ensure fairness, both test developers and those involved in the administration and scoring of an assessment need to ensure that test materials are secure.

Generalization

The generalization component of Kane's framework requires evidence that the observations (e.g., simulation scenarios, multiple-choice items, raters) were sampled adequately from the "universe" of available observations. In addition, evidence to suggest that the sample of observations is large enough to produce scores with reasonable precision is required. While the sampling of observations, and associated sources of measurement error, will necessarily vary as a function of the type of assessment, it is imperative that reasonably reliable estimates of ability can be derived. Take, for example, a short multiple-choice test of biomedical knowledge based on only four items. Clearly, the selection (sampling) of which four items to include will have some impact on how examinees perform.

Moreover, with so few items, it will be difficult to generalize any ability estimates (e.g., total score on the four items) to any other content-equivalent assessment or to the broader domain (biomedical knowledge). In effect, the sample of observations (items) is not sufficient to produce reliable ability estimates.

The sources of measurement error in assessment scores has been studied in detail.[56–60] Here, depending on the type of assessment used, some potential sources of "imprecision" are more relevant than others. For selected-response formats (e.g., MCQ tests) the sampling, and number, of items is key. Given that raters are not employed, and the time required for individual item responses is relatively small, MCQ tests can comprise a large number of items. Where this is the case, and item content is sampled appropriately from the domain (usually knowledge), precise measures of the targeted ability can be obtained. For other types of assessments (e.g., performance-based, constructed-response), other potential sources of measurement error come into play. As noted in the scoring section, raters are often employed to score performance-based assessments. Regardless of the scoring rubric employed, two raters watching the exact same performance may not provide the exact same scores. As a result, the choice and number of raters could have some impact on the precision of the ability estimates. It is important to note that task sampling plays a critical role in constructed-response formats. On an SP-based assessment, for example, it can take several minutes for an examinee to complete one task (e.g., interview the patient, perform a physical examination). Therefore, unlike an MCQ examination, it is impossible, without making the assessment inordinately long, to incorporate numerous simulation scenarios (tasks). As a result, the ability to generalize the scores from one set of tasks to another may be limited. While other potential sources of measurement error may exist (e.g., choice of assessment site, method of data collection), the primary ones, at least for health care-related assessments, pertain to choice of items (or tasks) and choice of raters.

While a detailed review of the techniques to explore sources of measurement error is beyond the scope of this chapter, it is important to note that the optimal conditions for test administration (e.g., test length, choice and number of raters), at least in terms of "maximizing" score precision, can be ascertained by estimating the magnitude of sources of variability in test scores.[61,62] Historically, various reliability measures (e.g., Cronbach's alpha, phi coefficient) were, and still are, used to estimate the internal consistency, inter-rater-consistency, and other precision-related properties of assessment scores. Unfortunately, in isolation, these measures are often inadequate at making relevant arguments about the overall generalizability of the scores (i.e., consistency of examinee performance over assessment conditions). Generalizability theory, detailed elsewhere,[63,64] has been advocated as a means to estimate, based on various potential sources of measurement error, the reproducibility of scores (association between the observed score—the score an examinee received on the assessment—and the universe score—the hypothetical score an examinee would receive if taking the assessment an infinite number of times). For example, in a multitask performance assessment, where raters provide scores, it is important to know that two examiners watching the same performance will provide reasonably equivalent scores. However, given the well-known effect of task specificity (i.e., the tendency of those being assessed to do well in one type of task, or content area, and not in another),[65] score precision can best be improved by adding additional relevant tasks, not raters per given task. Compared with knowledge-based examinations, it can be quite difficult to develop performance-based assessments with adequate score generalizability. Often, even though there is a desire to measure skills such as information gathering or clinical decision making, the choice of tasks (e.g., clinical scenarios) will have some impact on performance simply due to examinee familiarity with the specific content. As a result, examinees' performance may not reflect, or generalize to, their performance in another equivalent assessment (with different tasks) or, as discussed in the *extrapolation* section, to real-world performance.

Given that test content represents a sample from the knowledge or skill domain, those involved in assessment activities must take steps to ensure that the items (or tasks) are sampled sufficiently and, above all, are representative of the content domain. Defining the content domain can involve many steps, including consultations with experts, review of the curriculum (e.g., what is taught in medical, nursing), or various types of practice or job analyses.[66,67] In the health care professions, provider data can be used to delimit the scope of practice and types of patients, and associated conditions, that a practitioner is likely to encounter.[68] This information can subsequently be used to develop and validate relevant test content, including items for MCQs and simulation scenarios for performance-based assessments. Once this is accomplished, the assessment administration conditions that yield sufficiently reliable ability estimates (e.g., number of items or tasks, rating design if raters are employed) can be explored. Clearly, test developers must pay attention to what they intend to measure, the relevance of any test material to practice domain, and the adequacy of sampling (i.e., ensuring that there are enough items or cases or raters to yield reasonably precise scores). For example, if we produce a simulation-based assessment comprised entirely of critical care scenarios, it is not clear whether performance (assessment of clinical skills) on these scenarios will generalize to scenarios that focus on health mainte-nance. In terms of assessment quality, all things being equal, a short assessment with few items or tasks will yield less generalizable scores than a longer one.

Extrapolation

To the extent that assessment scores are obtained under standard conditions, and are reasonably precise, evidence to support that inferences based on these measures are meaningful comprise the next set of arguments in Kane's frame-work. If an assessment is not measuring what it is intended to measure, its quality, regardless of other measurement criteria, is necessarily poor. When collecting information that supports conclusions made about assessment results, determin-ing the relationship between assessment scores and actual behavior, proficiencies, or other relevant criterion measures is an important step in the inferential chain. Unfortunately, while research conducted on the validity of assessment scores yields some examples of studies that address the link between examination performance and real-world actions, these types of investigations are difficult to conduct. For example, if an examination is used for screening purposes, then any assessment-criterion relationships could be attenuated because those who do not meet selection criteria will not be eligible to move on to the next level of training or practice. However, other strategies to gather *extrapolation* evidence do exist. One can determine whether scores generated by assessments adequately or inadequately (construct underrepresentation) measure the targeted ability of interest or qualities other than those of interest (i.e., construct irrelevant vari-ance), the latter being a negative effect when viewed from an assessment quality perspective. In this section, we provide examples of studies that focus on the *extrapolation* argument and relate these to good assessment practices.

The key element of any assessment is the delineation of the trait, skill, or ability being measured. If the construct of interest (e.g., communication skills, clinical reasoning, knowledge) is not adequately defined and appropriately measured, then one cannot be certain of what is being assessed. As a result, relationships between the assessment scores and any criterion measures, either internal or external with respect to the assessment, could be confounded, ham-pering collection of evidence to support the *extrapolation* argument. For example, communication skills are often measured as part of SP assessments. If the assessment is based on checklists (e.g., maintained eye contact, introduced self, asked open-ended questions), then examinees may change their actual behavior to one that is more rote in order to capitalize on the scoring system. If this is the case, and the measure does not really reflect their "true" communication skills (introducing variability in scores based on something other than the construct of interest), then the assessment scores will have little meaning with respect to making inferences regarding "true" ability. Alternately, even if the communication skills are being measured adequately, performance may be idiosyncratic to the assessment environment. For example, one might expect that specific provider-patient communication, as measured in a standardized testing environment, might *not* be related to performance in the clinic, especially where the communication involves other health care workers and not simply patients. While often based on expert judgments, test developers also need to establish the relevance of assessment content (e.g., test items, simulation scenarios) for measuring the construct of interest. For health care workers, information about the requirements of practice, both in terms of skills required and typical practice conditions, can be gathered to inform assessment content. If the assessment context is not realistic or relevant, examinees may not be able to demonstrate their abilities, compromising the utility of the scores.

Provided the scores adequately represent the construct of interest (content validity), one can determine the extent to which the measures obtained are indicators of proficiency by identifying, and studying, other variables that are not related to the construct. For example, Swanson et al.[69] investigated the relationship between examinee and item characteristics and scores on a multiple-choice examination. They determined whether the difficulty of the item and presence of pictorial material affected examinee response time as part of the consideration of administering the examination in a computer-adaptive format. They concluded that there was an interaction between item difficulty and examinee proficiency. Under adaptive testing conditions, this could potentially introduce a factor that the examination was not intended to measure: speededness. This could result in inaccurate measurement of examinees' "true" proficiency, since more able examinees would be presented with more difficult items that take longer to read and complete, placing them at an unfair disadvantage. Because the examination was meant to assess knowledge of basic science rather than reading speed, the extent to which items increased in difficulty because of increased demand on a factor other than knowledge would introduce construct-irrelevant variance.

In contrast, studies that support assumptions about expertise in the construct of interest can provide evidence that the interpretations made about variability in scores are justified. An example of this is the work of Sawhill et al.,[70] who examined the relationship between medical licensure examination scores and postgraduate training of physicians. In the United States, for most jurisdictions, the license issued permits the general practice of medicine. The United States

Medical Licensing Examination (USMLE) Step 3 is the final examination in a series leading to licensure. The authors hypothesized that because the license issued in the United States is general in nature, those trainees who had begun to pursue a specialized medical career prior to taking USMLE Step 3 would not perform as well. The results of the study confirmed their hypothesis: those with more general training were more likely to obtain higher scores on the USMLE Step 3 examination. This would be expected, since the examination content would test knowledge across several clinical disciplines, and trainees who specialize may not have the same exposure to a broad range of patients. The results of their study provided additional evidence to support the *extrapolation* argument. Although not sufficient, at least on its own, for making any strong claims about the overall quality of the assessment, these types of studies can be used to support assertions that the examination content, given the purpose of the assessment, is appropriate for the intended test takers.

Using a performance-based (constructed-response) assessment, Boulet et al.[71] examined whether the medium used to collect post-encounter information affected ratings of content. Examinees were allowed to choose whether to write or type post-encounter notes as part of the administration of a high-stakes SP examination. The authors found that while there were differences in the characteristics of examinees choosing whether to write or type, there was no difference in the ratings awarded based on the medium used to complete the note. Because documentation and patient management skills are being assessed in the post-encounter exercise, handwriting should have minimal relationship to these skills. The findings of the study support the *extrapolation* argument: examinees receiving higher ratings on this measure were more able to document patient complaints and interpret findings than those who received lower ratings. In terms of the overall quality of the assessment, it was important to determine that the difference in media did not adversely impact (or provide an advantage) to either those who typed or those who handwrote their post-encounter notes. If administration conditions vary (e.g., mode of answering questions or responding to tasks, or timing), and this affects performance, the quality of the assessment results for making inferences about ability could be at risk.

There are also instances where examination scores are used for purposes that are not related to the construct of interest. Use of scores in this way may represent a "threat to validity" and can certainly hamper the *extrapolation* argument. An example of this possible misuse of scores (and potentially biased interpretations) was identified and reviewed by McGaghie and colleagues.[72] Although the USMLE series of examinations are clearly designed to provide licensing bodies with a common system of evaluation, and to ensure that examinees are sufficiently knowledgeable and have the proficiencies needed to practice general medicine in the United States, the same examination scores are often used to select postgraduate trainees. McGaghie et al.[72] correlated USMLE Step 1 (basic science) and Step 2 (clinical knowledge) scores with measures from clinical skills examinations taken by medical students and postgraduate trainees. They found that use of the scores for selection decisions was not supported by the study results; for the most part, scores from clinical skills examinations were only minimally related to scores from the knowledge (selected-response) examinations. While knowledge is likely to provide the basis for selection of appropriate techniques and procedures for patient care, it is not predictive of other skills needed to function as a practitioner. The findings of this study provide an indication that scores on basic science and clinical knowledge examinations are not sufficient to ensure that examinees have acquired the skills needed in supervised clinical practice (i.e., postgraduate medical education). It is important to note that the quality of an assessment is highly dependent on its purpose. An assessment that is designed to make criterion-referenced interpretations (e.g., establish minimal competence) may or may not be appropriate for norm-referenced interpretations (e.g., ranking candidates for selection into an advanced program).

As mentioned at the beginning of this section, it is challenging to accumulate evidence to support arguments associated with whether the assessment scores (or decisions) predict behavior in the workplace. Nevertheless, some work has been done in this area, including an investigation of the extent to which performance on the communication portion of a licensure examination predicted complaints filed with medical regulatory authorities. Tamblyn et al.[73] found that the risk of complaints was greatest for physicians whose performance was in the lowest quartile on the doctor-patient communication component of a national licensing examination using SPs. Also, poor performance on the clinical decision-making component of the examination was associated with the likelihood that complaints filed were due to errors affecting patient outcomes. This research supported the decision to include these measures in a national licensure examination. While the physicians included in the study had all passed the examination, these results still provide evidence that supports the *extrapolation* argument that better performance on the assessment is associated with better performance in actual practice. Given the purpose of certification and licensure assessments in the health professions (i.e., protect the public), these types of investigations are an essential part of the validity argument. Good assessments, especially those where the evaluation task closely approximates that encountered in the practice setting, require evidence that the scores appropriately represent, or predict, the proficiency, or proficiencies, of interest.

Interpretation/Decision

Assessments administered as part of the education, certification, and licensure of health professionals are frequently used to determine minimal competence (identify levels of knowledge or skill that are "good enough"). Using Kane's conception of validity, the evidence supporting the argument that decisions made based on the scores obtained are indicative of being "good enough" for progression, advanced training, or entry to practice provide the foundation of *interpretation/ decision* accuracy. The evidence in favor of decision and interpretation arguments also includes research conducted on the assessment scores to support theories, such as the nature of expert-novice differences in reasoning and clinical decision making. Whether the assessment is comprised of selected or constructed responses, decisions and interpretations made based on results are an integral part of the validity framework and, thus, a defining element of what constitutes a good assessment. Examples of evidence accumulation for this part of the framework will be presented for score interpretations based on theoretical constructs and for decisions made based on the assessment results obtained.

Theories from cognitive psychology can help explain how health professionals learn and develop problem-solving and clinical decision-making skills. Research has shown that the development of specialized problem solving routines is based on the opportunity to practice and repeat the process of finding solutions.[74] These theories assert that expertise is developed through experience and that experts differ from novices in measurable ways. Experts are thought to be more adept at identifying meaning, are less reliant on context, and are more adept at retrieving existing relevant knowledge from memory.[75] In order to develop consistent, accurate representations of knowledge, novices can benefit from connections made between biomedical and clinical knowledge.[76] It is likely, therefore, that those who perform well on assessments of biomedical knowledge are also more able when their clinical reasoning skills are assessed. It is also likely that the opportunity to practice and refine problem-solving routines varies with level of education. Research supports this assertion and several studies have been conducted that delineate performance differences between individuals with more and less experience.[77] The differences in performance, by education or experience, support the *interpretation* argument because the construct underlying performance should logically improve with additional training and practical experience. With respect to determining the quality of an assessment, the extent to which the scores align with some established theory (e.g., experiential learning) is certainly one criterion.

The scores from many assessments are used to establish minimal competence. To support the validity argument for these types of decisions, selection of the method to set the standard(s) is important. The process must be aligned with the purpose of the assessment (e.g., selection, progression, licensure), rely on the judgment of experts and stakeholders, require thoughtful effort on the part of the participants, be easy to explain and implement, and be supported by research.[78] Credibility of cut-scores, an integral component of assessments designed to categorize individuals, is based on the extent to which these criteria can be met. Evidence supporting the argument that results of standard setting meeting these requirements can be gathered before, during, and after the process. McKinley et al.[79] determined that standards on performance-based assessments could be established by having judges review and rate performances (e.g., videotaped encounters) based on an established definition of minimal competence. They found that reproducible, defensible, standards could be established by having judges determine whether the examination results they reviewed represented minimally adequate performance. Although standard-setting judgments are policy decisions, the methods used to derive the cut-scores were sensible and yielded credible classification decisions. It is also worthy to note that standards were set separately for various conjunctive elements of the examination. This is important because those individuals with poor performance in one area of the examination cannot compensate with better performance in another. The quality of the assessment, at least in terms of identifying those individuals with minimal competence in all important skills areas, would be compromised if a single pass/fail standard based on aggregate performance was embraced.

For licensure and certification examinations, where protection of the public is the primary purpose, it is often assumed that those passing the examination are competent to practice in their profession. This is a reasonable hypothesis if the standards were set and applied appropriately. Tamblyn et al.[80] examined whether performance on licensure/certification examinations was associated with improved patient outcomes (mammogram screenings, continuity of care, consultation/referrals, contraindicated prescribing, and disease-specific prescribing) among family physicians. They found that examinations taken as early as the end of medical school were predictive of patient outcomes 4–7 years after starting in practice. While not statistically significant, there was still a trend toward lower risk of contraindicated prescribing behaviors among those who achieved higher diagnosis and management subscores on the assessment. The results of the study suggest that, for the assessments included in this research, performance on the examination predicted behavior in practice. This evidence supports the decision that passing performance is positively associated with improved patient outcomes. For assessments where classification decisions are made, their quality, at least to some extent, will be based on the available evidence that supports the utility and meaningfulness of the decision rules.

Conclusion

There are numerous frameworks, and resultant criteria, that can be used to define good assessment practices. Based on Kane's idea of building a validity argument, several key components of good assessments are clear. First, the assessment administration conditions need to be standardized, the scoring system must be aligned with the purpose of the assessment, and the scoring rules must be explicit; also, special care must be taken to develop items and scales that allow for accurate data capture. Second, even if accurate scores can be obtained, it is important that the content domain be sampled sufficiently. For any examinee, the precision of our ability estimate, as derived from the assessment scores, is related to the number of times we measure the relevant construct, or constructs. In general, the greater the sampling (number of items on an MCQ test, number of tasks on a performance-based assessment, number of raters for a given task), the greater the generalizability of the scores. Good assessments, by employing designs that minimize potential sources of measurement error, will yield reasonably precise measures of ability. Third, good assessments should employ measurement tools that adequately cover the domain of interest. If the domain (skills, competencies) is underrepresented, any inferences that one makes based on the test scores may be flawed. Where assessments are employed to select or screen examinees, one needs to gather evidence to support the ranking or categorization process. For performance-based assessments, especially those that employ high-fidelity simulations, performance on the assessment should be related to real-world performance. For all assessments, evidence also needs to be gathered to indicate that the scores are not unduly influenced by factors unrelated to the construct of interest. Here, various research studies can be conducted to explore whether assessment scores are influenced by factors such as the administrative setting, examinee demographics, or the interaction between examinee and rater characteristics. Finally, when assessments are used to make decisions, evidence needs to be procured to support the accuracy of any categorizations.

Gathering this evidence can take many forms, but initially rests with the use of sensible standard-setting procedures. Likewise, for the scores to have any value with respect to quantifying specific skills or proficiencies, a theory-based inter-pretation of their meaning is essential. Whether one posits (based on theory) that individuals with more relevant experience should perform better, that some constructs are hierarchically related to others (e.g., knowledge, clinical decision making), or that certain skills (e.g., thoroughness and efficiency) are integral parts of proper patient care, the analysis of scores from an assessment should support these relationships.

References

1. Accreditation Council for Graduate Medical Education, American Board of Medical Specialties. *Toolbox of Assessment Methods: version 1.1*. Chicago, IL: Accreditation Council for Graduate Medical Education and American Board of Medical Specialties; 2000.
2. Boulet J, Errichetti A. Training and assessment with standardized patients. In: Riley RH, editor. *Manual of Simulation in Healthcare*. 1st ed. London: Oxford University Press; 2008. pp. 181–97.
3. Carraccio C, Englander R. Evaluating competence using a portfolio: a literature review and web-based application to the ACGME competencies. *Teach Learn Med*. 2004; **16**(4): 381–7.
4. Stringer KR, Bajenov S, Yentis SM. Training in airway management. *Anaesthesia*. 2002; **57**(10): 967–83.
5. Hambleton RK. Advances in performance assessment methodology. *Appl Psychol Meas*. 2000; **24**(4): 291–3.
6. Holmboe ES. Assessment of the practicing physician: challenges and opportunities. *J Cont Educ Health Prof*. 2008; **28**(Suppl. 1): S4–10.
7. Howley LD. Performance assessment in medical education: where we've been and where we're going. *Eval Health Prof*. 2004; **27**(3): 285–303.
8. Lammers RL, Davenport M, Korley F, et al. Teaching and assessing procedural skills using simulation: metrics and methodology. *Acad Emerg Med*. 2008; **15**(11): 1079–87.
9. Norcini JJ, McKinley DW. Assessment methods in medical education. *Teach Teach Educ*. 2007; **23**: 239–50.
10. Veloski J, Boex JR, Grasberger MJ, et al. Systematic review of the literature on assessment, feedback and physicians' clinical performance: BEME Guide No. 7. *Med Teach*. 2006; **28**(2): 117–28.
11. Case SM, Swanson DB. *Constructing Written Test Questions for the Basic and Clinical Sciences*, 3rd ed. Philadelphia, PA: National Board of Medical Examiners; 2010.

12. Boulet JR. Summative assessment in medicine: the promise of simulation for high-stakes evaluation. *Acad Emerg Med.* 2008; **15**(11): 1017–24.

13. Boulet JR, Murray DJ. Simulation-based assessment in anesthesiology: requirements for practical implementation. *Anesthesiology.* 2010; **112**(4): 1041–52.

14. Boulet JR, Smee SM, Dillon GF, et al. The use of standardized patient assessments for certification and licensure decisions. *Simul Healthc.* 2009; **4**(1): 35–42.

15. Hawkins RE, Swanson DB, Dillon GF, et al. The introduction of clinical skills assessment into the United States Medical Licensing Examination (USMLE): a description of USMLE Step 2 Clinical Skills (CS). *J Med Licen Dis.* 2005; **91**(3): 22–5.

16. Melnick DE, Dillon GF, Swanson DB. Medical licensing examinations in the United States. *J Dent Educ.* 2002; **66**(5): 595–9.

17. Dillon GF, Boulet JR, Hawkins RE, et al. Simulations in the United States Medical Licensing Examination (USMLE). *Qual Saf Health Care.* 2004; **13**(Suppl. 1): i41–5.

18. Dillon GF, Clyman SG, Clauser BE, et al. The introduction of computer-based case simulations into the United States Medical Licensing Examination. *Acad Med.* 2002; **77**(Suppl. 10): S94–6.

19. Swanson DB, Norcini JJ, Grosso LJ. Assessment of clinical competence: written and computer-based simulations. *Assess Eval Higher Educ.* 1987; **12**(3): 220–46.

20. Patil NG, Saing H, Wong J. Role of OSCE in evaluation of practical skills. *Med Teach.* 2003; **25**(3): 271–2.

21. Riley RH, editor. *Manual of Simulation in Healthcare.* Oxford: Oxford University Press; 2008.

22. Nestel D, Kneebone R, Black S. Simulated patients and the development of procedural and operative skills. *Med Teach.* 2006; **28**(4): 390–1.

23. Norcini J, Burch V. Workplace-based assessment as an educational tool: AMEE Guide No. 31. *Med Teach.* 2007; **29**(9): 855–71.

24. Norcini JJ. Work based assessment. *BMJ.* 2003; **326**(7392): 753–5.

25. Nestel D, van Herzeele I, Aggarwal R, et al. Evaluating training for a simulated team in complex whole procedure simulations in the endovascular suite. *Med Teach.* 2009; **31**(1): e18–23.

26. Kneebone R, Baillie S. Contextualized simulation and procedural skills: a view from medical education. *J Vet Med Educ.* 2008; **35**(4): 595–8.

27. Wright MC, Phillips-Bute BG, Petrusa ER, et al. Assessing teamwork in medical education and practice: relating behavioural teamwork ratings and clinical performance. *Med Teach.* 2009; **31**(1): 30–8.

28. Kirkpatrick DL. *Evaluating Training Programs: the four levels.* 2nd ed. San Francisco, CA: Berrett-Koehler; 1998.

29. American Educational Research Association, American Psychological Association, National Council on Measurement in Education. *Standards for Educational and Psychological Testing.* Washington, DC: American Educational Research Association; 1999.

30. McDonald RP. *Test Theory: a unified treatment.* Mahwah, NJ: Lawrence Erlbaum Associates; 1999.

31. Kane M. An argument-based approach to validation. *Psychol Bull*. 1992; **112**: 527–35.
32. Kane MT. Validating interpretive arguments for licensure and certification examinations. *Eval Health Prof*. 1994; **17**(2): 133–59.
33. Kane M, Crooks T, Cohen A. Validating measures of performance. *Educ Meas Issues Pract*. 1999; **18**(2): 5–17.
34. Messick S. Meaning and values in test validation: the science and ethics of assessment. *Educ Res*. 1989; **18**(2): 5–11.
35. Messick S. The interplay of evidence and consequences in the validation of performance assessments. *Educ Res*. 1994; **23**(2): 13–23.
36. Crocker L, Algina J. *Introduction to Classical and Modern Test Theory*. New York, NY: Harcourt Brace Jovanovich College Publishers; 1986.
37. Downing SM, Haladyna TM. Validity threats: overcoming interference with proposed interpretations of assessment data. *Med Educ*. 2004; **38**(3): 327–33.
38. Downing SM. Validity: on the meaningful interpretation of assessment data. *Med Educ*. 2003; **37**(9): 830–7.
39. Downing SM. Reliability: on the reproducibility of assessment data. *Med Educ*. 2004; **38**(9): 1006–12.
40. Cook DA, Beckman TJ. Current concepts in validity and reliability for psychometric instruments: theory and application. *Am J Med*. 2006; **119**(2): 166.e7–16.
41. Norcini J, Anderson B, Bollela V, et al. Criteria for good assessment: consensus statement and recommendations from the Ottawa 2010 Conference. *Med Teach*. 2011; **33**(3): 206–14.
42. Clauser BE, Margolis MJ, Swanson DB. Issues of validity and reliability for assessments in medical education. In: Holmboe ES, Hawkins RE, editors. *Practical Guide to the Evaluation of Clinical Competence*. Philadelphia, PA: Mosby/Elsevier; 2008. pp. 10–23.
43. Bennett RE, Bejar II. Validity and automated scoring: it's not only the scoring. *Educ Meas Issues Pract*. 1998; **17**(4): 9–17.
44. Clauser BE, Margolis MJ, Clyman SG, et al. Development of automated scoring algorithms for complex performance assessments: a comparison of two approaches. *J Educ Meas*. 1997; **34**(2): 141–61.
45. Clauser BE. Recurrent issues and recent advances in scoring performance assessments. *Appl Psych Meas*. 2000; **24**(4): 310–24.
46. De Champlain AF. A primer on classical test theory and item response theory for assessments in medical education. *Med Educ*. 2010; **44**(1): 109–17.
47. Hawkins RE, Margolis MJ, Durning SJ, et al. Constructing a validity argument for the mini-clinical evaluation exercise: a review of the research. *Acad Med*. 2010; **85**(9): 1453–61.
48. Ringsted C, Østergaard D, Ravn L, et al. A feasibility study comparing checklists and global rating forms to assess resident performance in clinical skills. *Med Teach*. 2003; **25**(6): 654–8.
49. Whelan GP, Boulet JR, McKinley DW, et al. Scoring standardized patient examina-

tions: lessons learned from the development and administration of the ECFMG Clinical Skills Assessment (CSA). *Med Teach*. 2005; **27**(3): 200–6.

50. Boulet JR, van Zanten M, De Champlain A, et al. Checklist content on a standardized patient assessment: an ex post facto review. *Adv Health Sci Educ Theory Pract*. 2008; **13**(1): 59–69.

51. Melnick D, editor. *The Use of Holistic Scoring for Post-Encounter Written Exercises*. Philadelphia, PA: National Board of Medical Examiners; 2000.

52. Clauser BE, Clyman SG, Swanson DB. Components of rater error in a complex performance assessment. *J Educ Meas*. 1999; **36**(1): 29–45.

53. McIntyre RM, Smith DE, Hassett CE. Accuracy of performance ratings as affected by rater training and perceived purpose of rating. *J Appl Psychol*. 1984; **69**(1): 147–56.

54. Boulet JR, McKinley DW, Whelan GP, et al. Quality assurance methods for performance-based assessments. *Adv Health Sci Educ Theory Pract*. 2003; **8**(1): 27–47.

55. Downing SM, Haladyna TM. Test item development: validity evidence from quality assurance procedures. *Appl Meas Educ*. 1997; **10**(1): 61–82.

56. Donoghue A, Nishisaki A, Sutton R, et al. Reliability and validity of a scoring instrument for clinical performance during pediatric advanced life support simulation scenarios. *Resuscitation*. 2010; **81**(3): 331–6.

57. Iramaneerat C, Yudkowsky R, Myford CM, et al. Quality control of an OSCE using generalizability theory and many-faceted Rasch measurement. *Adv Health Sci Educ Theory Pract*. 2008; **13**(4): 479–93.

58. Raymond MR, Clauser BE, Swygert K, et al. Measurement precision of spoken English proficiency scores on the USMLE Step 2 Clinical Skills examination. *Acad Med*. 2009; **84**(Suppl. 10): S83–5.

59. Swanson DB, Norcini JJ. Factors influencing reproducibility of tests using standardized patients. *Teach Learn Med*. 1989; **1**(3): 158–66.

60. Roberts C, Newble D, Jolly B, et al. Assuring the quality of high-stakes undergraduate assessments of clinical competence. *Med Teach*. 2006; **28**(6): 535–43.

61. Clauser BE, Harik P, Margolis MJ. A multivariate generalizability analysis of data from a performance assessment of physicians' clinical skills. *J Educ Meas*. 2006; **43**(3): 173–91.

62. Lawson DM. Applying generalizability theory to high-stakes objective structured clinical examinations in a naturalistic environment. *J Manip Physio Ther*. 2006; **29**(6): 463–7.

63. Boulet JR. Generalizability theory: basics. In: Everitt BS, Howell DC, editors. *Encyclopedia of Statistics in Behavioral Science*. Chichester, UK: John Wiley & Sons; 2005. pp. 704–11.

64. Brennan RL. *Generalizability Theory*. New York, NY: Springer-Verlag; 2001.

65. Turnbull J, Danoff D, Norman G. Content specificity and oral certification exams. *Med Educ*. 1996; **30**(1): 56–9.

66. Crocker L. Assessing content representativeness of performance assessment exercises. *Appl Meas Educ*. 1997; **10**(1): 83–95.

67. Murphy DJ, Bruce D, Eva KW. Workplace-based assessment for general practitioners: using stakeholder perception to aid blueprinting of an assessment battery. *Med Educ.* 2008; **42**(1): 96–103.

68. Boulet JR, Gimpel JR, Errichetti AM, et al. Using National Medical Care Survey data to validate examination content on a performance-based clinical skills assessment for osteopathic physicians. *J Am Osteopath Assoc.* 2003; **103**(5): 225–31.

69. Swanson DB, Case SM, Ripkey DR, et al. Relationships among item characteristics, examinee characteristics, and response times on USMLE Step 1. *Acad Med.* 2001; **76**(Suppl. 10): S114–16.

70. Sawhill AJ, Dillon GF, Ripkey DR, et al. The impact of postgraduate training and timing on USMLE Step 3 performance. *Acad Med.* 2003; **78**(Suppl. 10): S10–12.

71. Boulet JR, McKinley DW, Rebbecchi T, et al. Does composition medium affect the psychometric properties of scores on an exercise designed to assess written medical communication skills? *Adv Health Sci Educ Theory Pract.* 2007; **12**(2): 157–67.

72. McGaghie WC, Cohen ER, Wayne DB. Are United States Medical Licensing Exam Step 1 and 2 scores valid measures for postgraduate medical residency selection decisions? *Acad Med.* 2011; **86**(1): 48–52.

73. Tamblyn R, Abrahamowicz M, Dauphinee D, et al. Physician scores on a national clinical skills examination as predictors of complaints to medical regulatory authorities. *JAMA.* 2007; **298**(9): 993–1001.

74. Norman G. Research in clinical reasoning: past history and current trends. *Med Educ.* 2005; **39**(4): 418–27.

75. Regehr G, Norman GR. Issues in cognitive psychology: implications for professional education. *Acad Med.* 1996; **71**(9): 988–1001.

76. Woods NN. Science is fundamental: the role of biomedical knowledge in clinical reasoning. *Med Educ.* 2007; **41**(12): 1173–7.

77. Murray DJ, Boulet JR, Avidan M, et al. Performance of residents and anesthesiologists in a simulation-based skill assessment. *Anesthesiology.* 2007; **107**(5): 705–13.

78. Norcini J, McKinley D. Standard setting. In: Dent JA, Harden RM, editors. *A Practical Guide for Medical Teachers.* 3rd ed. New York, NY: Elsevier Churchill Livingstone; 2009. pp. 311–17.

79. McKinley DW, Boulet JR, Hambleton RK. A work-centered approach for setting passing scores on performance-based assessments. *Eval Health Prof.* 2005; **28**(3): 349–69.

80. Tamblyn R, Abrahamowicz M, Dauphinee WD, et al. Association between licensure examination scores and practice in primary care. *JAMA.* 2002; **288**(23): 3019–26.

3

Technology-Enabled Assessment of Health Professions Education*

Zubair Amin, John R. Boulet, David A. Cook,
Rachel Ellaway, Ahmad Fahal, Roger Kneebone,
Moira Maley, Doris Østergaard, Gominda Ponnamperuma,
Andy Wearn, and Amitai Ziv

Introduction

We live in a world suffused with information and communication technologies (ICTs). It is increasingly difficult now to remember a time without high-quality, synthesized electronic information at our fingertips. However, such technologies did not deliver on their promise immediately: systems were slow and data trustworthiness was uncertain.[1] Yet, the last decade has seen such technologies become an integral part of the instruction, assessment, and clinical practice of health professionals. Fundamental challenges remain as we seek to make appropriate and well-informed use of technologies in support of health professional assessment. This chapter presents a series of consensus recommendations to educators, administrators, and organizations about the use of different technologies in support of assessment practices.

This chapter is divided into three parts: the first part describes the role of ICT in assessment, the second part highlights challenges in using technology in

---

* Amin Z, Boulet JR, Cook DA, et al. Technology-enabled assessment of health professions education: consensus statement and recommendations from the Ottawa 2010 conference. *Med Teach.* 2011; **33**(5): 364–9. Reprinted by permission of Informa Healthcare.

assessment with a specific consideration of threats to the valid interpretation of assessment scores and associated outcomes, and the third part considers issues for research in this area. The chapter concludes with recommendations in general, for institutions and policy makers, for assessors and test developers, and about future research initiatives.

Technology in Context

New assessment technologies should be considered in the larger context of health care and health professions education. This section will explore change as a defining attribute of technology, the increasingly ubiquitous presence of technology in health professions education, and current applications of ICTs in assessment.

Change and Technology

Technologies tend not only to subvert their predecessors but also, in most cases, to immediately suggest further advances.[2] Nevertheless, not everything changes when a new technology is introduced into a given situation. We can consider three essential aspects of change associated with the use of technology in assessment: (1) transmediation, (2) innovation, and (3) prosthesis.

Transmediation involves moving existing information, practices, and tools to new media while retaining their essential qualities. For example, traditional end-of-course paper-based examinations that involve whole classes sitting down together are often transmediated by replicating the same examination on a computer. Although the medium has changed (computer has replaced paper), the fundamental content and process remains the same.

Innovation refers to forms and processes that could not exist without technology. Recent innovations in assessment include technology-enhanced simulation and dynamic media such as interactive images and video.[3,4] The relative proportions of transmediation and innovation indicate how much of the original has been translated through using ICT. The extent of real innovation tends to be low, following evolutionary rather than revolutionary trajectories. While this is not necessarily problematic, we may inadvertently introduce artifacts and enforce inappropriate orthodoxies in the design and use of the technology in question if we only transmediate current practice.[5] For instance, many online examinations unnecessarily still now follow the limitations of paper-based examination materials.

Prosthesis occurs when ICT extends action beyond human limits, allowing us to do things faster, more accurately, and in more places simultaneously than would be possible without the technology. For instance, ICTs can extend and enhance assessment workflows and logistics by facilitating the development of questions and examinations, managing security, and marking and providing feedback. Indeed, in many cases efficiency and quality control are the primary reasons for institutions to adopt e-assessment.[6]

Technology in Health Professional Education

Both medicine and education are intrinsically technology-enabled phenomena.[7,8] Modern medicine involves a large systematized knowledge base and a vast armamentarium of diagnostic tools, treatments, and other technologies. Becoming a doctor is in many ways synonymous with becoming a technocrat with humanistic goals of care and altruism. Doctors are caregivers whose authority comes in large part from an appropriate use and control of technology (e.g., tools, medicines, devices, and knowledge repositories). Similarly, education is founded on system-based learning, education structured using technologies such as computers, smart classrooms, and simulation.[9]

ICT is clearly fundamental to any health care system. It is currently manifested as electronic medical records, electronic ordering systems, picture archival and communication systems, billing systems, and more generally through PubMed, online journals, databases, and handheld and mobile technologies. The uptake of new technologies remains rapid, with two-thirds of physicians and 42% of the public using smartphones as of late 2009.[10] The creation of ICT applications related to health and health care is also moving quickly. Since February 2010, there were nearly 6000 medical applications available from Apple's iTunes App Store. The number is still growing.[10]

Higher education is loaded with technologies including PowerPoint and learning management systems such as Blackboard or Moodle. Contemporary student learning involves using Google and Wikipedia equal to an institutional library.[11,12] Most of the ICTs used in health profession education are generic. In addition, many health care-specific technologies can be employed for both formative and summative assessment. The technologies include applications of simulation ranging from low-fidelity task trainers to high-fidelity mannequins.[6,13]

Clearly, the applications and significance of technologies in health care and education are broad-based, inherent, and pervasive.[12,14] It is in this context that technology in assessment of health professions education must be considered, in part because it defines what is normative, acceptable and sustainable, and in part because good assessment practice should faithfully reflect the clinical environment.[15,16]

Technology in Health Professions Education Assessment

Although the use of ICT in assessment is not new,[17,18] major developments of technology in health profession education assessment are largely centered on computer-based assessment,[4] use of simulation,[19,20] and management of assessment processes. Not surprisingly, some of the strongest evidence supporting the use of technology comes from these areas.[21]

Computer-Based Assessments

Over the past 2 decades, improvements in ICTs have led to many enhancements in item and test construction, test delivery, and scoring. The use of paper-and-pencil multiple-choice examinations has gradually been transmediated into computer-based delivery of test content, often over the internet via secure, encrypted, connections. Computers also offer innovation and prosthesis: provided the item pool is sufficiently large and a detailed blueprint exists, automated test construction software can be used to generate multiple test forms.[20,22] Moreover, the use of computers enables rapid scoring, including the generation of adaptive testing and the provision of tailored feedback. The use of technology also allows for the construction of computerized virtual patient cases where those being assessed are tasked with managing a patient (or patients) in simulated real time on the computer.[23,24]

Simulation and Simulators

There have also been many innovations in simulator technology, including part-task trainers and various electromechanical mannequins.[13,20,25–27] Simulation and simulators create a safe, learner-centered environment where mistakes do not result in harm to the patient.[13,19,25,28] Appropriate use of technologies allows easier sampling of a much broader domain of physician competencies.[29] In addition to the focused assessment of individual skills, innovative procedures have been developed such as the use of part-task trainers together with standardized patients (e.g., suturing using a skin pad attached to a real human being) to allow concurrent assessment of both procedural and communication skills.[26] Crisis events can also be modeled, allowing health care teams to be evaluated in a realistic environment including rare but important clinical events essential for teaching patient safety.[30,31] Distributed simulation using a portable, low-cost, and highly immersive environment offers a new avenue of testing clinical skills in authentic setting.[16] Onscreen simulations, such as virtual patients, are another growing form and one that has been found to have utility in assessment as well as learning.[32,33] Overall, advancements in simulator technology have opened the door for more authentic assessments that can be used to assess a much wider range of skills that were previously difficult to measure.[13]

Management of Assessment Processes

Prosthesis by virtue of improved logistics (i.e., enhanced efficiency, tracking, and quality assurance) is a vitally important yet often overlooked advantage of ICTs in health professional assessment—perhaps because students are not directly involved. It is often in this area that the greatest benefits are to be found.[15] Examples of technology in assessment resource management include item banking, plagiarism detection, data monitoring and reporting, result analysis, remote tracking, and telemetry. In addition, planned integration of assessment processes with the clinical environment allows linking of patient outcome-related data to the performance of clinicians.[34,35]

Challenges in the Use of Technology for Assessment

Critical evaluation of the evidence supporting the use of ICTs in assessment is essential but not the only requisite for informed decision making. We must also appreciate the many challenges that can result from using ICTs in assessment. These challenges include factors such as resource limitation (e.g., expensive simulators), a lack of trained faculty, ethical challenges (e.g., balancing commercial interest with educational needs), and organizational inertia. While these factors are important, this section will focus on potential validity threats associated with using technologies in assessment, not least because validity is central to any good assessment.[36]

Assessing the Wrong Construct

Assessment fundamentally involves making inferences about the learner—inferences about their knowledge, attitudes, general competence, communication skills, and so forth. This intended inference is called a construct. Unfortunately, ICTs can sometimes interfere in unintended ways to alter the construct that is actually measured, and this of course adversely impacts the meaning of the assessment results. For instance, a poorly designed assessment tool might measure the candidate's ability to use the technology rather than (or in addition to) measuring the intended clinical performance (i.e., the intended construct). Of course, if the purpose of the assessment is to assess candidates' ability to the use of technology (such as working with an electronic medical record) then the construct is, in part, the use of technology.[37]

Deviation from Real-Life Experiences

Many technology-based assessments attempt to emulate real-life experiences. Since clinical practice is complex and influenced by multiple variables,[22] the scripts for such assessments must be carefully developed.[26] Using simple assessment activities that minimize the interactions among key variables may make the process easier to handle, but this will also widen the gap between the assessment activity and the clinical reality that it represents. Conversely, an instructor might design an assessment that contains details or requires actions that unnecessarily increase the complexity of the exercise beyond the learner's current level of training. This complexity, particularly if it is not germane or intrinsic to the construct being assessed, can increase cognitive load, which in turn can cause measured performance to suffer. Finally, there is a risk that the designers of technology-enhanced assessment activities might select topics that do not reflect situations encountered in a typical practice.[38] One should ensure that the measures of assessment are well linked to the practical context rather than what the "simulator" can effectively model and measure.

Tension between Learner Assessment and Course/Technology Evaluation

The educators implementing a new assessment technology will often be interested in evaluating the performance of the technology itself. To the degree that this evaluation interferes with the optimal assessment process, this could invalidate any inferences concerning the ability of the learners. For example, the act of measurement could directly affect trainees' performance (Hawthorne effect), or could paradoxically cause them to pay more attention to the simulation than they otherwise would. Identifying and balancing these confounders is critically important when applying study findings to real-life applications.

Inappropriate Levels of Fidelity

Validity and reliability are linked to the fidelity of representation of clinical contexts and candidates' actions within technology-enhanced assessment. While greater fidelity enhances the perceived realism of the assessment activity, it can also increase the complexity and cognitive load associated with the assessment exercise. High-fidelity assessments (e.g., simulation) may be poorly suited for assessing some learning objectives (e.g., knowledge) or may not be well suited for certain specialties. For example, full immersion simulation with human patient simulators works well for anesthetic teams, but may be less appropriate when the focus is on surgeons and others doing procedural interventions.[26] Also, higher fidelity usually comes at a price—both the monetary cost of the technology itself and the cost in instructor time to develop and conduct the assessment.[39] Thus, assessors should target appropriate levels of fidelity for the given assessment task to ensure that this study is both meaningful and sustainable.

Future Research

It is beyond the scope of this chapter to outline a specific research agenda related to technology-enabled assessment. There are, however, some general issues that must be addressed to ensure that any new technology-based developments used for formative or summative purposes yield valid and defensible scores or decisions.

Validity

As technology improves, offering more ways to assess candidates, we must continue to be concerned with the validity of the inferences we make based on the assessment scores. Although technological improvements can provide more efficient delivery of assessments, yield higher-fidelity test content, and enable rapid scoring and tailored feedback, we still need to ensure the validity of the assessment results. As outlined earlier, one can focus research efforts on investigating potential threats to validity.[40] These types of studies could include looking at the impact of candidate familiarity with the assessment method on ability estimation, timing and pacing issues, and, more broadly, the relationship between the fidelity of the assessment and performance. However, the most salient validity issue is establishing the relationship between performance on the assessment and, for health care practitioners, the performance with "real" patients. Longitudinally, we need to determine whether advances in assessment technologies lead to better patient outcomes or other benefits such as cost savings. Also, given the prevailing literature on impact of assessment on learning,[41,42] and the enhancements in the fidelity of various assessments, comparative research aimed at quantifying the educational impact of new assessment formats is certainly needed.

Reliability

Technological advances, including the development of computer-based delivery of test content and the evolution of part-task trainers, objective structured clinical examinations, and electromechanical mannequins, have allowed for the construction of many new and different types of assessment processes. Like all assessments, however, the sources of measurement error need to be investigated and quantified. For objective structured clinical examinations, especially those involving standardized patients, computer-based training of patient actors can enhance the fidelity of their portrayal and minimize scoring errors, thus yielding more reliable estimates.[43] Additional research concentrating on the application of technology for the training of those involved in health care-related performance assessments, including raters, is needed. Finally, with the introduction of physical and onscreen simulators into the assessment domain, test developers have been challenged with the construction of new scoring rubrics.[4] For some assessments, such as those involving procedural skills, the evaluation tools tend to be case specific, potentially limiting the generalizability of the scores. For others, including simulation scenarios keyed to measuring more generic skills such as teamwork and ethical behavior, the evaluation tools and scoring criteria can be difficult to interpret, even for experts, resulting in evaluations that can be subject to rater effects. As advances in technology broaden the assessment domain, it is important that research be conducted to determine the specific sources of measurement error in the scores.

Other Research Areas

While research concerning the validity and reliability of assessment scores is paramount, technological advancements in test delivery, test construction, and simulation for assessment also provide other opportunities for targeted studies. One of the most important research areas rests in ascertaining the comparative efficiency of competing testing approaches. While higher-fidelity assessment models may be perceived to be more effective in measuring educational outcomes, they are costly, can be logistically complex, and may not yield appreciably better measures of ability.[39] Likewise, if ICTs are used to deliver formative assessments, research is needed to best align educational models with the learning needs of the participants. These outcome measures can eventually be used to validate prior assessment scores.

Conclusions

The deliberations of this research group have highlighted the changing nature of ICTs, their near-ubiquitous presence in health care and education, the importance of integrating technology-enabled assessment within health professional education as a whole, the evidence supporting use of technologies in health profession education assessment, the educational challenges related to use of technologies in assessment, and directions for future research.

Because of the rapid change associated with ICTs, institutions and assessment planners should remain vigilant and should develop necessary expertise in technology-enabled education and assessment, along with a coherent and responsible institutional use of technology. Assessment planners should ensure that the basic tenets of quality education and assessment are adequately met and are not compromised through the use of ICTs.

Judicious use of ICTs can greatly improve assessment practices across the spectrum of health profession education. We hope that this chapter will help raise awareness of the scope and capability of using ICTs in support of assessment, to stimulate collaboration around their development, and to incorporate ICTs in assessment in a planned, supported and sustainable manner. The following set of consensus recommendations is intended to support these goals.

Consensus Statement and Recommendations

General Recommendations

1. Institutional leaders, teachers, and other stakeholders should understand and follow general principles of quality assessment when using technology-enabled assessment.

2. Educators and leaders should employ technologies that serve a demonstrable purpose or otherwise enable or extend current capabilities. Contextual considerations such as educational needs, resource efficiency, and relevance to local health care should be the primary deciding factors in choosing the appropriate technologies for enabling or enhancing assessment.

3. Technology-enabled assessment needs to be integrated within the larger ecosystem of health professional education through a coherent and comprehensive approach to its planning, implementation, and management.

Recommendations for Institutions and Policy Makers

1. Curriculum and assessment committees should include member(s) with

---

expertise in technology-enabled assessment to facilitate the appropriate planning, integration, and implementation of technology-enabled assessment.

2. Institutional leaders should facilitate appropriate faculty and student development in using technology-enabled assessment for their current and future needs. Conversely, individual teachers and developers should take a proactive approach toward personal and professional development in the use of rapidly changing technology in assessment.

3. Institutions should capitalize on available technologies for the entire life cycle of management of assessment processes including examination development, administration, data acquisition, analysis, reporting, storage, and quality assurance.

Recommendations for Assessors and Test Developers

1. Assessors and test developers should ensure validity of technology-enabled assessment through careful attention to the constructs being measured, and through selecting appropriate realistic scenarios and activities.

2. Assessors and test developers should take into account local technological contexts and should make appropriate use of available technologies in designing assessments.

3. Assessors and test developers should actively devise assessment strategies to include broader competencies such as teamwork, monitoring of practitioners' performance, and patient-safety through the appropriate usage of technologies.

Future Research

1. Researchers should study the relationships between assessment of performance in a simulated environment and performance in real-life practice settings.

2. Researchers should study the application of different technologies to specific contexts to better inform the selection of technologies they use.

3. Researchers should develop scoring methods that automate the collection, integration, and analysis of the vast and often novel information available through technology-enabled assessment.

4. Researchers should establish better and more robust links between workplace systems and patient outcome data and their use for assessment, including, but not limited to, data from electric medical records and clinical charts.

References

1. Hersh W. Relevance and retrieval evaluation: perspectives from medicine. *J Am Soc Inform Sci*. 1994; **45**(3): 201–6.
2. Graham G. *The Internet: a philosophical inquiry*. London: Routledge; 1999.
3. Gesundheit N, Brutlag P, Youngblood P, et al. The use of virtual patients to assess the clinical skills and reasoning of medical students: initial insights on student acceptance. *Med Teach*. 2009; **31**(8): 739–42.
4. Margolis MB, Clauser BE, Harik P. Scoring the computer-based case simulation component of USMLE Step 3: a comparison of preoperational and operational data. *Acad Med*. 2004; **79**(Suppl. 10): S62–4.
5. Scarborough H, Corbett JM. *Technology and Organization: power, meaning and design*. London: Routledge; 1992.
6. Bennett RE. Using new technology to improve assessment. *Educ Meas*. 2005; **18**(3):5–12. Available at: www3.interscience.wiley.com/journal/119079459/abstract?CRETRY=1&SRETRY=0 (accessed June 4, 2010).
7. Wireless health care: when your carpet calls your doctor. *Economist*. 2010, April 8. Available at: www.economist.com/business-finance/displaystory.cfm?story_id=15868133&source=hptextfeature (accessed April 10, 2010).
8. Reiser SJ. *Technological Medicine: the changing world of doctors and patients*. New York, NY: Cambridge University Press; 2009.
9. Kress G. *Multimodality: a social semiotic approach to contemporary communication*. London: Routledge; 2010.
10. Sarasohn-Kahn J. *How Smartphones are Changing Health Care for Consumers and Providers*. Oakland: California HealthCare Foundation; 2010. Available at: www.chcf.org/publications/2010/04/how-smartphones-are-changing-health-care-for-consumers-and-providers (accessed June 23, 2010).
11. Ellaway R, Martin R. What's mine is yours: open source as a new paradigm for sustainable healthcare education. *Med Teach*. 2008; **30**(2): 175–9.
12. Ellaway R, Masters K. AMEE Guide 32: e-learning in medical education, part 1. Learning, teaching and assessment. *Med Teach*. 2008; **30**(5): 455–73.
13. Issenberg SB, McGaghie WC, Hart IR, et al. Simulation technology for health care professional skills training and assessment. *JAMA*. 1999; **282**(9): 861–6.
14. Greenhalgh T. Computer assisted learning in undergraduate medical education. *BMJ*. 2001; **322**(7277): 40–4.
15. Ellaway RH, Kneebone R, Lachapelle K, et al. Practica continua: connecting and combining simulation modalities for integrated teaching, learning and assessment. *Med Teach*. 2009; **31**(8): 725–31.
16. Kneebone R, Arora S, King D, et al. Distributed simulation: accessible immersive training. *Med Teach*. 2010; **32**(1): 65–70.
17. Bradley P. The history of simulation in medical education and possible future directions. *Med Educ*. 2006; **40**(3): 254–62.
18. Tekian A, McGuire CH, McGaghie WC. *Innovative Simulations for Assessing*

Professional Competence: from paper-and-pencil to virtual reality. Chicago: Department of Medical Education, University of Illinois at Chicago; 1999.

19. Boulet JR, Murray D, Kras J, et al. Reliability and validity of a simulation-based acute care skills assessment for medical students and residents. *Anesthesiology.* 2003; **99**(6): 1270–80.

20. Norcini JJ, McKinley DW. Assessment methods in medical education. *Teach Teach Educ.* 2007; **23**: 239–50.

21. Norcini JJ, Anderson B, Bollela V, et al. Criteria of good assessment consensus statement and recommendations from the Ottawa 2010 Conference. *Med Teach.* 2011; **33**(3): 206–14.

22. Epstein RM, Hundert EM. Defining and assessing clinical competence. *JAMA.* 2002; **287**(2): 226–35.

23. Dillon GF, Boulet JR, Hawkins RE, et al. Simulation in the United States Medical Licensing Examination (USMLE). *Qual Saf Health Care.* 2004; **13**(Suppl. 1): i41–5.

24. Schuwirth LWT, van der Vleuten CPM, De Kock CA, et al. Computerized case-based testing: a modern method to assess clinical decision making. *Med Teach.* 1996; **18**(4): 294–9.

25. Gordon JA, Wilkerson WM, Shaffer DW, et al. Practicing medicine without risk: students' and educators' responses to high-fidelity patient simulation. *Acad Med.* 2001; **76**(5): 469–72.

26. Kneebone R, Kidd J, Nestel D, et al. An innovative model for teaching and learning clinical procedures. *Med Educ.* 2002; **36**(7): 628–34.

27. Ziv A, Wolpe PR, Small SD, et al. Simulation-based medical education: an ethical imperative. *Acad Med.* 2003; **78**(8): 783–8.

28. Fried MP, Satava R, Weghorst S, et al. Identifying and reducing errors with surgical simulation. *Qual Saf Health Care.* 2004; **13**(Suppl. 1): i19–26.

29. Dev P, Youngblood P, Heinrichs WL, et al. Virtual worlds and team training. *Anesthesiol Clin.* 2007; **25**(2): 321–36.

30. Sica GT, Barron DM, Blum R, et al. Computerized realistic simulation: a teaching module for crisis management in radiology. *AJR Am J Roentgenol.* 1999; **172**(2): 301–4.

31. Wong SH, Ng KF, Chen PP. The application of clinical simulation in crisis management training. *Hong Kong Med J.* 2002; **8**(2): 131–5.

32. Fischer M, Kopp V, Holzer M, et al. A modified electronic key feature examination for undergraduate medical students: validation threats and opportunities. *Med Teach.* 2005; **27**(5): 450–5.

33. Round J, Conradi E, Poulton T. Improving assessment with virtual patients. *Med Teach.* 2009; **31**(8): 759–63.

34. Scalese RJ, Obeso VT, Issenberg SB. Simulation technology for skills training and competency assessment in medical education. *J Gen Intern Med.* 2007; **23**(Suppl. 1): 46–9.

35. Shavit I, Keidan I, Hoffmann Y, et al. Enhancing patient safety during pediatric sedation: the impact of simulation-based training of non-anesthesiologists. *Arch Pediatr Adolesc Med.* 2007; **161**(8): 740–3.

36. Cook DA, Beckman TJ. Current concepts in validity and reliability for psychometric instruments: theory and application. *Am J Med.* 2006; **119**(2): 166.e7–16.

37. Shachak A, Hadas-Dayagi M, Ziv A, et al. Primary care physicians' use of an electronic medical record system: a cognitive task analysis. *J Gen Intern Med.* 2009; **24**(3): 341–8.

38. Downing SM, Haladyna TM. Validity threats: overcoming interference with proposed interpretations of assessment data. *Med Educ.* 2004; **38**(3): 327–33.

39. Reznick RK, MacRea H. Teaching surgical skills: changes in the wind. *N Engl J Med.* 2006; **355**(25): 2664–9.

40. Wiggins G. *Assessing Student Performance: exploring the purpose and limits of testing.* San Francisco, CA: Jossey-Bass; 1993.

41. Galvagno SM Jr., Segal BS. Critical action procedures testing: a novel method for test enhanced learning. *Med Educ.* 2009; **43**(12): 1182–7.

42. Larsen PD, Butler A, Roediger III HL. Repeated testing improves long-term retention relative to repeated study: a randomised controlled trial. *Med Educ.* 2009; **43**(12): 1174–81.

43. Errichetti A, Boulet JR. Comparing traditional and computer-based training methods for standardized patients. *Acad Med.* 2006; **81**(10): S91–4.

4

Research on Assessment Practices

Lambert Schuwirth, Jerry Colliver, Larry Gruppen,
Clarence Kreiter, Stewart Mennin, Hirotaka Onishi,
Louis Pangaro, Charlotte Ringsted, David Swanson,
Cees van der Vleuten, and Michaela Wagner

RESEARCH IN MEDICAL EDUCATION AND ASSESSMENT IS A YOUNG discipline that seeks its identity. Medical education research did not take off as an independent field until the 1960s. It has roots in two older disciplines: educational psychology and (bio) medical science. As an emerging research field, medical education benefits because it draws on the scientific approaches and traditions of both disciplines. However, it also suffers due to the differences between the research legacies of educational psychology as a social science and (bio) medical research as a natural science. Medical education research seeks its niche and aims to establish its own scholarly traditions that will likely employ a range of scientific approaches and methods. Medical education scholars are responsible for making well-informed methodological choices about the questions, theoretical frameworks, research designs, and measurement metrics that they use.

This chapter argues for the development of medical education and assessment as a scientific discipline. We describe the important facets of medical education research in general, and research into assessment in particular and offer a set of concrete ideas and recommendations. We describe where the field is at the moment and report what is needed for assessment research to advance. We also seek to inform medical and social science readers why medical assessment research is not a perfect fit with either biomedical or psychological research. Instead, medical assessment research is a hybrid discipline of its own.

Definitions
• • • • • • • • • • • • • •

This chapter features three terms whose definitions vary in the professional literature. We provide operational definitions of these terms to reduce ambiguity.

Theory

Theory refers to rational assumptions about the nature of phenomena, based on observations, and is subject to scientific studies aimed at their falsification. A theory is not necessarily useful on practical grounds but it should provide a framework for understanding phenomena. Classical test theory is a good example. The backbone of this theory is the notion that an observed score is the sum of a true score (the score a candidate would have obtained if he or she had answered all the possible relevant items of a certain domain) and measurement error.

Theoretical Framework

A theoretical framework implies a set of related theories that together explain a complicated professional problem or phenomenon (in this case, assessment). Examples of theoretical frameworks include various approaches to validity and validation. Validity has been defined by Messick[1] as the minimization of construct underrepresentation and construct-irrelevant variance and by Kane[2] as an argument-based rationale. Both views are theoretical frameworks.

Note that we avoid using the term "paradigm." Paradigm has a distinct meaning with important implications that are dependent on the specific philosophy of science stream in which it is embedded.

Conceptual Framework

Where a theoretical framework tries to organize a set of related theories to explain complicated phenomena, a conceptual framework helps to interpret findings and give directions. An example of a conceptual framework is assessment *for* learning rather than assessment *of* learning. Assessment for learning is a framework in which assessment is seen as a key part of the educational process and in which the assessment program serves to collect and collate information from various sources (tests and assessments) to support optimal education and to allow optimal progress for each student. In an assessment *of* learning framework, case-to-case variance is seen as measurement error. In an assessment *for* learning framework the same type of variance is judged meaningful because it enables the teacher to stimulate student learning by identifying strengths and weaknesses.

Types of Research

The fact that medical education and assessment have biomedical and social scientific research as its legacy leads to a wide array of possible methods and approaches. This section describes four scientific categories in medical education and assessment: (1) ideographic description; (2) developmental, design-based research; (3) justification research; and (4) theoretical or clarification research. Although these four streams are different, one of the connecting issues is the use of theory in research. Medical education research in this regard is unique. For example, if a biomedical scientist finds that a bacterium can use nitrogen for metabolism, it does not matter if the lab is in Vancouver, Toronto, Washington, London, Maastricht, Tokyo, or Mumbai. But when an educational or assessment intervention is studied it generally *does* matter where the intervention took place and researchers are responsible for supporting with theory why they believe the intervention worked and what generalizable lessons can be inferred from their study. Ideally, they will also address the contextual factors that may influence the success of replication studies elsewhere.

Ideographic Description or "Case Report"

The case report is chiefly drawn from the medical scientific literature. The medical literature contains many descriptive papers reporting new phenomena or disease entities. This is one reason why so many eponyms exist in medicine. Although it is now routine for authors to describe general lessons, in many reports they do not get beyond the level of "beware of these signs and symptoms."

Such "lessons" are insufficient for descriptive papers in medical education and assessment. This is not to say there is no room for descriptive articles in medical education. We also argue that scientific research should not be seen exclusively as experimental research consisting of planned and controlled experiments. Instead, we consider any planned and structured inquiry involving data collection with the intent to add to generalizable knowledge as central to scientific research.[3] The idea of general relevancy and applicability are epitomized in two questions implicit in this view: "who cares?" and "so what?"[4]

There are many examples of ideographic description of assessment methods and approaches. One of the earliest examples in general education was by William McCall[5] who introduced the true-false question format. Such descriptions are analogous to case reports in the medical literature. They may not agree with the definition of "a planned and structured collection of data" mentioned earlier but they certainly serve a purpose.

Educational "case reports" describe innovations without providing much supporting data. They may describe new instructional methods or assessment tools. For example, one can regard the first publication about the objective structured clinical examination (OSCE) as a case report.[6] This article has had enormous impact on educational practice because OSCEs are the most widely used approach to assessment of clinical skills. More important, however, the article has sparked a line of research that has increased our understanding of the influence of different sources of measurement error on test scores, demonstrating the relationship between interobserver unreliability and inter-case unreliability.[7] Without this line of research, it would have been difficult to endorse new assessment approaches such as the mini-clinical evaluation exercise.[8] Descriptions of local educational innovations can be valuable when authors report the implications of their instruments, methods, and approaches. What uses does the case have, how can it be used, which of its elements make it useful, and how should it be used in other contexts? Authors should also outline directions for further research. Although these publications originate as ideographic reports, their nomothetic aspects should be made plain.

A recent example of such a study is reported in an article about the multiple mini-interview by Eva et al.[9] in 2004. This presentation of a new approach is firmly rooted in the admission, selection, and OSCE literature. The article bridges all three areas. The article provides the rationale for the multiple mini-interview approach, initial information about its psychometric characteristics, and the implications for its use.

Developmental, Design-Based Research

Most scholarship in medical education and assessment is applied research. Many studies describe attempts to develop new educational interventions or assessment methods. These are reports about curriculum development, creation of new tests, and studies of faculty enrichment. Developmental research is needed because the changing context of medicine and social demands about doctors require better approaches to medical education.

Pediatrician Mark Adler and colleagues[10] provide a useful example of developmental research. These investigators created and tested a novel curriculum in pediatric emergency medicine in two phases. The first, *design* phase featured a case-based curriculum design, case presentations, and rater training. The second, *curriculum evaluation* phase involved a randomized trial with a simulation-based educational intervention, involving pediatric residents from two academic medical centers using outcome measures that yield reliable data with simple, straightforward data analyses. Results show that the new curriculum has valid content, that the curriculum improves resident clinical learning, but that measured educational outcomes would be stronger with a more powerful dose of teaching time. Adler et al.[10] conclude that "medical education cannot be done 'on the cheap.'" Powerful educational results come from powerful educational programs that are not compromised by such variables as resident duty schedules. Developmental research in medical education needs to be designed, conducted, reported, and understood, with attention to the practical context where it is embedded.

Justification Research

The most common form of medical education scholarship is justification research. A justification research project typically seeks to prove that one educational approach is better than another. This is analogous to clinical research comparing a new drug to conventional therapy. There are, of course, many research questions where such an approach is not suitable. These include many failed attempts to demonstrate the superiority of one curricular approach (e.g., problem-based learning) over another. There are reasons for failure. The issues involved (e.g., choice of outcome measures, quality and consistency of curriculum implementation) are often so complex that a simple justification study cannot answer the question adequately. Just as no single study can demonstrate that the use of MRI and CT scans has improved the population health of a country, no single study can demonstrate that current educational methods produce better (or worse) doctors than 20 years ago. Yet, plausible arguments can be made, and these arguments can lead to smaller, more focused justification studies.

Good examples of this in assessment research are studies that investigate whether open-ended questions are superior to multiple-choice questions.[11] Such research can be important in the context of convincing stakeholders to use an assessment approach, but it also has limitations. Justification research is not useful if the research goal is to disclose underlying processes. Justification research results do not reveal why an approach works or does not work. A second limitation is that a local justification research finding may not apply to other schools and settings. Thus, a clear description of the theory underlying a justification research study is essential to allow others to interpret the applicability of its results for their own situation.

An example will clarify this condition. Many studies in medical assessment have tried to determine whether the open-ended or multiple-choice question format is better. Investigators have correlated scores on multiple-choice tests with those on open-ended tests covering the same topic. Moderate correlations ranging from 0.40 to 0.50 are typically found.[12] However, these correlations are uninterpretable results because it is unclear whether the glass is half full or half empty. By contrast, if the study had been done from the framework of validity and cognitive psychology, the research goal might address whether question content or format determines the memory pathways a question activates. Such comparisons show that when the content is similar and the format is different, true (disattenuated) correlations are high, and when the content differs and the format is the same, correlations are low.[13] A deeper probe using a think-aloud protocol grounded in the theory on expertise and its development shows that the stimulus type (case-based or plain factual knowledge) directly influences the quality of the thinking processes.[14]

Limitations of justification research are often overlooked because in medicine the randomized controlled trial is frequently considered the "gold standard" scientific approach. Yet in medical education, justification research can only establish one link in the chain connecting theoretical scientific findings with practice. This is similar to studies that demonstrate the superiority of one cancer drug over usual therapy but do not provide insight into the fundamental mechanisms of cancer. The limits of justification research have been discussed vigorously in the medical educational literature.[15–17]

Typical justification research questions are: is assessment approach A more valid than B, does assessment approach A lead to better learning than B, and is assessment approach A more feasible than B? Such studies are often done without a clear conception of the assessment purpose or a clear specification of the skills to be assessed.

Fundamental Theoretical or Clarification Research

Every scientific discipline needs to build theory and expand on it, or seek to falsify old theories and replace them with new and better ones. Theory is essential. Without fundamental theoretical research to clarify the mechanisms of learning and assessment, actions justified by these studies would be poorly understood and there would be no foundation to build on. Fundamental theoretical research can be qualitative or quantitative but seeks to understand how things work or why things work.[18]

A good medical education research project on any topic depends on a thorough review of existing literature. Many presumably "new ideas" reported in a publication have been presented earlier. Recent discussions about penalty for guessing are not new. The first article on the subject dates from 1923.[19] Poor knowledge of the existing literature will often lead to unnecessary duplication. Replication studies provide a new example of a condition already demonstrated. Replication is essential for scientific advancement. Knowledge of the existing literature on a topic will sharpen one's research questions and place a focus on unknowns instead of current knowledge.

Literature descriptions in a research report are often limited to citations to a few journals within the investigator's specialty. We urge researchers to also scan adjacent or comparative scientific fields. Research on assessment in recent decades has profited greatly from research in cognitive psychology. The current scope of health sciences research and workplace-based assessment (*see* Chapter 12, this volume) has a broader reach than earlier studies because it cites scholarship in psychology and business. Well-read researchers are more knowledgeable and precise about what their studies add to existing knowledge. These scientists can report whether their work is something completely new, is a replication of findings in a different field, or is a replication study in a different context.

Theoretical Frameworks/Context

Research in educational assessment is rooted in social science research. In (bio) medical research theoretical assumptions and implications are almost universally known and accepted. To illustrate, we know that high blood pressure is a risk factor for cardiovascular disease and that sodium and potassium levels are measures of kidney function. Authors do not have to explain to readers why they use such parameters as scientific outcome measures even though these values—like constructs in the social sciences—are not directly visible. In social scientific research, by contrast, a clearly explained choice among specific theoretical frameworks is needed to understand the motivation for a study, interpret its results, and understand the implications. There are numerous examples of this. An assessment example is the use of human judgment in workplace-based assessment. Research questions can be approached from such theories as naturalistic decision making,[20] cognitive load theory,[21] or theories on the actuarial value of human judgment.[22]

There are several reasons why such theoretical frameworks are needed. Theoretical frameworks help focus research questions and underpin the operational definitions of variables or constructs. They are also essential to interpret research results and understand their implications. In addition, theoretical frameworks help focus and define hypotheses than can be falsified or retained. Most important, however, they serve to link various studies to a coherent overarching theory or paradigm, either by using studies founded in the same theoretical framework or different studies comparing or connecting different frameworks. This helps medical assessment research grow into a coherent scientific domain where studies are planned to form a research program rather than a domain with detached individual studies.

Another important issue is the theoretical and practical context in which a study is performed. Two mainstream contexts at the moment are assessment *of* learning versus assessment *for* learning.[23] The former is aimed at establishing whether student learning activities make them competent; the latter includes the close relationship between assessment and learning. The former approaches assessment as a psychometric measurement problem; the latter sees assessment as an educational design problem.

Study Design, Choices of Methods

Medical education scholarship uses a broad range of research methods because it draws on many scientific disciplines. There is a widespread misconception that some research methods are better than others. The causal comparative design and the randomized controlled trial are frequently cited here. We argue that *the best method is the one that is most suited to answer one's research question unambiguously.* So, rather than simply endorsing a specific method uncritically, researchers must provide a coherent and defensible rationale about why a chosen method is best. This is not always easy to reach. Most investigators learn a research tradition that has its own language and idioms. We suggest investigators think through their methodological choice, imagine the possible outcomes of a study, and then consider critically which conclusions could be drawn. The investigator should use another method if the presumptive results are inconclusive or if there are plausible rival explanations for the research outcomes.

Instrument Characteristics: Validity and Reliability

Data collection instruments used in many scientific domains already exist and rarely need adaptation or redesign. In assessment research, however, instruments frequently have to be created or redesigned for a specific purpose. Thus instrument development and description must be conducted with great care.

Unfortunately, in many studies insufficient attention is given to ensure the quality of measurement instruments. Investigators must realize that just as a group of questions do not make a good questionnaire, a good research measure is more than a simple collection of items. We are concerned that many current research results have been published despite poor instrumentation. Two elements are key to establishing the value of research instruments: validity and reliability.

Validity

The study of validity in assessment has matured over the past century. A central idea in the discussion is that educational scientists aim to assess constructs that are not directly visible but that are assumed to exist and have theoretical characteristics. A validation program for an assessment instrument or procedure involves a series of studies evaluating the extent to which the scores from the instrument provide information about the unseen construct. A validation program is, much like a scientific theory, never finished. Instead, it consists of a series of thematic studies to determine whether the test actually assesses the construct it intends to measure. Such an extensive validation program is not needed for all measures that are used in practice. It is not only impractical but also impossible to spend years on validation studies for every measure. However, a careful validation procedure must be followed for measures used in scientific research.

A principal idea about validation concerns criterion validity. Criterion validity is addressed when assessment scores predict performance on another measure consistently. For example, in North America scores on the Medical College Admission Test are strong predictors of scores on the United States Medical Licensing Examination Step 1, a partial criterion of readiness for medical practice. This is a convenient approach to test validation because it is practical and convincing to stakeholders and policy makers. However, because the aim is to assess an invisible and intangible construct, a tautological problem can arise. The problem is that the criterion measure also needs validation. If we are validating scores from an assessment instrument, which is intended to predict whether someone will become a good professional, we also need a criterion measure of "good professionalism." The criterion is also a construct and needs validation research as well. This would then invariably lead to a circular problem needing another criterion to validate the primary criterion, ad infinitum. This is one of the main reasons why criterion validation has diminished as the dominant scientific approach.

A second approach to validation is content validity. In content validity, expert judges carefully study assessment items and features to determine the extent to which its content covers the construct of interest. This is an obvious approach to validation that is easy to explain and defend. However, its reliance on human judgment poses problems. If the judges in the content validation process are also the test developers they cannot be neutral. Presumably independent judges are also not free from bias[24] and the specific choice of content judges may influence the outcome of the validation process as shown in the formation of Angoff panels.[25]

The currently dominant idea of construct validation is analogous to the empirical scientific method beginning with theory generation and moving to data collection, data analysis, interpretation, and refinement or rejection of the theory. Construct validation is a process of first making the construct one aims to assess plain and clear and then collecting and evaluating scientific data to see if an assessment instrument captures the assumed characteristics of the construct. An assessment instrument cannot be valid in itself. Instead, scores from an assessment instrument are judged to be valid for a specific purpose. Construct validation is currently popular among medical education scholars. However, like other problems in inductive science, one never knows if there are enough observations to substantiate validity decisions. Conversely, scientists need to determine if data that can falsify a validity argument can be collected and analyzed.

Current views about validity are comparable with modern ideas in philosophy of science. Validity is best seen as an argument process built on several inferences and theoretical notions. Kane[2] describes validity as a set of inferences and their strengths. First, there is the inference from observation to score—that is, how students' observed actions are converted to a scorable variable. The second inference is one from observed score to universe score. This is similar but not identical to the meaning of reliability. Before an inference can be made about generalization from an observed score to a universe score, one must make assumptions about the nature of the universe. Internal consistency reliability indexes (alpha, split-half, Kuder-Richardson) are all useful approaches to judge the observed score to universe score consistency. This also assumes the universe from which the sample was drawn is internally consistent. Content specificity is a source of measurement error in this situation. However, if the theoretical notion of the construct is one of heterogeneity, internal consistency of the sample is an indication of construct underrepresentation and poor generalizability to the universe score. In this situation, content specificity is innate to the construct. If one were to take the blood pressure of a group of patients during the day and found clear differences among the patients but no variation between measurements within patients, it would be highly internally consistent. However, the data would not be considered a generalizable sample because the construct of blood pressure is assumed to vary with time of day or previous activities.

A third inference is from universe scores to target domain. This asks, "Is the generalizable score on this test representative of the construct or does it measure only one element of the construct?"

Messick[1] highlights the consequences of an assessment procedure as another element to include in thinking about validity. This is an important notion because assessment never occurs in a vacuum and can never be disentangled from its (educational) consequences.

Validity is never a static but always a dynamic process of collecting and analyzing data, interpreting results, and refining an instrument to better match the target construct. Research that uses an instrument that was validated elsewhere in a different context needs to include a sound rationale and new data to argue that the instrument is also valid for the right reason in the current situation.

Reliability

Even though generalization of the observed score to the universe score is part of the validation process, the concept of reliability is usually treated separately. Therefore, this chapter warrants a separate section on reliability.

Assessing individual differences regarding competencies, knowledge, skills, and attitudes requires assessment instruments that are capable of capturing these differences and translating the empirically observable differences in the domain of interest into meaningful numbers. The basic requirements for scores from any measure used in an educational context are validity and reliability. Validity, as stated earlier, addresses the degree to which evidence and theory support the indented interpretation of test scores. Reliability refers to the consistency of measurement when it is repeated. Psychometric analysis provides statistics that can contribute to validity evidence. Psychometrics also offers statistics to quantify the consistency of scores from an instrument when it is administered repeatedly. Three types of reliability inferences are studied frequently:

1. Would the student obtain the same score on a parallel test as he or she did on the actual test?
2. Would the student take the same place in the rank ordering from best to worst performing on the parallel test as he or she did on the actual test?
3. Would the student receive the same pass-fail decision as he or she did on the actual test?

Knowing the reliability of scores derived from a measurement is important because reliability determines the extent to which different measures can correlate (for instance to estimate the disattenuated correlations) which is relevant in research settings. Reliability coefficients are also used to calculate a confidence interval around a score, thus determining the score range that takes reliability into account.

Three theoretical approaches to reliability are currently popular: (1) classical test theory, (2) generalizability theory, and (3) probabilistic theories (item response theory and Rasch modeling).

The basic principle of *classical test theory* (CTT) is that an observed score is the sum of a true score (the score candidates receive based on their competence) plus error. This is expressed as the association between the observed score and the score on a so-called parallel test (an equally difficult test covering the same topic).

The most popular reliability estimate within CTT is Cronbach's alpha, expressing the consistency of the assessment items used, assuming each item being a "parallel-test" (Kuder-Richardson reliability estimates are functionally equivalent to Cronbach's alpha). However, reliability estimates based on the alpha coefficient are not always the best approach.[26] Cronbach's alpha is based on the notion of a test-retest correlation and is only useful in estimating the replicability of the rank order of candidates' scores. As such, it is an overestimate of the reliability if a criterion-referenced (absolute norm) approach is used. A general rule of thumb for the interpretation of alpha coefficients is that 0.80 is a minimum for high-stakes testing. On some occasions it is advisable to use alpha to evaluate the quality of test results and decisions based on these results. For example, if pass-fail decisions are made using a cutoff score the reliability coefficient can be used to calculate a standard error of measurement. The standard error of measurement is used to derive a 95% confidence interval around the cutoff score to determine the students for whom a pass-fail decision is uncertain. Here, the reliability is compared with actual data and the robustness of the pass-fail decisions is established. Based on the score distribution and the cutoff score there are some situations where an alpha of 0.60 gives more reliable pass-fail decisions than in other situations (with other distributions and other cutoff scores) with an alpha of 0.80.

CTT is a special case of *generalizability theory* (G-theory). G-theory is more flexible because it allows the user to dissect and estimate error variance from multiple sources. Under the assumption that differences in examinees' scores are partly based on differences in assessed competence (true variance) and partly the result of unwanted sources (error variance), generalizability theory enables the calculation of reliability as the ratio of true score variance to total score variance.

G-theory has additional flexibility because it allows researchers to specifically include or exclude sources of error variance in calculations. It provides a conceptual framework for both criterion- and norm-referenced score interpretation. In criterion-referenced assessment, systematic variance related to certain facets of measurement (e.g., systematic item variance) is included in measurement error. In norm-referenced assessment this source is not included. But flexibility comes at a price. Researchers must be careful in thinking about which measurement designs they use, which sources of variance are included and not included, and which sources to treat as random versus fixed factors. G-theory also requires researchers to completely describe a chosen design in any publication and report complete variance component G study tables. Without detailed reporting, readers cannot interpret or evaluate results and the results cannot be used in meta-analytic syntheses.

G-theory also enables calculation of the reproducibility of pass-fail decisions using a so-called D-cut analysis similar to procedures mentioned under CTT. In simple high-stakes summative competency assessments this can be a better approach to estimating reliability.

A final feature of G-theory is the possibility of performing a decision study (D-study). With such a study, generalizability coefficients can be estimated for any desired number of items, judges, or occasions. This is important because it enables researchers to make informed implementation decisions (hence the name decision study) about alternate test designs.

Like CTT, *probabilistic measurement models* (PMMs) are used to capture individual differences and translate the empirically observable differences in the domain of interest into meaningful numbers. PMMs do this in a different way, addressing CTTs' disadvantages of sample dependent item difficulty and item consistency (Cronbach's alpha) estimates.

A probabilistic measurement framework also allows investigators to statistically test the assumption that items contribute meaningfully to a raw score expressing ability, which cannot be done within CTT. For example, the Rasch model, the simplest PMM model, expresses item difficulties relative to each other. Its mathematical formula combines the answers a person gave to a set of items with ideas about the relative strength of persons and items. The Rasch model absorbs inevitable irregularities and uncertainties of experience systematically by specifying the occurrence of an event as a probability rather than a certainty.[27]

Item difficulty is estimated independent from the persons' ability and simultaneously for multiple-item/multiple-person sets with overlapping items. Thus, items are equated and one can make an objective comparison of item difficulties estimated using data from different person samples. Person ability is expressed using the same scale as with item difficulty. For example, solving nine out of ten items gives a lower ability measure with easier items but a higher measure for more difficult items.

Item consistency in contributing meaningfully to the score is tested statistically with coefficients expressing the degree of fit between the empirical data matrix and the theoretical, model-based data matrix. A standard error of measurement is calculated individually for each person accounting for the items' difficulty and the individual outcome (correct/incorrect).

Items can be characterized by more than their difficulty so other models include more parameters to describe how persons respond to items. A two-parameter model includes discriminatory power. In this model the probability of a correct answer is not only influenced by a the test taker's ability but also by the power of the item to discriminate between two test takers of different ability levels.

The more parameters that are included in a PMM model the more data are needed to obtain reasonable item difficulty estimates and fit statistics. As a rule of thumb, 200 test takers are enough when working with a Rasch model, whereas up to 1000 are needed when working with PMM models with more parameters.

Cost/Acceptability

Research on assessment frequently focuses on validity and reliability issues. There are many other assessment research issues that have nothing to do with the measurement properties of instruments and the data they yield. They include political and legal issues surrounding assessment programs, technical support issues, documenting and publishing assessment program results, research and development approaches, change management, audit methods, cost-effectiveness, accountability issues, and many others.[28,29] Research about these issues is difficult to publish yet is extremely important. Given current developments involving workplace-based assessment (*see* Chapter 12, this volume), the value of assessments for users (both assessors and students) is essential. Assessments that are too costly, time-consuming, or difficult to understand will not live long or will be trivialized by users.

Research on stakeholder acceptability is necessary because current assessment instruments rely heavily on human observation and judgment. In standardized tests (e.g., a multiple-choice test) opportunities for reliability and validity estimation can be built into the test paper document or screen-based procedure. However, such qualities have to be accounted for by the user in observation-based tests. In fact, in the observational measurements, the "paper part" of the assessment is only to record data. The real assessment is captured in the interaction between observer and student. Quality of assessment depends on rater training, calibration, and feedback on performance. If the stakeholders are not convinced about the added value of the assessment procedure and are not carefully instructed in its use the results can never be valid or reliable.

Ethical Issues

Research involving human subjects has to conform to minimum ethical standards. Assessment research has even more ethical requirements. There is also a risk due to inequality, or a hierarchical relationship, between the researcher and study participants. Assessment is an issue of high importance for both students and faculty.

Different countries have distinct cultural approaches and procedures regarding ethical consent. In some countries ethical committees rule educational research exempt automatically. By contrast, other countries insist on a full ethical review, sometimes by medical ethics committees. In countries where ethical review of education research is not institutionalized, the onus is on the researcher to ensure that adherence to minimum ethical standards is maintained even if these may not be legally binding.

Recommendations

We conclude with a set of six "best practices" concerning research on assessment practices.

1. A scientific study must be aimed at building or adding to generalizable knowledge. As such it must be thoroughly informed theoretically and must be able to generate general (nomothetic) lessons. This is the case for any type of study ranging from descriptive studies to fundamental research.

2. No single scientific approach is intrinsically best. There is always need for descriptive, design-based, justification, and fundamental research. This applies to methods as well. There is no single superior research method.

The best method is the one most suitable to answer one's research question clearly.

3. Conducting medical education research is not easy. Important medical education research is usually performed by teams of scholars who have functionally diverse skills.

4. Care must be taken to ensure the measurement or assessment instruments are of sufficient quality for the study. Always evaluate the reliability, validity, feasibility, and cost-effectiveness of data derived from the instruments used and the associated score interpretations.

5. In assessment research, investigators should not disregard topics outside validity and reliability. They should also study issues such as acceptability, stakeholder use and expertise, cost-effectiveness, and acceptability to fill the currently existing gaps in the literature.

6. When an ethical review committee exists with sufficient knowledge and jurisdiction to judge the ethical status of a research project it should be consulted. If there is no such committee, the researcher must provide information about the ethical care taken in the research project.

References

1. Messick S. The interplay of evidence and consequences in the validation of performance assessments. *Educ Res.* 1994; **23**(2): 13–23.
2. Kane MT. Validation. In: Brennan RL, editor. *Educational Measurement.* 4th ed. Westport, CT: American Council on Education and Praeger Publishers; 2006. pp. 17–64.
3. Miser WF. Educational research: to IRB, or not to IRB? *Fam Med.* 2005; **37**(3): 168–73.
4. Bligh J. "Nothing is but what is not." *Med Educ.* 2003; **37**(3): 184–5.
5. McCall WA. A new kind of school examination. *J Educ Res.* 1920; **1**(1): 33–46.
6. Harden RM, Gleeson FA. Assessment of clinical competence using an objective structured clinical examination (OSCE). *Med Educ.* 1979; **13**(1): 41–54.
7. Swanson DB. A measurement framework for performance-based tests. In: Hart I, Harden R, editors. *Further Developments in Assessing Clinical Competence.* Montreal, Canada: Can-Heal Publications; 1987. pp. 13–45.
8. Norcini J, Blank LL, Arnold GK, et al. The mini-CEX (clinical evaluation exercise): a preliminary investigation. *Ann Intern Med.* 1995; **123**(10): 795–9.
9. Eva KW, Rosenfeld J, Reiter HI, et al. An admissions OSCE: the multiple mini-interview. *Med Educ.* 2004; **38**(3): 314–26.
10. Adler MD, Vozenilek JA, Trainor JL, et al. Development and evaluation of a

simulation-based pediatric emergency medicine curriculum. *Acad Med.* 2009; **84**(7): 935–41.

11. Schuwirth LW, van der Vleuten CP, Donkers HH. A closer look at cueing effects in multiple-choice questions. *Med Educ.* 1996; **30**(1): 44–9.

12. Norman GR, Swanson DB, Case SM. Conceptual and methodological issues in studies comparing assessment formats. *Teach Learn Med.* 1996; **8**(4): 208–16.

13. Norman GR, Tugwell P, Feightner JW, et al. Knowledge and clinical problem-solving. *Med Educ.* 1985; **19**(5): 344–56.

14. Schuwirth LW, Verheggen MM, van der Vleuten CP, et al. Do short cases elicit different thinking processes than factual knowledge questions do? *Med Educ.* 2001; **35**(4): 348–56.

15. Regehr G. It's NOT rocket science: rethinking our metaphors for research in health professions education. *Med Educ.* 2010; **44**(1): 31–9.

16. Torgerson CJ. Educational research and randomised trials. *Med Educ.* 2002; **36**(11): 1002–3.

17. Norman G. RCT = results confounded and trivial: the perils of grand educational experiments. *Med Educ.* 2003; **37**(7): 582–4.

18. Bordage G, Caelleigh AS, Steinecke A, et al.; for Joint Task Force of Academic Medicine and the GEA-RIME Committee. Review criteria for research manuscripts. *Acad Med.* 2001; **76**(9): 897–978.

19. West PV. A critical study of the right minus wrong method. *J Educ Res.* 1923; **8**(1): 1–9.

20. Klein G. Naturalistic decision making. *Hum Factors.* 2008; **50**(3): 456–60.

21. Van Merriënboer J, Sweller J. Cognitive load theory and complex learning: recent developments and future directions. *Educ Psychol Rev.* 2005; **17**(2): 147–77.

22. Dawes RM, Faust D, Meehl PE. Clinical versus actuarial judgment. *Science.* 1989; **243**(4899): 1668–74.

23. Shepard L. The role of assessment in a learning culture. *Educ Res.* 2000; **29**(7): 4–14.

24. Plous S. *The Psychology of Judgment and Decision Making.* New York, NY; McGraw-Hill; 1993.

25. Verhoeven BH, Verwijnen GM, Muijtjens AM, et al. Panel expertise for an Angoff standard setting procedure in progress testing: item writers compared to recently graduated students. *Med Educ.* 2002; **36**(9): 860–7.

26. Cronbach LJ, Shavelson RJ. My current thoughts on coefficient alpha and successor procedures. *Educ Psychol Meas.* 2004; **64**(3): 391–418.

27. Wright BN, Masters GN. *Rating Scale Analysis: Rasch measurement.* Chicago, IL: MESA Press; 1982.

28. Dijkstra J, van der Vleuten CP, Schuwirth LW. A new framework for designing programmes of assessment. *Adv Health Sci Educ Theory Pract.* 2010; **15**(3): 379–93.

29. Van der Vleuten CPM. The assessment of professional competence: developments, research and practical implications. *Adv Health Sci Educ.* 1996; **1**(1): 41–67.

5

Assessment for Selection for the Health Care Professions and Specialty Training*

David Prideaux, Chris Roberts, Kevin Eva, Angel Centeno, Peter McCrorie, Chris McManus, Fiona Patterson, David Powis, Ara Tekian, and David Wilkinson

Introduction: Assessment for Selection

The term assessment is usually associated with the process of examining or testing candidates once admitted to a course or program. Yet, the principles that underlie assessment are every bit as important when applied upfront to the very process of selecting those to be admitted to the course. Indeed, universally in the health professions, whether at initial or subsequent phases of training, there are many more applicants than places available. Careers in the health professions are satisfying and financially rewarding. Furthermore, attrition rates in health professional courses are low and, once selected, most entrants graduate. As a result, in common with much in-course assessment, the stakes can be high. Selection processes therefore need to be credible and fair, valid and reliable, and, above all, publicly defensible. By conceptualizing selection as "assessment for selection,"

* Prideaux D, Roberts C, Eva K, et al. Assessment for selection for the health care professions and specialty training: consensus statement and recommendations from the Ottawa 2010 Conference. *Med Teach.* 2011; **33**(3): 215–23. Reprinted by permission of Informa Healthcare.

the well-developed quality assurance mechanisms associated with high-stakes assessment can be applied to the selection process. These include:

- proceeding from a clear blueprint of the content for selection
- using evidence from psychometric studies and a theory base to inform the selection process
- developing congruity between selection, curriculum, and assessment
- using clear standard-setting and decision-making procedures
- providing a focus on the impact of selection (a variant of the adage that assessment drives learning).

This chapter summarizes the current state of the findings on selection measures. Yet, despite the importance of selection, there are limitations in the literature. Like much of medical education research, few studies proceed from an explicit theoretical focus or even from a strong conceptual framework. Rather, there is a concentration on the properties of individual selection measures. Most of the studies originate from North America, where the graduate entry mode has resulted in greater emphasis on written tests and non-test selection measures. There is an emerging literature from the United Kingdom and Australia as new medical schools have opened in those countries, some of which have adopted graduate entry approaches. There is a small comparative literature from the Netherlands as alternatives are adopted to the national lottery system.

While the title of this chapter includes reference to health care professionals and specialty training, most of the literature concentrates on the selection of medical students for the initial phase of education. There is one study cited here on selection for Canadian Dental Schools[1] and, in Australia, the Graduate Australian Medical Schools Admission Test (GAMSAT) and Undergraduate Medical Admission Test (UMAT) are used for selection to health professional programs such as dentistry, optometry, and physiotherapy. Salvatori[2] has produced a review entitled "The reliability and validity of admissions tools used to select students for the health professions." While the literature is drawn from across the health professions, many of the findings of the review are drawn from medical education.

Additionally, there are few studies of selection for postgraduate training and only three such studies are included in this review.[3,4,5] Selection at this level has not been subject to the same scrutiny as for initial medical education. The numbers of entrants are small and practices tend to be less openly discussed and investigated.

The literature, however, does fall into three categories of significance. The first two categories are commonly represented by a so-called cognitive-noncognitive divide. The former consists of written tests and ratings of academic achievement such as grade point average (GPA) or equivalent. These are discussed in sections "The Current Position: Written Tests" and "The Current Position: Achievement Ratings." The so-called noncognitive measures include interviews and their objective structured clinical examination (OSCE)-inspired variant multiple mini-interviews (MMIs) and are discussed in sections "The Current Position: Interviews," "The Current Position: Multiple Mini-Interviews," and "The Current Position: Other Measures." Nevertheless, it is maintained that the cognitive-noncognitive dichotomy is flawed and is not used further in this chapter. While the constructs underlying OSCEs and MMIs are not always clear, it is inconceivable that these forms of selection have no cognitive components.

The other area of considerable importance in selection is the question of widening access to medical and health professional courses to include greater representation of ethnic minorities, low socioeconomic or disadvantaged groups or indigenous peoples. This is a different dimension from that of the comparative merits of different types of selection measures. It is a values question, not a technical question, and it has strong local and political dimensions. The term "political validity" is important here. Widening access is discussed in section "The Current Situation: Widening Access."

The final sections of the document provide a consensus statement and recommendations both for implementation and for further study to advance the understanding of this important endeavor in the medical and health professions.

The Current Position: Written Tests

This section introduces another flawed dichotomy: that between aptitude and achievement tests. Aptitude tests purport to measure potential for achievement while achievement tests purport to measure actual achievement. The most well-known selection test is the North American Medical College Admission Test (MCAT). The MCAT was developed out of the more general Scholastic Aptitude Test in the post-Flexner reforms of North American medical education. Its use is now ubiquitous in that context. It contains four main sections: (1) physical sciences, (2) verbal reasoning, (3) a writing sample, and (4) biological sciences. While the MCAT had its origins in an aptitude test, at least the physical and biological sciences sections purport to measure achievement. It is less clear for the remaining sections. The GAMSAT is now used in Australia and the United Kingdom. It is modeled on the MCAT and has three sections: (1) reasoning in the humanities and social sciences, (2) written communication, and (3) reasoning in the biological and physical sciences. It purports to be an achievement test at least for the first and third sections.

A second test is used in Australia for courses taking school-leaver students: the UMAT. It has three sections: (1) logical reasoning, (2) understanding people, and (3) nonverbal reasoning. From 2006, some medical schools in the United Kingdom have used the United Kingdom Clinical Aptitude Test (UKCAT), which comprises measures of verbal reasoning, quantitative reasoning, abstract reasoning, and decision analysis. These tests purport to measure potential or aptitude for medical study.

The predictive validity of the MCAT is reasonably well established. Donnon et al.[6] conducted a meta-analysis of 23 studies investigating the predictive validity of the MCAT as it related to performance in medical schools and Step 1 of the United States Medical Licensing Examination (USMLE). They found a predictive validity coefficient of 0.39 for the MCAT for performance in the preclinical years of the medical course and 0.6 for performance in Step 1 of the USMLE. The biological sciences section was the best predictor on both measures. Julian's[7] study involved two cohorts of entrants from 14 medical schools. Again, the predictive validity of the MCAT was measured against medical school and USMLE performance, the latter involving all three steps. Medical school performance was predicted best by combining the MCAT and the GPA from prior degree studies. The MCAT provided a substantial increment over the prior GPA, particularly in year 3 studies. MCAT scores provided superior prediction of scores in the steps of the USMLE. The MCAT had the advantage of being a standard score while the determination of GPA scores varied by school.

Studies by Koenig et al.[8] and Tekian[9] report on the positive predictive validity of the MCAT but with some caveats. Koenig et al.[8] found that MCAT scores were predictive of medical school and USMLE Step 1 performance, and that there was no difference in prediction between men and women. The performance of three designated ethnic groups was "overpredicted." The study concluded that the MCAT was not a perfect predictor and other variables such as "diligence," "motivation," and "communication skills" need further investigation. Tekian[9] used a combination of medical school performance factors including withdrawal and graduation status, USMLE performance, and students with "significant events" to examine MCAT and prior GPA predictive validity with underrepresented minority (URM) and non-URM groups. MCAT and prior GPA scores were correlated with success in medical schools but did not have sufficient ability to define or differentiate the success or failure of students considered "at risk."

The use of large-scale testing outside of North America is a relatively recent phenomenon. The number of studies of the GAMSAT is small. As in the North American context, Coates[10] found that GAMSAT and GPA scores were the best predictors of medical school performance in year 1. The author also demonstrated high levels of divergence in GAMSAT, initial GPA, and interview scores in relation to year 1 performance. In a study of two Australian medical schools, Groves et al.[11] found significant correlations with year 2 medical school assessments only for the physical and behavioral sciences section of the GAMSAT. There was a negative correlation with scores in clinical reasoning tests. More recently, Wilkinson et al.[12] found in a single medical school study that the school's selection criteria, prior GPA, interview, and the GAMSAT were only modestly predictive of performance in examinations in years 1 and 4 of a 4-year course.

No published studies of the UMAT were located for this article. Lynch et al.[13] in a study of two Scottish medical schools found that the UKCAT did not predict performance in the first year of medical school. Further studies are required before definite statements can be made about the utility of this test.

While the properties of the MCAT are well known, there are simply not enough studies as yet to make conclusions about the other tests or the relative merits of so-called achievement or aptitude tests. Further, not enough is known about the underlying constructs of the tests to confidently classify them as achievement or aptitude and whether it is even possible to do so. Much work remains to be done.

Much work also remains to be done on predictive validity. Most studies are focused on the relation between selection tests and in course assessment, "tests predicting tests," and do not proceed from strong theoretical foundations. Not much is known about the relationships with other qualities on selection blueprints or indeed with eventual practice as a health professional. This requires more sophistication in measurement methods and in choice of outcome variables.

The Current Position: Achievement Ratings

The academic achievement of potential candidates prior to selection is commonly incorporated into selection processes. In the North American graduate entry context, this means the GPA achieved in the preselection degree. The predictive utility of the GPA in combination with the MCAT has already been presented as part of findings in the previous section. Kreiter and Kreiter's[14] meta-analysis has shown that there are positive correlations between initial GPA and subsequent performance. There is no clear evidence about the relative merits of the GPA in science compared with non-science subjects. Didier et al.[15] reported on a method to adjust the GPA to equate for differences between institutions. The adjusted GPA showed improved relation to MCAT scores and better prediction of USMLE and medical school performance, but only when large adjustments to institutional scores were necessary. Again, the same limitations about predictive validity from a narrow range of potential selection blueprint attributes apply.

There are few studies of the utility of school leaving scores despite their widespread use internationally. McManus et al.[16] found that A-level grades for UK schools were predictive of medical career choice but the results of a general intelligence test were not. In a study from one school from the Netherlands, the school-leaving GPAs of students within the national lottery selection system were associated with shorter times for graduation, greater success in achieving preferred specialist training and greater scientific output.[17] In a study of universities and colleges admission scores (UCAS) in the United Kingdom, Powis et al.[18] found that higher scores were associated with being younger and male and were related to ethnic origin and type of school. This has implications for discussions in "The Current Situation: Widening Access" section of this chapter.

The Current Position: Interviews

The interview, face-to-face contact with single interviewer or a panel with varying degrees of structure, is a common part of selection processes. Despite its ubiquity, there are very few studies defining its psychometric properties. Those that do exist do not indicate that the interview is a robust selection measure.

Kreiter et al.[19] conducted a review of studies of interviewer reliability since 1990. Nine studies were reviewed in total. Reported reliability was varied widely, which the authors attribute to the differing definitions of reliability. They concluded that there was not sufficient evidence to establish the reliability of interviews. Their own study investigated 92 applicants who were interviewed over 2 consecutive years having failed to gain a place in the medical school the first time around. Reliability was established using multivariant and univariant generalizability theory. Their estimates of reliability ranged from 0.27 to 0.38 and they concluded that this range was not sufficient to establish the reliability of the interview in question.

In their review of the assessment of personal qualities for selection for medicine, Albanese et al.[20] reached a similar conclusion. They described the results of reliability and validity studies as "equivocal." Furthermore, they indicated a high degree of variability among interview formats, particularly the characteristics that they purport to measure. Stansfield and Kreiter[21] have indicated at least one way to improve reliability. In their study in one medical school, they found higher reliability for ratings at the high or low ends of a rating scale rather than middle levels. As a result, they argue that a three-point ranking scale may be as useful as the commonly used five-point scale.

A study for selection into orthopedic residency in one university indicates at least one of the potential problems of interview: interviewer bias.[4] In a study of 135 single interviewers, it was found that clinician interviewers gave candidates more favorable rankings when personality preferences, as measured by the Myers-Briggs scale, matched, notably the dimensions for extrovert-sensing, sensing-thinking, and sensing-judging. The matching did not occur for interviewers who were basic scientists or residents.

Meredith et al.[22] found significant correlations of interview scores with clinical assessments but the best defense of the interview has come from a study of applicants to Canadian Dental Schools using the Canadian Dental Association structured interview.[1] The interview was the result of extensive work by the association. The blueprint was based on a job analysis of dental work that defined eight essential competencies. Questions were based upon critical incidents that matched the competencies. All interviewers were trained. Two member panels of faculty members and dental practitioners were used. An inter-rater reliability coefficient of 0.81 has been established over five cycles of admissions with 1467 applicants. In a study of 573 applicants to four schools in 1 year, positive correlations were found between interview scores and years 3 and 4 clinical performance but academic performance was not predicted. The authors concluded that the interview has a place in the selection process along with the Dental Aptitude Test and other measures. What this study perhaps indicates is that some psychometric properties of the interview can be improved, provided sufficient attention is given to both its detailed construction and its operation.

The Current Position: Multiple Mini-Interviews

The MMI was first developed at the Michael G. DeGroote School of Medicine at McMaster University in Canada. It applies the principles of the OSCE to the interview context. The OSCE provides a series of short testing stations and has been shown to have superior reliability to the single long case. Similarly, the MMI employs a series of short interview scenarios with a single rater in each station or scenario. Eva et al.[23] indicate that, like the OSCE, the MMI overcomes the problem of poor test-retest reliability and context specificity where the measurement of an attribute in one context does not necessarily transfer to another. Test-retest reliability provides a better indication of the quality of a test than inter-rater reliability because it focuses on the overall test, not just a component of its operation.

Good predictive validity and reliability of the MMI have been established in studies by Eva et al.,[23–25] LeMay et al.,[26] Reiter et al.,[27] and Roberts et al.[28] Eva et al.[25] have found reliability coefficients of 0.78, 0.65, and 0.76 in three separate studies with a median reliability of 0.73 over eight administrations of a 12-station MMI at McMaster. They have also found significant correlations with the Canadian Qualifying Examination Part II, which employs an OSCE format for both postgraduate and undergraduate samples. The study by Reiter et al.[27] from the same institution involving 117 volunteers indicated that the MMI was a better predictor of success on clinical clerkship OSCE performance, clinical encounter cards, and performance ratings than prior GPA and other measures of noncognitive variables used in the admissions process. The MMI was also a better predictor of the ethical sections of Part I of the Canadian Qualifying Examination.[29] Importantly, these studies revealed a complementary relationship between the MMI and the GPA, with the GPA being more predictive of other academic outcomes such as progress test performance and the core rotations of the qualifying examination.

The study by Roberts et al.[30] is drawn from the Australian context—the University of Sydney. The authors report a reliability coefficient of 0.7 on an eight-station MMI for 485 candidates. There was a small but significant correlation with Section 1 of the GAMSAT, reasoning in the humanities and social sciences, but a small negative correlation with Section 3, reasoning in biological and physical sciences. Interviewer subjectivity was responsible for the majority of the measurement errors, and the authors recommended increased rater training to address this. Roberts et al.[28] have also subjected 39 items in their bank to item response theory analysis. No items were found to have differential item function, and the questions appeared to measure the unidimensional constant of "entry-level reasoning skills in professionalism."

Further studies have demonstrated other attributes of the MMI. The Eva et al.[23] study demonstrated that increasing the number of stations had a greater impact on reliability than increasing interviewers. Dodson et al.[31] demonstrated that reducing station length from 8 to 5 minutes had little impact on reliability and it has also been shown the results of the MMI appear not to be affected by security violations.[32] Kumar et al.[33] have provided some theoretical insights into how judges arrive at their decisions and the biases to which they are subject. There is also evidence for both interviewer and candidate support of the process[33,34] and that, while the MMI may require more physical space, it requires fewer planning hours.[35] The MMI has been shown to have high reliability when based as part of selection for international medical graduates into family medicine residencies[3] and gained support of candidates and interviewers when used as part of selection of senior house officers for a regional pediatrics program.[36]

The Current Position: Other Measures

Other measures used in the selection process include personal statements, autobiographical statements, or letters of recommendation. However, there is no evidence that they are necessarily reliable or have predictive validity. In Albanese et al.'s[20] review of personal qualities in selection, no research papers could be located on such measures and no evidence that they measured anything different from interviews could be found.

Lievens et al.[37] and Lievens and Sackett[38] provide studies of a situational judgment test based on written or video-based responses to hypothetical scenarios. Responses are selected from a list of alternatives. The method is used as part of a centralized selection system for medical and dental students in Belgium. The test showed greater predictive validity for GPA than science-related and cognitive ability tests but only where curricula included specific interpersonal content.

There is growing interest in other measures. Carr[39] has investigated emotional intelligence. However, in the Australian context, she found no correlation between measures of emotional intelligence and the UMAT or Tertiary Entrance Rank, the Australian equivalent of GPA for school-leaving students. Based on negative correlations with a dysfunctional personality scale and final examinations, Knights and Kennedy[40] argue for the use of such a scale in selection. Ziv et al.[41] have produced evidence of reliability and content and face validity for a simulation-based selection test and Dore et al.[42] have demonstrated correlations with MMI and clinical performance scores for computer-based responses to video-based scenarios.

There is also growing interest in the application of personality testing used in business or commerce careers for selection. Albanese et al.'s[20] review points to one of the difficulties with this approach. The authors point to Price et al.'s[43] study indicating 87 qualities of successful doctors. There is great variability in the qualities currently assessed through interviews, MMIs, and other noncognitive measures. The psychology literature has shown some acceptance of the "big five" personality characteristics—openness, conscientiousness, extroversion, agreeableness, and neuroticism—but there have been few attempts to apply this to selection for the medical and health professions.

Powis,[44] Powis et al.,[45] and Lumsden et al.[46] have developed a Personal Qualities Assessment tool comprising a mental agility test, a moral orientation scale and a NACE scale (narcissism, aloofness, confidence, and empathy). It was administered to 507 volunteer applicants to Scottish medical schools in 2003 but played no part in the actual selection process. While good discrimination power was shown for the test, it was not possible to correlate with other measures to determine predictive validity. It remains an interesting area for further development.

The Current Situation: Widening Access

As indicated previously, widening access is a values question, not a technical question of choosing one selection method over another. Widening access is driven by sociopolitical concerns. These are real concerns. The competitive nature of entry to the medical and health professions has meant that certain groups within populations are not well represented in medical school cohorts. In the United States, widening access means attracting more students from URM groups. In the United Kingdom, there is a concern to attract socioeconomic diversity. In Australia, Canada, New Zealand, and South Africa, among other countries, there is an interest in ensuring that more indigenous students and more rural students are represented in medical school populations. The latter is tied to concerns about workforce distribution as well as equity issues. It is acknowledged that rural students are more likely to practice in rural locations after graduation. A common approach has been to institute quotas for such groups.

There is increasing interest in the social accountability mandate of medical schools,[47] including the formation of a Training for Health Equity network of medical schools. Social accountability requires responsiveness to the communities the medical school serves and ensuring that the communities are represented in the student population. From this derives the concept of political validity. How does the selection process meet the requirements of the communities served by the schools and what impact does it have on the success of community members in gaining admission? The measurement of this form of validity will be informed not by a psychometric discourse but by one derived from the social and political sciences.

Certainly, there is evidence from the United Kingdom to show that traditional methods of selection do discriminate against defined groups within the population. Powis et al.,[18] for example, found that the UCAS tariff scores in the United Kingdom, the equivalent of a school-leaving GPA, were associated with being young; being male; being less materially disadvantaged; being white, Chinese, or mixed ethnic origin; and the type of school attended. Similarly, James et al.[48] studied the new UKCAT for entrants to 23 UK medical and dental schools. They found that UKCAT scores could be used as a "proxy" for the A-levels school-leaving examinations but there were biases toward male candidates and candidates from higher socioeconomic classes and from independent schools. James et al.[49] are advocates for graduate entry as a means to widen access. They compared school leaver and graduate applications to the Nottingham Medical School in 2002/03. The applicant pool for graduate entry contained more males, lower socioeconomic students and students with low UCAS scores than the school-leaver programs. The differences were maintained in the actual entrants who gained places in the two programs.

Alternative selection processes aimed at widening access have not been extensively studied. Steinecke et al.[50] discuss the evidence for four main types of approaches: (1) traditional measures, (2) socioeconomic measures based on personal or family demographic data, (3) adversity indices based on assessment of current or prior disadvantage, and (4) community outreach strategies. Of the four approaches, the authors conclude that socioeconomic measures hold "promise," although requiring further study. Traditional measures have not been successful in widening access and the outcomes of the use of adversity indices and outreach are as yet not well studied.

One of the problems faced in selecting for widening access is how to make decisions based on the data collected during selection and the socioeconomic data or measures of disadvantage. In 1997, Tekian[51] surveyed 15 medical schools that admitted URM students. The author found that there were varied weightings for the various quantitative, qualitative, and student disadvantage data used. He described the admission polices as "secretive." Technical solutions to this have been provided by Kreiter[52] (constrained optimization), Bore et al.[53] (multiple cut-off scores in a regression model), and Reiter and Maccoon[29] (Hofstee standard setting). All claim that use of these methods can result in selection that increases student diversity.

One approach to widening access that is having some success is the development of special preparation programs through which members of underrepresented groups can gain the skills to be competitive at entry. Reeves et al.[54] have shown how a premedical certificate program has enabled previously rejected applicants to gain entry to the University of North Texas Health Sciences Center. Dalley et al.[55] report on a statewide approach in Texas. The Joint Admissions Medical Program applies to all nine Texas medical schools. Applicants to the Joint Admissions Medical Program must produce evidence of economic disadvantage and have completed some university studies at first-year level. They then follow an enrichment program throughout their studies including summer internships. The program has proved popular with 1230 applicants in the first 6 years of operation and 164 of 288 participants gaining places in medical schools.

As indicated previously, some schools have developed community outreach programs as part of their commitment to underserved populations in the communities they serve. These involve "pipeline" and special preparation programs within comprehensive strategies of recruitment, retention and community service. Acosta and Olsen[56] report on the University of Washington's approach to attract and retain American Indian and native Alaskan physicians. The authors outline two recruitment programs involving attracting high school students into health courses and medical/dental summer schools. They combine this with retention, support, and curriculum strategies once students are admitted. From 1989 to 2005, 477 students have participated in the programs, with 34 entering the University of Washington and 102 other medical schools.

Baylor College of Medicine has developed a partnership with the University of Texas-Pan American, a largely Hispanic University.[57,58] The Preclinical Honors Program involves an enriched program at the University of Texas-Pan American. Importantly, conditional entry at Baylor is granted subject to GPA requirements being met. The program has resulted in an average of 12 students per year gaining entry since 1994, which represents a significant increase over previous figures. This community outreach and special program approach is being adopted elsewhere, especially in Australia to recruit Indigenous Australians, many of whom reside in underserved communities and whose participation rate in health professional courses is low. These programs are not yet represented in the literature.

Outreach may well represent a promising development in addressing the question of widening access, especially as more medical schools are embracing their social accountability mandates. Entry through a preparation program with conditional places overcomes the significant issue of combining different types of entry data. Combining selection with support and curriculum measures could well have the potential to add strength to this approach.

Consensus and Conclusion

Consensus

What this chapter shows is that there is a consensus about assessment for selection for the health professions and specialty programs but the areas of consensus are small. There is evidence for the predictive validity of the MCAT and the GPA. There is not strong evidence as yet for the credibility of newer tests introduced in countries outside of North America such as the GAMSAT, the UMAT, or the UKCAT. Nor is there much evidence outside North America about the GPA of prior study, whether it be in the form of high school-leaving grades or prior university study. There is an obvious need for more studies in these areas.

For other measures, there is evidence of the test-retest reliability and predictive validity of the MMI but not much else. Furthermore, there is evidence on this issue from outside North America. There is not much evidence of the credibility of interviews, personal statements and letters of reference.

Next Steps

What was made clear from the outset in this chapter is that the study of selection for assessment is largely atheoretical. Only one article located in this review proceeded from a strong theoretical background. Sternberg[59] used the theory of intelligence to examine current approaches to selection, although the theory itself lacks current credibility. Interestingly, however, he draws many of his examples from outside of medical education. The discipline of medical education as a whole has been served well by looking outside the discipline's boundaries, which are at best loose in any case. The adoption of outcome-based curriculum from mainstream education is a good case in point.

Thus, the study of selection measures could benefit from an examination from other literature, notably that in psychology and the social sciences. The aforementioned study by Price et al.[43] included 87 qualities that could be assessed for selection. Measurement of them all is not feasible. At the other end of the scale, the "big five" factors have been identified for personal qualities in the psychology literature. Powis,[44] Powis et al.,[45] and Lumsden et al.[46] have developed Personal Qualities Assessment, drawing from the psychological and moral development literature. The area may prove to be of promise.

There are caveats. There may be dangers in moving to an overly psychometric view of the measurement of personal qualities in selection. Models of selection drawn from career selection and business and commerce may not transfer across into the professional world of health care providers. A view from across the social sciences, not just psychology, is necessary. It may be useful to take a step backward from the pursuit of unifying theory to consider Regehr's[60] concept of programmatic research where "communities" of researchers work together toward an eventual goal of consensus. He claims research on the OSCE as one such example of programmatic research. This could also be applied to its selection-related variant, the MMI, where there is an emerging consensus about its credibility, feasibility, and acceptability.

The development of the MMI has taken the key concept of context specificity and applied it to a recasting of the traditional interview into a new format just as the OSCEs recast the traditional long case. In turn, context specificity has a theoretical basis in social psychology and instance-based models of cognition. Are there other benefits to be gained from examining key concepts in other parts of our assessment processes and applying them to assessment for selection? Van der Vleuten and Schuwirth[61] have argued that thinking about assessment should be moved from a consideration of methods to programs; another use of the term "programmatic," this time in programmatic assessment. Programmatic assessment concentrates on the overall program of assessment with a combination of methods, each with their differing psychometric properties, to make decisions about student performance. This may prove profitable for medical schools in making decisions based on the variety of selection measures in use. There is perhaps one limitation in that the sheer numbers of applicants for places in medical and health professional programs would limit the number of measures that can be used. Nevertheless, consideration of assessment for selection as a program rather than a collection of methods may well strengthen our understanding of this area.

Comparative studies of different programs of selection and their effects could provide important data for this endeavor. Given the high-stakes nature of selection, it is not practical nor defensible to divide applicants into different groups for selection for research purposes. However, there are opportunities for natural experimentation where alternative selection measures exist side by side, such as in the Netherlands where individual schools are introducing alternative pathways for selection to the national lottery system.[17,62] There have been further studies of different tracks within individual medical schools.[63,64]

Before concluding this section, it is appropriate to turn to the title of this chapter and again point out the lack of evidence for selection outside of medical education and for specialty training. These too are areas for further activity and will bring new perspectives in the current debate. How does the selection of medical students differ from their health care colleagues, particularly in environments where interprofessional teamwork is the norm? What is the effect of raising the stakes even higher as in specialty training?

Widening Access

Adopting a programmatic approach to admission for selection may assist in one of the dilemmas in widening access: how to make decisions on the complex combination of merit, equity, fairness, and social accountability issues represented on health professional selection blueprints. However, it is also useful to remember that widening access is a values-based, not a technically based, decision and hence it should be treated as such. Removing it from the technical domain should not be seen as downgrading its importance. Rather, the reverse is true. It should be seen as a central point of a medical or health professional school's mission requiring different approaches to selection. This should be underpinned by the further development of the concept of political validity, a discourse derived from social sciences rather than psychometrics.

Widening access should not be seen as solely the domain of technical experts on the selection committee or medical education units. It requires the whole school to define its values position, particularly with respect to the communities it purports to serve. Where the communities are underserved or disadvantaged, there are compelling reasons for schools to select and retain students from those communities.

The outreach approach combined with targeted enrichment or preparation programs and conditional selection has been outlined in the text of this article. This approach is not new. It has some demonstrated success and deserves more attention as a fundamental part of assessment of selection.

Conclusion

A consensus statement on assessment for selection is important. Indeed, conceptualizing selection within an assessment framework gives it the possibility of additional intellectual scrutiny. The stakes for selection are every bit as high as for assessment for competence within a program, if not higher. Psychometric concepts like validity and reliability apply. Like in-course assessment, there is a consensus on assessment for selection, but only around a small number of methods. Again like in-course assessment, alternative methods are used, many without the evidence base that is desirable.

Keeping selection within the purview of assessment and applying concepts of programmatic selection will make it an effective area of study within medical and health professional education. Selection is, after all, the very first step in developing a competent and caring medical and health professional.

Recommendations

1. Admissions committees and all who have an interest in selection processes should adopt the principles of good assessment in defining the purpose of selection; blueprinting of assessable domains and attributes, selecting appropriate formats, employing transparent standard setting and decision making, and including an evaluation cycle in a programmatic manner.

2. An integrative approach should apply the principles of good assessment and curriculum alignment along the education and training pathway, including the progression hurdles between health professional degrees, prevocational practice, and basic and advanced specialty training.

3. There should be a focus on multi-method programmatic approaches in collecting, analyzing, interpreting and reporting data from a range of selection instruments, which are fit for purpose.

4. There needs to be an emphasis on developing interdisciplinary theoretical frameworks that underpin development of both policy and the research agenda.

5. There is an urgent need for the development of sophisticated measurement models from the family of regression methods which will require application to multisite high-quality data sets, for increasing the sophistication of predictive validity studies using a range of attributes from selection blueprints, and for a focus on test-retest reliability.

6. The social accountability of universities demands that social inclusion, workforce issues, consumer choice, and widening of access to students of promise are embedded in the principles of good assessment for selection, with recognition that there are political (and nonuniversal) issues that need to be considered in the definition of optimal decisions.

7. Outreach, targeting strategies, preparation programs, and conditional selection should be considered as core strategies for medical and health professional schools to achieve their widening access missions.

References
•••••••••••••••

1. Poole A, Catano V, Cunningham D. Predicting performance in Canadian dental schools: the new CDA structured interview, a new personality assessment, and the DAT. *J Dent Educ.* 2007; **71**(5): 664–76.

2. Salvatori P. Reliability and validity of admission tools used to select students for the health professions. *Adv Health Sci Educ Theory Pract.* 2001; **6**(2): 159–75.

3. Hofmeister H, Lockyer J, Crutcher R. The multiple mini-interview for selection of international medical graduates into family medicine residency education. *Med Educ.* 2009; **43**(6): 573–9.

4. Quintero AJ, Segal LS, King TS, et al. The personal interview: assessing the potential for personality similarity to bias the selection of orthopaedic residents. *Acad Med.* 2009; **84**(10): 1364–72.

5. Thordarson DB, Ebramzadeh E, Sangiorgio SN, et al. Resident selection: how we are doing and why? *Clin Orthop Relat Res.* 2007; **459**: 255–9.

6. Donnon T, Paolucci E, Violato C. The predictive validity of the MCAT for medical school performance and medical board licensing examinations: a meta-analysis of the published research. *Acad Med.* 2007; **82**(1): 100–6.

7. Julian ER. Validity of the Medical College Admission Test for predicting medical school performance. *Acad Med.* 2005; **80**(10): 910–17.

8. Koenig JA, Sireci SG, Wiley A. Evaluating the predictive validity of MCAT scores across diverse applicant groups. *Acad Med.* 1998; **73**(10): 1095–106.

9. Tekian A. Cognitive factors, attrition rates, and underrepresented minority students: the problem of predicting future performance. *Acad Med.* 1998; **73**(Suppl. 10): S38–40.

10. Coates H. Establishing the criterion validity of the Graduate Medical Schools Admission Test (GAMSAT). *Med Educ.* 2008; **42**(10): 999–1106.

11. Groves MA, Gordon J, Ryan G. Entry tests for graduate medical programs: is it time to re-think? *Med J Aust.* 2007; **186**(3): 120–3.

12. Wilkinson D, Zhang J, Byrne GJ, et al. Medical school selection criteria and the prediction of academic performance. *Med J Aust.* 2000; **188**(6): 349–54.

13. Lynch B, Mackenzie R, Dowell J, et al. Does the UKCAT predict Year 1 performance in medical school? *Med Educ.* 2009; **43**(12): 1203–9.

14. Kreiter CD, Kreiter Y. A validity generalization perspective on the ability of undergraduate GPA and the medical college admission test to predict important outcomes. *Teach Learn Med.* 2007; **19**(2): 95–108.

15. Didier T, Kreiter CD, Buri R, et al. Investigating the utility of a GPA institutional adjustment index. *Adv Health Sci Educ Theory Pract.* 2006; **11**(2): 145–53.

16. McManus IC, Smithers E, Partridge P, et al. A levels and intelligence as predictors of medical careers in UK doctors: 20 years prospective study. *BMJ.* 2003; **327**(7407): 139–42.

17. Cohen-Schotanus J, Muijtjens AM, Reinders JJ, et al. The predictive validity of grade point average scores in a partial lottery medical school admission system. *Med Educ.* 2006; **40**(10): 1012–19.

18. Powis D, James D, Ferguson E. Demographic and socio-economic associations with academic attainment (UCAS tariff scores) in applicants to medical school. *Med Educ*. 2007; **41**(3): 242–9.
19. Kreiter CD, Yin P, Solow C, et al. Investigating the reliability of the medical schools admissions interview. *Adv Health Sci Educ Theory Pract*. 2004; **9**(2): 147–59.
20. Albanese MA, Snow MH, Skochelak SE, et al. Assessing personal qualities in medical school admissions. *Acad Med*. 2003; **78**(3): 313–21.
21. Stansfield RB, Kreiter CD. Conditional reliability of admissions interview ratings: extreme ratings are the most informative. *Med Educ*. 2007; **41**(1): 32–8.
22. Meredith KE, Dunlap MR, Baker HH. Subjective and objective admission factors as predictors of clinical clerkship performance. *J Med Educ*. 1982; **57**(10 Pt. 1): 743–51.
23. Eva KW, Reiter HI, Rosenfeld J, et al. The relationship between interviewers' characteristics and ratings assigned during a multiple mini-interview. *Acad Med*. 2004; **79**(6): 602–9.
24. Eva KW, Rosenfeld J, Reiter HI, et al. An admissions OSCE: the multiple mini-interview. *Med Educ*. 2004; **38**(3): 314–26.
25. Eva KW, Reiter HI, Trinh K, et al. Predictive validity of the multiple mini-interview for selecting medical trainees. *Med Educ*. 2009; **43**(8): 767–75.
26. LeMay JF, Lockyer JM, Collin VT, et al. Assessment of non-cognitive traits through the admissions multiple mini-interview. *Med Educ*. 2007; **41**(6): 573–9.
27. Reiter HI, Eva KW, Rosenfeld J, et al. Multiple mini-interviews predict clerkship and licensing examination performance. *Med Educ*. 2007; **41**(4): 378–84.
28. Roberts C, Zoanetti N, Rothnie I. Validating a multiple mini-interview question bank assessing entry-level reasoning skills in candidates for graduate-entry medicine and dentistry programmes. *Med Educ*. 2009; **43**(4): 350–9.
29. Reiter H, Maccoon K. A compromise method to facilitate under-represented minority admissions to medical school. *Adv Health Sci Educ Theory Pract*. 2007; **12**(2): 223–37.
30. Roberts C, Walton M, Rothnie I, et al. Factors affecting the utility of the multiple mini-interview in selecting candidates for graduate-entry medical school. *Med Educ*. 2008; **42**(4): 396–404.
31. Dodson M, Crotty B, Prideaux D, et al. The multiple mini-interview: how long is long enough? *Med Educ*. 2009; **43**(2): 168–74.
32. Reiter HI, Salvatori P, Rosenfeld J, et al. The effect of defined violations of test security on admissions outcomes using multiple mini-interviews. *Med Educ*. 2006; **40**(1): 36–42.
33. Kumar K, Roberts C, Rothnie I, et al. Experiences of the multiple mini-interview: a qualitative analysis. *Med Educ*. 2009; **43**(4): 360–7.
34. Razack S, Fareno S, Drolet F, et al. Multiple mini-interviews versus traditional interviews: stakeholder acceptability comparisons. *Med Educ*. 2009; **43**(10): 993–1000.
35. Rosenfeld JM, Reiter HI, Trinh K, et al. A cost efficiency comparison between the multiple mini-interview and traditional admissions interviews. *Adv Health Sci Educ Theory Pract*. 2008; **13**(1): 43–58.

36. Humphrey S, Dowson S, Wall D, et al. Multiple mini-interviews: opinions of candidates and interviewers. *Med Educ.* 2008; **42**(2): 207–13.

37. Lievens F, Buyse T, Sackett PR. The operational validity of a video-based situational judgment test for medical college admissions: illustrating the importance of matching predictor and criterion construct domains. *J Appl Psychol.* 2005; **90**(3): 442–52.

38. Lievens F, Sackett PR. Video-based versus written situational judgment tests: a comparison in terms of predictive validity. *J Appl Psychol.* 2006; **91**(5): 1181–8.

39. Carr SE. Emotional intelligence in medical students: does it correlate with selection measures? *Med Educ.* 2009; **43**(11): 1069–77.

40. Knights JA, Kennedy BJ. Medical school selection: impact of dysfunctional tendencies on academic performance. *Med Educ.* 2007; **41**(4): 362–8.

41. Ziv A, Rubin O, Moshinsky A, et al. MOR: a simulation-based assessment centre for evaluating the personal and interpersonal qualities of medical school candidates. *Med Educ.* 2008; **42**(10): 991–8.

42. Dore KL, Reiter HI, Eva KW, et al. Extending the interview to all medical school candidates: Computer-Based Multiple Sample Evaluation of Noncognitive Skills (CMSENS). *Acad Med.* 2009; **84**(Suppl. 10): S9–12.

43. Price PB, Lewis EG, Loughmiller GC, et al. Attributes of a good practicing physician. *J Med Educ.* 1971; **46**(3): 229–37.

44. Powis D. Personality testing in the context of selecting health professionals. *Med Teach.* 2009; **31**(12): 1045–6.

45. Powis D, Bore M, Munro D, et al. Development of the personal qualities assessment as a tool for selecting medical students. *J Adult Cont Educ.* 2005; **11**(1): 3–14.

46. Lumsden MA, Bore M, Millar K, et al. Assessment of personal qualities in relation to admission to medical school. *Med Educ.* 2005; **39**(3): 258–65.

47. Boelen C, Woollard B. Social accountability and accreditation: a new frontier for educational institutions. *Med Educ.* 2009; **43**(9): 887–94.

48. James D, Yates J, Nicholson S. Comparison of A level and UKCAT performance in students applying to UK medical and dental schools in 2006: cohort study. *BMJ.* 2010; **340**: c478.

49. James D, Ferguson E, Powis D, et al. Graduate entry to medicine: widening academic and socio-demographic access. *Med Educ.* 2008; **42**(3): 294–300.

50. Steinecke A, Beaudreau J, Bletzinger RB, et al. Race-neutral admission approaches: challenges and opportunities for medical schools. *Acad Med.* 2007; **82**(2): 117–26.

51. Tekian A. Minority students, affirmative action, and the admission process: a survey of 15 medical schools. *Acad Med.* 1998; **73**(9): 986–92.

52. Kreiter CD. The use of constrained optimization to facilitate admission decisions. *Acad Med.* 2002; **77**(2): 148–51.

53. Bore M, Munro D, Powis D. A comprehensive model for the selection of medical students. *Med Teach.* 2009; **31**(12): 1066–72.

54. Reeves RE, Vishwanatha JK, Yorio T, et al. The post-baccalaureate premedical certification program at the University of North Texas Health Science Center strengthens admission qualifications for entrance into medical school. *Acad Med.* 2008; **83**(1): 45–51.

55. Dalley B, Podawiltz A, Castro R, et al. The Joint Admission Medical Program: a statewide approach to expanding medical education and career opportunities for disadvantaged students. *Acad Med.* 2009; **84**(10): 1373–82.

56. Acosta D, Olsen P. Meeting the needs of regional minority groups: the University of Washington's programs to increase the American Indian and Alaskan native physician workforce. *Acad Med.* 2006; **81**(10): 863–70.

57. Thomson WA, Ferry PG, King JE, et al. Increasing access to medical education for students from medically underserved communities: one program's success. *Acad Med.* 2003; **78**(5): 454–9.

58. Thomson WA, Ferry P, King J, et al. A baccalaureate-MD program for students from medically underserved communities: 15-year outcomes. *Acad Med.* 2010; **85**(4): 668–74.

59. Sternberg RJ. Assessing students for medical schools admissions: is it time for a new approach? *Acad Med.* 2008; **83**(Suppl. 10): S105–10.

60. Regehr G. Trends in medical education research. *Acad Med.* 2004; **79**(10): 939–47.

61. Van der Vleuten CP, Schuwirth LW. Assessing professional competence: from methods to programmes. *Med Educ.* 2005; **39**(3): 309–17.

62. Urlings-Strop LC, Stijnen T, Themmen AP, et al. Selection of medical students: a controlled experiment. *Med Educ.* 2009; **43**(2): 175–83.

63. Hulsman RL, van der Ende JS, Oort FJ, et al. Effectiveness of selection in medical schools admissions: evaluation of outcomes among freshmen. *Med Educ.* 2007; **41**(4): 369–77.

64. Paolo AM, Stites S, Bonaminio GA, et al. A comparison of students from main and alternate admission lists at one school: the potential impact on student performance of increasing enrolment. *Acad Med.* 2006; **81**(9): 837–41.

6

Clinical Competence Assessment*

*Katharine Boursicot, Luci Etheridge, Zeryab Setna,
Alison Sturrock, Jean Ker, Sydney Smee,
and Elango Sambandam*

The Theme in Context

Whatever exists at all exists in some amount, to know it thoroughly involves knowing its quantity as well as its quality.

—Thorndike, 1904

Definition of the Theme

A modern approach to defining performance assessment in medical education requires recognition of the dynamic nature of the perspectives and definitions. These changes result from the variations in which clinical practice and education are delivered and a lack of clarity in defining competence and performance.[1]

Competence describes what an individual is able to do in clinical practice,

---

* Boursicot K, Etheridge L, Setna Z, et al. Performance in assessment: consensus statement and recommendations from the Ottawa Conference. *Med Teach.* 2011; **33**(5): 370–83. Reprinted by permission of Informa Healthcare.

while performance should describe what an individual actually does in clinical practice. Clinical competence is the term being used most frequently by many of the professional regulatory bodies and in the educational literature.[2-4] There are several dimensions of medical competence including the scientific knowledge base and other professional practice elements; such as history taking, clinical examination skills, skills in practical procedures, doctor-patient communication, problem-solving ability, management skills, relationships with colleagues, and ethical behavior.[5-7] In the last 50 years, a wide range of assessment frameworks have been developed examining these different dimensions. Ensuring these are reliable and valid is, however, challenging.[8]

Theoretical Background

Miller's pyramid has been used over the last 20 years as a framework for assessing clinical competence.

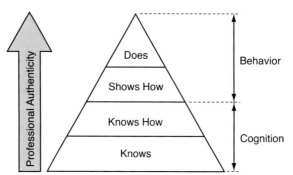

FIGURE 6.1 Miller's model of clinical competence

Source: Miller GE. The assessment of skills/competence/performance. *Acad Med*. 1990; 65(Suppl. 9): S63–7.

Here we address performance assessment defined as assessment of skills and behavior in academic and workplace settings. We recognize that there are many other perspectives that relate to required standards and credentialing. Performance assessment can be illustrated by building in a degree of complexity to Miller's pyramid, recognizing both the development of performance expertise[9] and the need for skills and behavior maintenance through deliberate practice.[10] This enhanced model recognizes, through the skills complexity triangle, some of the contextual factors that affect individual and systems performance measures including taking experience into account.

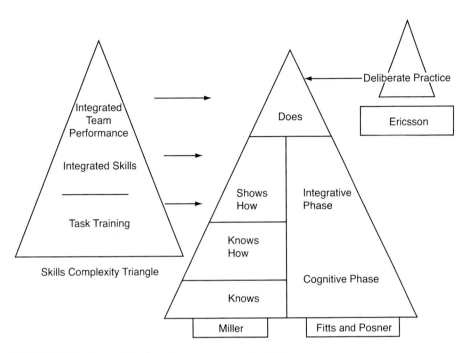

FIGURE 6.2 Miller's model of performance assessment

We will examine the assessment tools designed to test the top two levels of Miller's pyramid: the "shows how" and "does" aspects.

Challenges for assessing the individual performance of health care professionals recognize that health care is increasingly being delivered by teams. Even if patients have the same medical condition the complexity of their care makes it difficult to compare performance.

Assessment tools for clinical competence include the objective structured clinical examination (OSCE), the objective structured long case examination record (OSLER), and the objective structured assessment of technical skills (OSATS). These are undertaken outside the "real" clinical environment but have many aspects of workplace realism and are assessed at the "shows how" level of Miller's pyramid. Workplace-based assessments (WPBAs) include the mini-clinical evaluation exercise (mini-CEX), direct observation of procedural skills (DOPS), and case-based discussions (CbDs). WPBA tools assess at the "does" level of Miller's pyramid (*see* Chapter 12).

Historical Perspective
••••••••••••••••••••••••••

The assessment of clinical performance has historically involved direct observation of learners by professional colleagues. This stems from the traditional apprenticeship model whose legacy stems from antiquity (*see* Chapter 1). Medical knowledge and skills were passed down from one person to another. The apprentice learned from the master by observing and helping him treat patients.[11] The first medical schools in Greece and southern Italy were formed by leading medical practitioners and their followers.[4] Hippocrates, widely regarded as the father of medicine, was born about 460 BCE on the island of Cos, Greece,[12] and is credited with suggesting changes in the way physicians practiced medicine. They were encouraged to offer reasonable and logical explanations concerning the cause of a disease rather than explanations based on superstitious beliefs.[4] The medical school in Alexandria established around 300 BCE was considered a center of medical excellence. Its best two teachers were Herophilus, an anatomist, and Erasistratus, who is considered by some to have founded physiology. Medical education in this school was based on the teaching of theory followed by practical apprenticeship under one of the physicians.[4]

In the United Kingdom medieval records identify that guilds maintained control of entry to the medical profession. Prior to the Medical Act of 1858, which established the medical professional regulatory body the General Medical Council, doctors in the United Kingdom were virtually autonomous practitioners and assessment was not the norm.[13] Aspiring doctors could pursue their studies at one of the three universities[14] that offered undergraduate medical courses in the United Kingdom and would receive a university degree in medicine. Alternatively, they could follow an apprenticeship with a senior practitioner and eventually join one of the licensing corporations: the Royal Colleges of Physicians and of Surgeons, which were established by royal charters in the mid-sixteenth century, or the Society of Apothecaries, which was established in the early seventeenth century.[15] There were no formal examinations for entry to the medical profession. Apprentices were deemed satisfactory by their master and could then practice independently, or were awarded medical degrees within the universities.

The current situation in relation to performance assessment and national regulatory standards are that Canada, China, and Japan have established national licensing examinations and the United States has national assessment for entry into postgraduate training. Several other countries are exploring the use of national licensing examinations—for example, Korea, Indonesia, and Switzerland. There is currently no national licensing examination in the United Kingdom.

The Importance of the Theme

The current medical education world is dominated by discourse around accountability.[15,16] Along with the perceived loss of trust between society and professionals, including doctors,[17] no one can be assumed to be competent. Clinical performance has to be proven by testing, measurement, and recording. It also needs to be psychometrically acceptable and defensible. One of the major challenges is to ensure that performance assessment is aligned to clinical teaching in the workplace and that it is feasible to deliver. A three-stage model for assessing clinical performance has been suggested.[18] This includes a screening test to identify doctors at risk who then undergo a more detailed assessment. Those who pass the screening test pursue a quality improvement pathway to enhance their performance, which may require different degrees of psychometric rigor. Hays et al.[19] suggested three domains of performance assessment that take account of experience and context: (1) doctors as managers of patient care, (2) doctors as managers of their environment, and (3) doctors as managers of themselves.

There is increasing acknowledgment of the need to explore the role of knowledge in competence and performance assessment. There is also a concern that competence and performance are not seen as two opposing entities but rather as part of a continuous spectrum. There needs to be recognition of the complexities between performance and competence to achieve this.[20]

The increasing use of simulation is another area that requires debate and development of new evidence. The level of simulation used in competency and performance assessment varies from the use of part-task trainers and standardized patients (SPs) in OSCEs to the use of covert simulated patients as "mystery shoppers" in primary care in the Netherlands.[21] The international movement in quality improvement and patient safety has seen increasing use of simulation for performance assessment, led by anesthesiology,[22] but increasingly being used in other health care contexts. This has been led by the experience of simulation in other high-reliability organizations, such as the aviation nuclear, and oil industries.[23] Governments and regulatory authorities have developed national strategies in skills and simulation, recognizing that consistent standards of practice enhance patient outcomes and experience of health care services. Developing performance assessments using simulation may be the most defensible method of ensuring reliability and validity for individual practitioners' health care teams and organizations. The role of virtual reality and the use of technology will also need to be considered in performance assessment.

There is a need to develop international consensual standards of professional practice. By developing uniform standards in performance assessment we can begin to ensure consistency across national borders. The remainder of this chapter provides an overview and background of some of the commonly used tools for competence and performance assessment.

Section A: Competence Assessment

Competence describes what an individual is able to do in clinical practice. The London Deanery booklet *Structured Assessments of Clinical Competence*[24] summarizes the competence assessment tools which are being used. The following is based on this booklet. The tools described are the OSLER, the OSCE, and the OSATS.

Objective Structured Long Case Examination Record

In the traditional long case examination, candidates spend 1 hour with a patient, during which they are expected to take a full formal history and perform a complete physical examination. The assessee is not observed. On completion of this task, the assessee is questioned for 20–30 minutes about the case, usually by a pair of examiners, and is occasionally taken back to the patient to demonstrate clinical signs. Holistic appraisal of the assessee's ability to interact, assess, and manage a real patient is a laudable goal of the long case. However, in recent years, there has been much criticism of this approach due to reliability issues caused by examiner bias, variation in examiner stringency, unstructured questioning, and global marking without anchor statements.[25] Measurement consistency in the long case encounter is also diminished by variability in degree and detail of information disclosure by the patient and variability in patient demeanor, comfort, and health. Furthermore, some patients' illnesses are straightforward whereas others are complex. Assessees' clinical skills also vary significantly across tasks,[26] so that assessing on one patient may not provide generalizable estimates of an assessee's overall ability.[25,27]

Validity of the inferences from a long case examination is one of the strengths of the genre. However, inferring assessees' overall clinical skills from a 1-hour-long case encounter is debatable. Given the evidence of the importance of history taking in achieving a diagnosis,[28] and the need for students to demonstrate good patient communication skills, the omission of direct observation of this process is a deficiency.

The OSLER was developed to address the shortcomings of the long case while attempting to retain the concept of seeing a "new" patient in a holistic way.[29]

The OSLER has 10 key features:

1. It is a 10-item structured record.
2. It has a structured approach—there is a prior agreement on what is to be examined.
3. All learners are assessed on identical items.
4. Construct validity is recognized and assessed.
5. History process and product are assessed.
6. Communication skill assessment is emphasized.
7. Case difficulty is identified by the examiner.
8. OSLER can be used for both criterion and norm referenced assessments.
9. A descriptive mark profile is available where marks are used.
10. It is a practical assessment with no need for extra time over the ordinary long case.

The OSLER has ten items, including four on history, three on physical examination and three on management and clinical acumen. For any individual item examiners decide on their overall grade and mark for the learner and then discuss this with the coexaminer, agreeing on a joint grade. This is done for each item and also for the overall grade and final mark. Thirty minutes is recommended for this examination.[30]

There is evidence that the OSLER is more reliable than the standard long case.[31] However, to achieve a predicted Cronbach's alpha of 0.84 requires 10 separate cases and 20 examiners, and thus raises issues of practicality.[32]

Objective Structured Clinical Examination

In addition to the long case, learners classically undertook between three and six short cases. Here learners were taken to a number of patients with widely differing conditions, asked to examine individual systems or areas and give differential diagnoses of their findings, and demonstrate abnormal clinical signs or produce spot diagnoses. However, students rarely saw the same set of patients, cases often differed greatly in their complexity, and the same two assessors were not present at each case. The cases were not meant to assess communication skills but instead concentrated on clinical examination skills. The assessment was not structured and the assessors were free to ask any questions. Like the long case, there was no attempt to standardize the expected level of performance. The lack of consistency and fairness led to the development and adoption of the OSCE.

In an OSCE the learner rotates sequentially around a series of structured cases. Specific tasks have to be performed at each OSCE station usually involving clinical skills such as history taking, examination of a patient, or practical skills. Stations can include simulation. The marking scheme for each station is structured and determined in advance. There is a time limit for each station, after which the learner must move to the next task.

The basic structure of an OSCE may be varied in the timing for each station, use of checklists or rating scales for scoring, and the use of clinician or SP as assessor. Assessees often encounter different simulation fidelities, e.g., simulated patients, part-task trainers, charts and results, resuscitation manikins or computer-based simulations where they can be tested on a range of psychomotor and communication skills. High levels of reliability and validity can be achieved in OSCE assessments.[33] The fundamental principle is that every assessee has to complete the same task in the same amount of time and is marked according to a structured marking schedule.

Terminology associated with the OSCE format can vary. They are consistently known as OSCEs in undergraduate assessment. However, a variety of terminologies are used in postgraduate settings. For example, in the United Kingdom the Royal College of Physicians' membership clinical examination is called the Practical Assessment of Clinical Examination Skills while the Royal College of General Practitioners' membership examination is called the Clinical Skills Assessment (CSA).

The use of OSCEs in summative assessment has become widespread in the field of undergraduate and postgraduate medical education since they were originally described,[33–38] mainly because of the improved reliability of this assessment format. This has resulted in a fairer test of learners'clinical abilities because the score is less dependent on who is examining and which patient is selected.

The criteria used to evaluate any assessment method are well described and summarized in the Association for the Study of Medical Education booklet *How to Design a Useful Test: the principles of assessment*.[39] These cover reliability, validity, educational impact, cost-efficiency, and acceptability.

Reliability

OSCEs are more reliable than unstructured observations in four main ways:

1. Structured marking schedules allow for more consistent scoring by assessors, using predetermined criteria.
2. Wider sampling across different cases and skills results in a more reliable

picture of overall competence. The more stations or cases each assessee has to complete, the more generalizable the test.

3. Increasing number and homogeneity of stations or cases increases the reliability of the overall test score.
4. Multiple independent observations are collated by different assessors at different stations. Individual assessor bias is thus attenuated.

The most important contribution to reliability is sampling across different cases. More stations boost OSCE reliability. However, increasing the number of OSCE stations has to be balanced with practicality. In practical terms, to enhance reliability it is better to have more stations with one assessor per station than fewer stations with two assessors per station.[40,41]

Validity

Validity asks, "What is the degree to which evidence supports the inference(s) made from the test results?" Each separate inference or conclusion from a test may require different supporting evidence. Note that it is the inferences that are validated, not the test itself.[42,43]

Inferences about ability to apply clinical knowledge to bedside data gathering and reasoning, and to effectively use interpersonal skills, are most relevant to the OSCE model. Inferences about knowledge are less well supported by this method than inferences about the clinically relevant application of knowledge, clinical and practical skills.[44]

Types of validity evidence include content validity and construct validity. Content validity of an OSCE is determined by how well the sampling of skills matches the learning objectives of the course for which that OSCE is designed.[44,45] The sampling should be representative of the whole testable domain, and the best way to ensure an adequate spread of sampling is to use a blueprint.

Construct validity of an OSCE is the implication that those who performed better at this test had better clinical skills than those who did not perform as well. We can only infer an assessee's clinical skills in actual practice, because the OSCE is an artificial situation.

The length of any OSCE station should be fitted to the task to achieve the best authenticity possible to enhance OSCE validity inferences. For example, a station in which blood pressure is measured could authentically be achieved in 5 minutes whereas taking a history of chest pain or examining the neurological status of a patient's legs would be done more authentically in 10 minutes.[46]

Educational Impact

The impact on learning from a testing process is known as consequential validity. The design of an assessment system can reinforce, augment, or undermine learning.[47,48] It is well recognized that learners focus on assessments rather than the learning objectives of the course. By aligning explicit, clear learning objectives with assessment content and format, learners are encouraged to learn the desired clinical competences. By contrast, an assessment system that measures learners' ability to answer multiple choice questions about clinical skills will encourage them to focus on knowledge acquisition. Neither approach is wrong—they simply demonstrate that assessment drives education and that assessment methods need to be thoughtfully applied. There is a downside in using detailed checklists because they may encourage learners to memorize checklist steps rather than learn and practice the skills in different contexts. Rating scale marking schedules encourage persons to learn and practice skills holistically. Hodges and McIlroy[49] identified the positive psychometric properties of using global rating scales in OSCEs, such as a higher internal consistency and construct validity than using checklists. These scholars also endorse the need to be explicit about global ratings because some are sensitive to learners' levels of training.

OSCEs may be used for formative or summative assessment. When teaching and improvement is a major goal of an OSCE, time should be built into the schedule to allow the assessor to give feedback to the assessee on his or her performance, providing a very powerful opportunity for learning. For summative certification examinations, expected competences should be clearly communicated to the assessees so they have an opportunity to learn the skills before taking such assessments.

Cost-Efficiency

OSCEs can be very complex to organize. They require meticulous and detailed forward planning, engagement of considerable numbers of assessors, real patients, simulated patients, and administrative and technical staff to prepare and manage the examination. It is most cost-effective to use OSCEs to test clinical competence and not knowledge. Knowledge is tested more efficiently in a different format. Effective implementation of OSCEs requires thoughtful use of resources and logistics with attention to production of assessment material, timing of sittings, suitability of facilities, catering, and collating and processing results. Other critical logistics include assessor and SP recruitment and training. This is possible even in resource-limited environments.[50]

Acceptability

The increased reliability of the OSCE over other formats, and its perceived fairness by learners, has helped to engender the widespread acceptability of OSCEs among test takers and testing bodies. Since Harden and Gleeson's[36] original description, OSCEs have also been used to replace traditional interviews in selection processes in both undergraduate and postgraduate settings[51,52]—for example, for recruitment to general practice training schemes in the United Kingdom.

Objective Structured Assessment of Technical Skills

Another variation on this assessment tool is the OSATS. This was developed as a classroom test for surgical skills by the Surgical Education Group at the University of Toronto.[53] The OSATS assessment is designed to test a specific procedural skill—for example, caesarean section, diagnostic hysteroscopy, or cataract surgery. The OSATS has two parts. The first part assesses specifics of the procedure. The second part is a generic technical skill assessment which includes judging competences such as knowledge and handling of instruments and documentation. OSATS are gaining popularity among surgical specialties in many other countries.

Reliability

Data regarding the reliability of OSATS are limited. Many studies have been carried out in laboratory settings rather than in clinical settings. There is a high reported inter-observer reliability for the checklist part of OSATS in gynecological procedures and surgical procedures.[54,55]

Validity

OSATS have a high face validity and strong construct validity, with significant correlation between surgical performance scores and level of experience.[56,57]

Acceptability

Most of the studies looking at OSATS have been done in simulated settings; therefore, the evidence for acceptability is low. The majority of assessees and assessors report that the OSATS is a valuable tool that would improve a trainee's surgical skill and it should be part of the annual assessment for trainees.[56]

Issues on Competency Assessment that Merit Discussion

There are several issues that merit further discussion or research in relation to competency assessment:

- use of different scoring systems
- who should be doing the scoring
- use of different standard-setting methods
- developing national assessments of competence
- use of high-fidelity simulation
- assessor training.

Use of Different Scoring Systems

There is continued debate in the literature about the merits of checklist or global scoring for OSCEs. The consensus is that checklists are more suitable for early, novice-level stages, while global scoring more appropriately captures increased clinical expertise.

Who Should Be Doing the Scoring

In the United States, SPs score the candidates. Clinician assessors are prevalent in most other world locations. The fundamental debate is whether the clinical competence of a professional should be judged by other professionals or whether it can be scored by a highly trained nonprofessional person.

Use of Different Standard-Setting Methods

There are a variety of standard-setting methods described in the OSCE literature, but most of these were designed for multiple-choice questions rather than OSCEs. The "gold standard" method is the Borderline Group/Borderline Regression Method, which was developed specifically for OSCEs by the Medical Council of Canada.

Developing National Assessments of Competence

In 1992, the Medical Council of Canada added an SP component to its national licensing examination because of the perception that important competences expected of licensed physicians were not being assessed.[58] Since inception, approximately 2500 assessees per year have been tested at multiple sites throughout the country at fixed time periods.

In 1998, the United States Educational Commission for Foreign Medical Graduates instituted an assessment of clinical and communication skills expected of foreign medical graduates seeking to enter residency training programs. From 1998 to 2004, when it was incorporated into the United States Medical Licensing Examination (USMLE), there were 43 642 administrations making it the largest high-stakes clinical skills examination in the world.[59] The assessment had a standardized format of 11 scored encounters with a trained simulated patient. Competence was evaluated by averaging scores across all encounters and determining the mean for the integrated clinical encounter and communication. Generalizability coefficients for the two conjunctively scored components were approximately 0.70–0.90.[60] In 2004, the USMLE adopted the Educational Commission for Foreign Medical Graduates CSA model and began testing all US medical graduates.

Use of High-Fidelity Simulation

Simulation has been integral to competency assessment, enabling individual competences of history-taking examination and professional skills to be measured reliably in the OSCE format.[33] One of the concerns in using high-fidelity simulation is that it may engender abnormal risk-taking behaviors in a risk- and harm-free environment. Some assessees may form a comfort zone within the simulated environment and use this as their normal standard in the face of a challenging clinical workplace—"simulation seeking behavior."

A systematic review of assessment tools for high-fidelity patient simulation in anesthesiology identified a growing number of studies published since 2000. While there is good evidence for face validity of high-fidelity simulation there is less evidence for its reliability and predictive validity, which is important in high-stakes assessments.[61]

Potential benefits of high-fidelity simulation in assessment include the ability to assess both technical and nontechnical skills and the ability to assess teams.

The use of simulation is expensive but can be cost-effective but may help reduce adverse events, thus providing long-term cost-effectiveness.

Assessor Training

Despite extensive research into assessment formats, little research has been carried out to determine the qualities of a "good" assessor. Trainers and assessors are usually the same people, although extensive understanding of a training program may not equate to the ability to use assessment tools fairly, objectively, and in the manner intended. Inter-rater reliability is known to be a major determinant of the reliability of assessments. However, while several approaches to assessor training have been suggested, there is little evidence of the impact of these on performance.[62]

Section B: Assessment of Clinical Performance
• •

Performance describes what an individual actually does in clinical practice. AMEE Guide No. 31, *Workplace Based Assessment as an Educational Tool*[63] was another key background document.

WPBA is a form of authentic assessment testing of performance in the real environment facing doctors in their everyday clinical practice. It is structured and continuous, unlike the opportunistic observations previously used to form judgments about competence. By using repeated evaluations, an assessor has the opportunity to collect documentary evidence of the progression of individual learners. This evidence may then be used to identify "gaps" in practice that will allow the assessor and learner to mutually plan individual development needs. Using a wide range of WPBA tools helps identify strengths and weaknesses in different areas of practice including technical skills, professional behavior, and team working (*see* Chapter 12).

There are various types of WPBA tools currently in use. A summary is given here, covering format, reliability, validity, acceptability, and educational impact.

Mini Clinical Evaluation Exercise

The mini-CEX is a method of CSA developed by the American Board of Internal Medicine to assess residents' clinical skills.[64] It was particularly designed to assess those skills that doctors most often use in real clinical encounters. It is now being increasingly used in undergraduate assessment as well.[65] The mini-CEX involves direct observation by the assessor of a candidate's performance in "real" clinical encounters in the workplace. The assessee is judged in one or more of six clinical domains (history taking, clinical examination, communication, clinical judgment, professionalism, organization/efficiency) and overall clinical care, using a seven-point rating scale. The assessor then gives feedback. The mini-CEX is performed on multiple occasions with different patients and different assessors.[63]

The average mini-CEX encounter takes around 15–25 minutes. There is opportunity for immediate feedback,[66] which not only helps identify strengths and weaknesses but also helps improve skills. The time reported in the literature for feedback can vary from 5[67] to 17 minutes.[68]

Reliability

Although there is good evidence of the reliability of the mini-CEX in the literature, a large proportion of these data come from studies that employ the mini-CEX in experimental settings rather than in naturalistic settings. Experimental settings make it possible for a performance to be assessed by multiple assessors, a situation that is not practical in real clinical settings. The reported inter-rater reliability of the mini-CEX is variable even among same assessor groups.[69] In addition, there is variation in scoring across different levels of assessors, with studies showing that residents tend to score mini-CEX encounters more leniently than consultants.[65] Inter-rater variations in marking can be reduced with more assessors rating fewer encounters, rather than few assessors rating multiple encounters. Between 10 and 14 encounters are needed to show good reliability, if assessed by different raters and on multiple patients.[64]

In practical terms the number of mini-CEX encounters possible in real clinical practice settings needs to be balanced against the need for reliability. One possible method of reducing assessor variation in scoring is through formal assessor training in using these tools. The evidence for reducing this variation through assessor training is, however, variable, with some studies showing that training makes little difference to scoring consistency,[70] whereas others report more stringent marking and greater confidence while marking following assessor training.[71]

Validity

Strong concurrent validity has been reported between mini-CEX and CSA in the USMLE.[69] Any assessment tool that measures clinical performance over a wide range of clinical complexity and level of training must be able to discriminate between junior and senior doctors. In addition, senior doctors should be performing more complex procedures and performing more procedures independently. The mini-CEX is able to discriminate, with the senior doctors attaining higher clinical and global competence scores.[64] The domains of history taking, physical examination, and clinical judgment within the mini-CEX correlate highly with similar domains of the American Board of Internal Medicine evaluation form.[71]

Acceptability

One measure of acceptability is to record the uptake of forms by both assessors and assessees, with the assumption that higher uptakes will reflect greater acceptability for the assessment method. Some studies report a high uptake of mini-CEX,[65] whereas other studies report a lower uptake.[68] A reduced uptake of forms may be related to time constraints and lack of motivation to complete these forms in busy clinical settings. Assessees may find completing WPBAs time-consuming, difficult to schedule, or even stressful and unrealistic.[72] However, both assessors and assessees have reported high satisfaction rates with regard to the ability of the forms to provide opportunities for structured training and feedback.[72]

Educational Impact

The perceived educational impact of the mini-CEX is related to the formative use of the assessment to monitor progress and identify educational needs. Appropriate and timely feedback allows assessees to correct their weaknesses and to mature professionally.[73] Assessees find the mini-CEX beneficial because it reassures them of satisfactory performance and increases their interaction with senior doctors.[72] However, it is important to train assessors to give good-quality observation and feedback.

Direct Observation of Procedural Skills

DOPS is a method of assessment developed by the Royal College of Physicians in the United Kingdom specifically for assessing practical skills.[73] DOPS is mainly used for postgraduate doctors but many medical schools are planning to use it as part of their undergraduate assessments. It requires the assessor to:
- directly observe the trainee undertaking the procedure;
- make judgments about specific components of the procedure;
- grade the trainee's performance.

Reliability

As with the mini-CEX, DOPS needs to be repeated on several occasions for it to be a reliable measure. Subjective assessment of competences done at the end of a rotation has poor reliability and unknown validity. A wide variety of skills that can be assessed with DOPS, from simple procedures such as venipuncture to more complex procedures such as endoscopic retrograde cholangiopancreatography. The DOPS specifically focuses on procedural skills and pre/post-procedure counseling carried out on actual patients.[73]

Validity

The majority of assessees feel that DOPS is a fair method of assessing procedural skills.[73] It has also been established that DOPS scores increase between the first and second half of the year, indicating validity.[74]

Acceptability

The majority of trainees feel that the DOPS is practical.[73] The mean observation time for DOPS varies according to the procedure assessed; on average feedback time took an additional 20%–30% of the procedure observation time. Davies et al.[74] have demonstrated that a mean of 6.2 DOPS were undertaken by first-year foundation trainees in the United Kingdom. The median times for observation and feedback where 10 and 5 minutes, respectively.

Educational Impact

There is little current research on the educational impact of DOPS, although the opportunity for timely feedback gives it the potential for high educational value.

Case-Based Discussion/Chart-Stimulated Recall

These are essentially case reviews, in which the assessee discusses particular aspects of a case in which they have been involved to explore underlying reasoning, ethical issues, and decision making. Repeated encounters are required to obtain a valid picture of an assessee's level of development.

Chart-stimulated recall (CSR)[75] was developed for use by the American Board of Emergency Medicine. The CbD tool is a UK variation. These tools can be used in a variety of clinical settings (e.g., clinics, wards, and assessment units). Different clinical problems can be discussed, including critical incidents. The CbD assesses seven clinical domains: (1) medical record keeping, (2) clinical assessment, (3) investigations and referrals, (4) treatment, (5) follow-up and future planning, (6) professionalism, and (7) overall clinical judgment. The assessee discusses with an assessor cases that they have recently seen or treated. It is expected that they will select cases of varying complexity. A CbD should take 15–20 minutes and 5–10 minutes for feedback.[74] The number of cases suggested during the first 2 years of training is a minimum of six per year.

Reliability

There are data available for the CSR that show good reliability.

Validity

A study using different assessment methods has shown that assessment carried out using CSR is able to differentiate between doctors in good standing and those identified as poorly performing, and correlates with other forms of assessment.

Acceptability

This has not been extensively reported. As with all WBPAs, evidence about the true costs of these assessments is scarce. Costs include assessor training because assessor bias reduces WPBA validity. There are also costs associated with assessor and assessee time in theaters, clinics, and wards. It has been calculated that the median time taken to do an assessment and provide feedback is about 1 hour per month for one trainee.[74]

Educational Impact

Again, there is little published research on the educational impact of these methods. However, as with DOPS, the opportunity for feedback on clinical reasoning and decision making is thought to be valuable in helping learners progress.

Mini Peer Assessment Tool

The mini-peer assessment tool (mini-PAT) is a modified version of the Sheffield peer review assessment tool, which is a validated assessment with known reliability and feasibility.[76] The mini-PAT is used by the Foundation Assessment Programme and various Royal Colleges in the United Kingdom.

There are a number of methods to collate the judgments of peers. The most important aspect of peer judgment is systematic and broad sampling across different individuals who are in a legitimate position to make evaluations. The mini-PAT is one example of the objective, systematic collection and feedback of performance data. The mini-PAT is useful for assessing behaviors and attitudes such as communication, leadership, team working, punctuality, and reliability. It asks peers to complete a structured questionnaire with 15 questions about the individual doctor's performance.[77] This information is collated anonymously and fed back to the trainee. A minimum of eight and up to 12 assessors can be nominated. The time taken to complete a mini-PAT assessment is between 1 and 50 minutes, with a mean duration of 7 minutes.[74]

Reliability

Good inter-item correlation in the mini-PAT has been reported but correlation between assessments is lower. Inter-rater variance has been reported, with consultants tending to give a lower score. However, the longer the consultants have known the learners, the more likely they are to score them higher.

Validity

The 15 questions within the mini-PAT assessment were modified and mapped against the UK Foundation Assessment Programme curriculum and the General Medical Council guidelines for Good Medical Practice, to ensure content validity. Strong concurrent validity has been reported between the mini-PAT, mini-CEX, and CbD. There is evidence of construct validity, with senior doctors achieving a small but statistically significantly higher overall mean score at mini-PAT compared with more junior doctors.[74,76]

Acceptability

As discussed earlier, acceptability may be inferred from the number of completed assessment forms. A high response rate of 67% was achieved in one study.[76] One of the main advantages of such assessments is that they can be kept anonymous, encouraging assessors to be more honest about their views. The main criticisms are that feedback is often delayed and that it is difficult to attribute unsatisfactory performance to specific clinical placements because of anonymous feedback.[78]

Educational Impact

The mini-PAT has been used primarily as a formative form of assessment rather than summative.[78] This allows the assessees to reflect on the feedback they receive in order to improve their clinical performance.

This method of assessment has been used in industry for approximately 50 years and in medicine within the last 10 years. The aim is to provide an honest and balanced view of the person being assessed from various people they have worked with. This can include colleagues, nurses, residents, administrative staff but also medical students and patients. However, this method has some disadvantages, including risk of victimization and potentially damaging harsh feedback.[72]

Issues that Merit Discussion on Performance Assessment

There are several issues that merit further discussion or research in relation to performance assessment:
1. reliability of WPBA tools and their alignment to learning outcomes
2. feasibility of tools in contemporary clinical workplaces
3. use of simulation in transferring performance to the workplace
4. use of feedback in performance assessment
5. development of tools to assess teamwork.

Reliability, Feasibility, and Predictive Validity

As discussed, there is good evidence for individual WPBA tools but less evidence regarding how these tools fit together into a coherent program of ongoing assessment. A major concern of clinicians is the impact the administration of these assessments will have on clinical workload for both assessors and learners. In addition, little is understood about how the results of these assessments predict the future clinical performance of individuals.

Simulation and Transfer

There is initial evidence that using simulation to train novices in surgical skills, such as laparoscopy, results in improved psychomotor skills during real clinical performance. However, the complexity of real clinical performance is often overlooked and a simulation program needs to be part of a comprehensive learning package[79] so that high-stakes decisions can be made.[61]

Feedback in Performance Assessment

There has been a tendency to move toward multisource feedback, as evidence of performance in the workplace.[77] Peer group feedback can give learners a realistic perspective about standards of performance.[80] In addition feedback can be given by simulators by collecting data of events and interactions and from attached monitors. Tutors and facilitators can provide feedback where the main focus is on striving for better professional performance.

Assessing Teamwork

While teamwork and professionalism are emphasized in many curricula documents,[7] the assessment of these "soft" skills is problematic. Formative assessments, such as multisource feedback, often incorporate these elements. The research foundation and its evidence base for formative and summative evaluation of health care teamwork is now growing in breadth and depth (*see* Chapter 9, this volume).

Draft Consensus Statements and Recommendations

Widespread use of competency assessments such as the OSCE, and of performance assessments such as the mini-CEX, grew out of assumptions and principles that are incorporated into the consensus statements from the 2010 Ottawa Conference in Miami and recommendations that follow.

Section A: Competency Assessments (OSCEs)

Consensus

1. Competency assessments are needed to assess at the "shows how" level of Miller's pyramid.

2. Competency assessments should be designed and developed within a theoretical framework of clinical expertise.
3. Competency assessments can generate scores with good reliability and validity.
4. Competency assessments can provide documented evidence of learning progress and readiness for practice.
5. Competency assessments should be designed using a wide range of methodologies.

Recommendations for Individuals (Including Individual Committees)

1. Articulate clearly the purpose of the competency assessment. Ensure that the purpose and the blueprinting criteria are congruent and that they reflect curriculum objectives.
2. Develop assessments that measure more than basic clinical skills; for example, assessment of clinical competence in the context of complex patient presentations, interprofessional and team skills, ethical reasoning, and professionalism.
3. Use scoring formats appropriate to the content and training level being assessed. No single scoring format is best for all.
4. Employ criterion-referenced methods for setting standards for decision making. Useful methods include contrasting groups, borderline group, or borderline regression.
5. Identify how competency assessment can be best linked to a remediation framework.

Recommendations for Institutions

1. Implement competency assessments, especially when summative, as a component of an overall assessment plan for the curriculum.
2. Engage in collaborations within and across institutions where common approaches can enhance standards of practice.
3. Provide appropriate levels of support to the faculty members who create and administer competency assessments. These assessments require support staff, equipment, space, and funds. Creating content, designing scoring instruments, setting standards, recruiting and training simulated patients or SPs and examiners, plus organizing the assessment itself, all require time and teamwork to a degree that is frequently underestimated and underappreciated.

4. Formalize the recognition of scholarly input to competency assessment.
5. Engage faculty who participate in competence assessments as content developers and examiners, with faculty development. Recognize their participation.

Outstanding Issues

1. Establishing a common language and criteria regarding scoring instruments to clarify what is meant by global rating (versus, for example, generic rating), checklists, and grids.
2. Ensuring all aspects of competence are assessed, including "softer" competences of leadership, professionalism, and so forth.
3. Ensuring assessment of competence but promotion of excellence.
4. Creating a wide range of scoring tools for scoring assessments based on complex content and tasks. Moving beyond a dichotomous discussion of checklists versus global rating scales to development of scoring formats keyed to the content and educational level of a specific assessment.
5. Ensuring consensus around use and abuse of terminology.
6. Promoting better understanding and use of existing standard-setting methods.
7. Developing feasible as well as psychometrically sound standard-setting methods for small cohorts.
8. Articulating guidelines and rationales regarding who should score assessments, including SPs and nonphysician and physician raters, as well as further establishing training requirements and methods for each.
9. Exploring integration of simulation and SP-based methodologies for assessment.
10. Gathering further information about the predictive validity of use of simulation in high-stakes assessments.
11. Developing and promoting more feasible equating methods for assessments.
12. Establishing the role of the OSCE as a "gatekeeper" for progression.
13. Engaging stakeholders in identifying key areas from assessment (e.g., patient groups).
14. Ensuring constituency of assessors by training and observation.

Section B: Performance Assessments (WPBAs)

Consensus

1. WPBAs assess the two behavioral levels at the top of Miller's model of clinical competence, shows how and does, because the workplace provides a naturalistic setting for assessing performance over time.
2. WPBAs can cover not only clinical skills but also aspects of skills such as professionalism, decision making, and timekeeping.
3. WPBAs, specifically the mini-CEX and multisource feedback, can generate sufficiently reliable and valid results for formative purposes.
4. WPBAs occur over multiple occasions and lead to documented evidence of developing clinical competence.
5. WPBAs should provide the timely feedback that is essential to learning and enhancing its acceptability among users.

Recommendations for Individuals (Including Committees)

1. Ensure assessments go hand in hand with learning and are not isolated exercises.
2. Encourage learners to receive assessments distributed regularly throughout the year rather than clustering the assessments as their final assessment is due.
3. Articulate and disseminate the purpose of the assessment clearly. Ensure that each assessment is appropriately driven by learning objectives, practice standards, and assessment criteria.
4. Create WPBAs within the framework of a program of assessment that incorporates the use of multiple methodologies, occasions, and assessors. This can reside within a portfolio.

Recommendations for Institutions

1. Ensure time and costs for training and assessments are included in workplace planning—for example, included in job plans, clinic schedules, and budgets.
2. Select methodologies that are appropriate for the intended purpose (summative or formative).
3. Use results in accordance with the intended purpose to protect assessment processes. For example, using formative outcomes for summative decision making pushes learners to delay assessment occasions until the end of the assessment period, thereby undermining the documentation of their development over time.

4. Educate assessors and assessees about the assessment method and the use of the rating tools to enhance the quality of feedback, reduce stress of both groups, and preserve the naturalistic setting.

5. Promote strong reliability by minimizing inter-rater variance (e.g., increasing number of assessors), providing clear assessment criteria and training to all assessors and minimizing case effect (e.g., drive wider sampling, take into account assessee level of expertise and set case selection criteria).

6. Enrich validity by incorporating use of external assessors to offset the effect of learners choosing their own assessors.

7. Combine WPBA with other forms of performance assessment to provide more comprehensive evaluations of competence, as occurs with a portfolio.

8. Individualize assessments based on learner performance. Individuals having difficulty may need more frequent assessments and feedback than those who are performing well.

9. Identify individuals in difficulty as early as possible with robust systems of assessment.

Outstanding Issues

1. Establishing the reliability and validity of outcomes from DOPS and CbD/CSR in workplace (naturalistic) settings.

2. Estimating the total number of DOPS/CbD/CSR required to achieve sufficient reliability and validity for decision making (guiding remediation) within specified contexts (e.g., specialty based).

3. Exploring how various workplace assessment tools, when combined, facilitate learning and meet the overall objectives of training or practice.

4. Exploring the role of WPBAs in summative assessment, including approaches to reporting outcomes (e.g., scores, profiles).

5. Researching further the concept of transfer between simulation and workplace-based performance.

6. Developing more feasible approaches to WPBAs and how these relate to portfolio assessment processes.

7. Conducting predictive validity studies on the impact of WPBAs on long-term performance.

8. Developing WPBAs for team working and professionalism.

References

1. Murphy DJ, Bruce DA, Mercer SW, et al. The reliability of workplace-based assessment in postgraduate medical education and training: a national evaluation in general practice in the United Kingdom. *Adv Health Sci Educ Theory Pract*. 2009; **14**(2): 219–32.
2. General Medical Council (GMC). *Tomorrow's Doctors*. London: GMC; 2009.
3. Miller GE. The assessment of clinical skills/competence/performance. *Acad Med*. 1990; **65**(9): S63–7.
4. Pikoulis E, Msaouel P, Avgerinos ED, et al. Evolution of medical education in ancient Greece. *Chin Med J (Engl)*. 2008; **121**(21): 2202–6.
5. Berk RA. Using the 360 degrees multisource feedback model to evaluate teaching and professionalism. *Med Teach*. 2009; **31**(12): 1073–80.
6. Epstein RM, Hundert EM. Defining and assessing professional competence. *JAMA*. 2002; **287**(2): 226–35.
7. General Medical Council (GMC). *Tomorrow's Doctors*. London: GMC; 2003.
8. Schuwirth LW, van der Vleuten CP. Challenges for educationalists. *BMJ*. 2006; **333**(7567): 544–6.
9. Fitts PM, Posner MI. *Learning and Skilled Performance in Human Performance*. Belmont, CA: Brock-Cole; 1967.
10. Ericsson KA. Deliberate practice and the acquisition and maintenance of expert performance in medicine and related domains. *Acad Med*. 2004; **79**(10, Suppl.): S70–81.
11. Bynum WF, Porter R. *Companion Encyclopedia of the History of Medicine*. London: Routledge; 1993.
12. Smith G. Toward a public oral history. In: Ritchie DA, editor. *The Oxford Handbook of Oral History*. Oxford: Oxford University Press; 2010. pp. 80–123.
13. Loudon I. The market for medicine: essay review. *Med Hist*. 1995; **39**(3): 370–2.
14. David TJ, Hargreaves A, Clerc D. Medical students and the juvenile court. *Lancet*. 1980; **8**(2): 1017–18.
15. Power M. *The Audit Society: rituals of verification*. Oxford: Oxford University Press; 1997.
16. Shore C, Selwyn T. The marketisation of higher education: management discourse and the politics of performance. In: Jary D, Parker M, editors. *New Higher Education: issues and directions for the post-Dearing university*. Stoke-on-Trent, UK: University of Staffordshire Press; 1998. pp. 153–72.
17. O'Neill O. A question of trust. Reith lectures. BBC Radio 4; April 3–May 1, 2002.
18. Rethans JJ, Norcini JJ, Barón-Maldonado M, et al. The relationship between competence and performance: implications for assessing practice performance. *Med Educ*. 2002; **36**(10): 901–9.
19. Hays RB, Davies HA, Beard JD, et al. Selecting performance assessment methods for experienced physicians. *Med Educ*. 2002; **36**(10): 910–17.
20. Ram P, van der Vleuten C, Rethans JJ, et al. Assessment in general practice: the

predictive value of written-knowledge tests and a multiple-station examination for actual medical performance in daily practice. *Med Educ.* 1999; **33**(3): 197–203.

21. Rethans JJ, Sturmans F, Drop R, et al. Assessment of the performance of general practitioners by the use of standardized (simulated) patients. *Br J Gen Pract.* 1991; **41**(344): 97–9.

22. Weller J, Wilson L, Robinson B. Survey of change in practice following simulation-based training in crisis management. *Anaesthesia.* 2003; **58**(5): 471–3.

23. Maran NJ, Glavin RJ. Low- to high-fidelity simulation: a continuum of medical education? *Med Educ.* 2003; **37**(Suppl. 1): S22–8.

24. London Deanery. *Structured Assessments of Clinical Competence.* Available at: www.faculty.londondeanery.ac.uk./e-learning/structured-assessments-of-clinical-competence (accessed December 3, 2012).

25. Norcini J. The validity of long cases. *Med Educ.* 2001; **35**(8): 720–1.

26. Swanson DB, Norman GR, Linn RL. Performance-based assessment: lessons learnt from the health professions. *Educ Res.* 1995; **24**(5): 5–11.

27. Norcini JJ. The death of the long case? *BMJ.* 2002; **324**(7334): 408–9.

28. Hampton JR, Harrison MJ, Mitchell JR, et al. Relative contributions of history-taking, physical examination, and laboratory investigation to diagnosis and management of medical outpatients. *BMJ.* 1975; **31**(2): 486–9.

29. Gleeson F. Assessment of clinical competence using the objective structured long examination record (OSLER). *Med Teach.* 1997; **19**: 7–14.

30. Gleeson F. The effect of immediate feedback on clinical skills using the OSLER. In: Rothman AI, Cohen R, editors. *Proceedings of the Sixth Ottawa Conference of Medical Education.* Toronto, Canada: Bookstore Custom Publishing, University of Toronto; 1994. pp. 412–15.

31. Van Thiel J, Kraan HF, van der Vleuten CPM. Reliability and feasibility of measuring medical interviewing skills: the revised Maastricht history-taking and advice checklist. *Med Educ.* 1991; **25**(3): 224–9.

32. Wass V, Jones R, van der Vleuten C. Standardized or real patients to test clinical competence? The long case revisited. *Med Educ.* 2001; **35**(4): 321–5.

33. Newble D. Techniques for measuring clinical competence: objective structured clinical examinations. *Med Educ.* 2004; **38**(2): 199–203.

34. Cohen R, Reznick RK, Taylor BR, et al. Reliability and validity of the objective structured clinical examination in assessing surgical residents. *Am J Surg.* 1990; **160**(3): 302–5.

35. Davis MH, Harden R. Competency-based assessment: making it a reality. *Med Teach.* 2003; **25**(6): 565–8.

36. Harden RM, Gleeson FA. Assessment of clinical competence using an objective structured clinical examination (OSCE). *Med Educ.* 1979; **13**(1): 41–54.

37. Reznick RK, Smee S, Baumber JS, et al. Guidelines for estimating the real cost of an objective structured clinical examination. *Acad Med.* 1993; **68**(7): 513–17.

38. Sloan DA, Donnelly MB, Schwartz RW, et al. The objective structured clinical examination: the new gold standard for evaluating postgraduate clinical performance. *Ann Surg.* 1995; **222**(6): 735–42.

39. Schuwirth LWT, van der Vleuten CPM. *How to Design a Useful Test: the principles of assessment.* Edinburgh, UK: Association for the Study of Medical Education; 2006.

40. Swanson DB. A measurement framework for performance based tests. In: Hart IR, Harden RM, editors. *Further Developments in Assessing Clinical Competence.* Montreal, Canada: Heal Publications; 1987. pp. 13–45.

41. Van der Vleuten CPM, Swanson DB. Assessment of clinical skills with standardized patients: state of the art. *Teach Learn Med.* 1990; **2**(2): 58–76.

42. Downing SM, Haladyna TM. Validity threats: overcoming interference with proposed interpretations of assessment data. *Med Educ.* 2004; **38**(3): 327–33.

43. Kane MT. Validation. In: Brennan RL, editor. *Educational Measurement*, 4th ed. Westport, CT: American Council on Education and Praeger Publishers; 2006. pp. 17–64.

44. Downing SM. Validity: on meaningful interpretation of assessment data. *Med Educ.* 2003; **37**(9): 830–7.

45. Biggs J. *Teaching for Quality Learning at University.* Buckingham, UK: Society for Research into Higher Education and Open University Press; 1999.

46. Petrusa ER. Clinical performance assessments. In: Norman GR, van der Vleuten CPM, Newble DI, editors. *International Handbook for Research in Medical Education.* Dordrecht, the Netherlands: Kluwer Academic Publishers; 2002. pp. 248–320.

47. Kaufman DM. ABC of learning and teaching in medicine: applying educational theory in practice. *BMJ.* 2003; **326**(7382): 213–16.

48. Newble DI, Jaeger K. The effect of assessments and examinations on the learning of medical students. *Med Educ.* 1983; **17**(3): 165–71.

49. Hodges B, McIlroy JH. Analytic global OSCE ratings are sensitive to level of training. *Med Educ.* 2003; **37**(11): 1012–16.

50. Vargas AL, Boulet JR, Errichetti A, et al. Developing performance-based medical school assessment programs in resource-limited environments. *Med Teach.* 2007; **29**(2–3): 192–8.

51. Lane JL, Gottlieb RP. Structured clinical observations: a method to teach clinical skills with limited time and financial resources. *Pediatrics.* 2000; **105**(4): 973–7.

52. Eva KW, Reiter HI, Rosenfeld J, et al. The ability of the multiple mini-interview to predict pre clerkship performance in medical school. *Acad Med.* 2004; **79**(10): 40–2.

53. Dath D, Reznick RK. Objectifying skills assessment: Bench model solutions; challenges of assessment in training and practice. In: *Surgical Competence.* The Royal College of Surgeons of England/The Smith and Nephew Foundation; 1999.

54. Fialkow M, Mandel L, van Blaricom A, et al. A curriculum for Burch colposuspension and diagnostic cystoscopy evaluated by an objective structured assessment of technical skills. *Am J Obstet Gynecol.* 2007; **197**(5): 1–6.

55. Goff B, Mandel L, Lentz G, et al. Assessment of resident surgical skills: is testing feasible? *Am J Obstet Gynecol.* 2005; **192**(4): 1331–8.

56. Bodle JF, Kaufmann SJ, Bisson D, et al. Value and face validity of objective structured assessment of technical skills (OSATS) for work based assessment of surgical skills in obstetrics and gynecology. *Med Teach.* 2008; **30**(2): 212–16.

57. Collins JP, Gamble GD. A multi-format interdisciplinary final examination. *Med Educ*. 1996; **30**(4): 259–65.
58. Reznick RK, Blackmore D, Dale Dauphinee W, et al. Large-scale high-stakes testing with an OSCE: report from the Medical Council of Canada. *Acad Med*. 1996; **7**(1): 19–21.
59. Whelan GP, Boulet JR, McKinley DW, et al. Scoring standardized patient examinations: lessons learned from the development and administration of the ECFMG clinical skills assessment (CSA). *Med Teach*. 2005; **27**(3): 200–6.
60. Boulet JR, Friedman BM, Ziv A, et al. Using standardized patients to assess the interpersonal skills of physicians. *Acad Med*. 1998; **73**(10): 94–6.
61. Edler AA, Fanning RG, Chen MI, et al. Patient simulation: a literary synthesis of assessment tools in anesthesiology. *J Educ Eval Health Prof*. 2009; **6**(1): 3.
62. Williams RG, Klamen DA, McGaghie WC. Cognitive, social and environmental sources of bias in clinical competence ratings. *Teach Learn Med*. 2003; **15**(4): 270–92.
63. Norcini J, Burch V. Workplace-based assessment as an educational tool: AMEE Guide No. 31. *Med Teach*. 2007; **41**(10): 926–34.
64. Norcini JJ, Blank LL, Arnold GK, et al. The mini-CEX (clinical evaluation exercise): a preliminary investigation. *Ann Intern Med*. 1995; **123**(10): 795–9.
65. Kogan JR, Bellini LM, Shea JA. Feasibility, reliability, and validity of the mini-clinical evaluation exercise (mCEX) in a medicine core clerkship. *Acad Med*. 2003; **78**(10): 33–5.
66. Holmboe ES, Hawkins RE. Methods for evaluating the clinical competence of residents in internal medicine: a review. *Ann Intern Med*. 1998; **129**(1): 42–8.
67. Norcini JJ. Work based assessment. *BMJ*. 2003; **326**(5): 753–5.
68. De Lima AA, Barrero C, Baratta S, et al. Validity, reliability, feasibility and satisfaction of the mini-clinical evaluation exercise (mini-CEX) for cardiology residency training. *Med Teach*. 2007; **29**(8): 785–90.
69. Boulet JR, McKinley DW, Norcini JJ, et al. Assessing the comparability of standardized patient and physician evaluations of clinical skills. *Adv Health Sci Educ Theory Pract*. 2002; **7**(2): 85–97.
70. Cook V, Sharma A, Alstead E. Introduction to teaching for junior doctors: 1. Opportunities, challenges and good practice. *Br J Hosp Med (Lond)*. 2009; **70**(11): 651–3.
71. Durning SJ, Cation LJ, Markert RJ, et al. Assessing the reliability and validity of the mini-clinical evaluation exercise for internal medicine residency training. *Acad Med*. 2002; **77**(9): 900–4.
72. Cohen SN, Farrant PB, Taibjee SM. Assessing the assessments: UK dermatology trainees' views of the workplace assessment tools. *Br J Dermatol*. 2009; **161**(1): 34–9.
73. Wilkinson JR, Crossley JGM, Wragg A, et al. Implementing workplace-based assessment across the medical specialties in the United Kingdom. *Med Educ*. 1998; **42**(4): 364–73.

74. Davies H, Archer J, Southgate L, et al. Initial evaluation of the first year of the Foundation Assessment Programme. *Med Educ*. 2009; **43**(1): 74–81.

75. Maatsch JL, Huang R, Downing S, et al. *Predictive Validity of Medical Specialist Examinations*. Final report for Grant HS 02038-04, National Center of Health Services Research. East Lansing, MI: Office of Medical Education Research and Development, Michigan State University; 1983.

76. Archer J, Norcini J, Southgate L, et al. Mini-PAT (Peer Assessment Tool): a valid component of a national assessment programme in the UK? *Adv Health Sci Educ Theory Pract*. 2008; **13**(2): 181–92.

77. Archer JC, Norcini J, Davies HA. Use of SPRAT for peer review of paediatricians in training. *BMJ*. 2005; **330**(7502): 1251–3.

78. Patel JP, West D, Bates IP, et al. Early experiences of the mini-PAT (Peer Assessment Tool) amongst hospital pharmacists in South East London. *J Pharm Pract*. 2009; **17**(2): 123–6.

79. Gallagher AG, Ritter EM, Champion H, et al. Virtual reality simulation for the operating room. *Ann Surg*. 2005; **241**(2): 364–72.

80. Norcini JJ. Peer assessment of competence. *Med Educ*. 2003; **37**(6): 539–43.

7

Evaluation of Knowledge Acquisition

Dorthea Juul

KNOWLEDGE IS THE FOUNDATION OF PROFESSIONAL PRACTICE. AS illustrated graphically by the Miller pyramid,[1] the professional has to know and know how in order to do. Hence, assessment at all levels of training and practice almost always includes evaluation of knowledge acquisition.

This chapter will review the steps in building knowledge assessments, including development of test specifications, selection of item formats, item writing, test administration, test scoring and analysis, standard setting, and reporting results.

The item formats most commonly used to measure knowledge are constructed-response items such as short-answer items and essay questions and selected-response items such as multiple-choice questions (MCQs). The item-writing section will focus on these formats.

Steps in Test Development

There are several commonly agreed upon steps in test development. Following the steps increases the likelihood of producing knowledge evaluations that yield reliable data, which promote valid decisions. These steps are:
- specify the purposes of the test
- develop test specifications
- select item formats
- write the items

- administer the test
- score the test and analyze the results
- set pass-fail standard, if needed
- report results.

The procedures associated with each of these steps will be described.

Specify the Purposes of the Test

Tests serve many purposes in the health professions. They often play a role in admission to a training program, are administered throughout training for formative and summative evaluation of student progress, and may be required for licensure to practice and for certification. Health professionals are being assessed throughout their careers as a component in documenting continued competency.

The first step in developing a test is to specify its purpose. The main educational issue is whether the test will be used to give feedback to learners (formative assessment) or to assign a grade or final judgment (summative assessment). Formative tests used to guide student learning usually have a narrow focus, are brief, and may not have a pass-fail standard. They may be combined with other evaluation results such as performance ratings and final examination scores to produce a final course grade.

Develop Test Specifications

Test specifications are the test plan. Test specifications are also known as a content outline or blueprint. The content outline specifies the topics to be covered and the number of items allotted to each topic. The total number of items is primarily determined by the purpose of the test and the amount of content to be covered. Practical considerations such as available testing time also influence test length.

Test developers often find it useful to add a second dimension to their test: blueprints that reflect cognitive complexity in addition to content coverage. The objectives of education in the health professions are rarely limited to recall of factual information. Trainees are expected to use their knowledge in the context of patient problems. If item writers are not guided to write questions at higher levels of cognitive complexity, the result is often a mismatch between teaching and testing. In addition to guiding item writers, test blueprints may also be shared with examinees to inform their test preparation.

Bloom and his colleagues[2] developed a six-level hierarchical taxonomy: (1) knowledge, (2) comprehension, (3) application, (4) analysis, (5) synthesis, and (6) evaluation. This taxonomy has been modified to three levels, defined as follows:

1. *recall*: ability to remember previously learned material
2. *application*: ability to use previously learned material in a new situation
3. *problem solving*: ability to analyze and synthesize information and apply knowledge to produce a solution to a problem, typically a patient's problem in the health professions.[3]

An example of a two-dimensional test blueprint for a 100-item test in clinical cardiology appears in Table 7.1. The number of items represents relative emphasis in the curriculum/instructional objectives. Heart sounds has the most items allotted to it (35%), and preventive cardiology has the least (5%). Across all content areas, 10% of the items should test recall, 45% should test application, and 45% should test problem solving. Within content areas, there are differences in how the items are allotted across the taxonomic levels with, for example, no preventive cardiology items at the problem-solving level, four classic valve lesions weighted more toward application, and heart sounds weighted more toward problem solving.

TABLE 7.1 Clinical Cardiology Test Blueprint with Five Content Areas and Three Cognitive Levels

Content Area	Cognitive Level			Total
	Recall	Application	Problem Solving	
Normal cardiovascular physiology	2% (n = 2)	5% (n = 5)	8% (n = 8)	15% (n = 15)
Cardiac anatomy	2% (n = 2)	6% (n = 6)	7% (n = 7)	15% (n = 15)
Heart sounds	2% (n = 2)	10% (n = 10)	23% (n = 23)	35% (n = 35)
Four classic valve lesions	2% (n = 2)	21% (n = 21)	7% (n = 7)	30% (n = 30)
Preventive cardiology	2% (n = 2)	3% (n = 3)	0% (n = 0)	5% (n = 5)
Total	10% (n = 10)	45% (n = 45)	45% (n = 45)	100% (n = 100)

Select Item Formats

The two broad categories of items used to assess knowledge are constructed-response items, such as short-answer items and essay questions and selected-response items, such as true/false questions and MCQs. Both formats can be used to assess at all cognitive levels, and each has advantages and disadvantages.

Constructed-response items are less time-consuming to develop than selected-response items. They are, however, more time-consuming to score. This is because, in addition to developing the scoring key, experts have to read and score examinee responses. An advantage of constructed-response items is that they measure if examinees can recall the correct information, not just recognize it. There is evidence that recall is often more difficult than recognition yet performance on content-matched items in both formats is highly correlated.[4] However, if the objective is to assess an examinee's ability to produce a coherent piece of writing, then essay questions should be used.

Selected-response items, specifically MCQs, dominate knowledge assessment in the health professions. MCQs are popular because of the wide range of objectives that can be tested and the relative ease of scoring either by hand or via computer. Computer administration of MCQs is now widespread, further facilitating scoring as well as eliminating printing costs and enhancing security.

A disadvantage of MCQs is that they are difficult to construct and often require training in item-writing principles to avoid common "mistakes" or "flaws" in their presentation.

The four components of the United States Medical Licensing Examination provide examples of both constructed- and selected-response items.[5] The Step 1 (basic sciences), Step 2 clinical knowledge (clinical sciences for supervised practice), and Step 3 (clinical sciences for unsupervised practice) examinations all use MCQs to assess learner understanding and application. Step 2 also includes a clinical skills examination based on encounters with 12 standardized patients and as part of that assessment, examinees produce patient notes (short-answer items) that are scored by experts (physicians). In addition to MCQs, Step 3 includes simulations of patient cases that require entry of data gathering and treatment options. These can be computer scored because extensive lists of options have been developed and entries that do not match are not allowed.

Write the Items

Health professions' faculty have no formal preparation for their work as test developers. Faculty development is needed to ensure that faculty test item writers understand expectations. This is usually done in a workshop where participants are taught item-writing guidelines and learn common item-writing flaws. Workshop participants are also given suggestions for writing items at higher cognitive levels. Most important, faculty participants receive feedback about their items from the workshop leader and from each other.

Descriptions of different item types and some common guidelines for item writing are outlined here. Because MCQs have come to dominate assessment of knowledge acquisition, they will be discussed first and in more detail than other test item formats.

Multiple-Choice Questions

MCQs have a stem followed by 3–5 options, one of which is the one best answer. The goal is for all lettered or numbered options to be plausible. The stem can be in the form of a question or an incomplete statement. If the latter is the case, each of the options completes the sentence. An example of an MCQ is as follows:

> The first step in test development is to
> a. determine the purpose of the test
> b. develop test specifications
> c. write items
> d. set the pass-fail standard
> e. conduct an item-writing workshop.

The discussion of cognitive levels highlights the issue of writing MCQs that test at the application and problem-solving levels. Joorabchi[6] suggests beginning with a database. Data can be presented in nonverbal formats as well—for example, in pictures, video and audio clips, charts, and graphs. The information should be "unprocessed"—that is, it should be presented as realistically as possible without interpretations and labels. The cases should be unfamiliar to the examinees; otherwise, their answers may represent recall rather than problem solving.

There are many guidelines for writing MCQs. Here is a summary of some of the most common. Those who are interested in exploring this area in more depth should obtain (free of charge) the National Board of Medical Examiners comprehensive guide developed by Case and Swanson.[7]

● The stem should clearly convey the question being asked. For example,

"Ascorbic acid" as a stem is inadequate because examinees have almost no idea what this question is about until they read the responses.

- Negative stems (e.g., Which of the following is *in*correct?) are not recommended because examiners usually want to determine if examinees know what to do in a given situation. Asking about what *not* to do does not elicit a correct response. If negative stems are used, the negative phrase should be emphasized in some way (e.g., highlighting, underlining), or examinees may misread the question.
- The item should be focused. In the example given earlier, the options might refer to different properties of ascorbic acid—dietary sources, metabolism in the body, consequences of deficiencies. The recommendation is to focus on the most important aspect—for example, "What is the most significant sequela of inadequate consumption of ascorbic acid?" followed by five choices.
- Avoid excess verbiage. Phrase the stem and options as simply as possible. Put words that are common to all options in the stem.
- All options should be about the same length. The correct answer should not "stand out" because it is longer or shorter than the others.
- Place the options in logical sequence. For example, if the distracters are drug dosages, they should be placed in ascending or descending order.
- Options should be independent and should not overlap.
- Combination options (e.g., all of the above) should not be used because it is possible for the examinee to get the answer correct with only partial information.
- "None of the above" should not be used as a distracter. If this is the correct answer, the examinees have not demonstrated that they know what is correct in this situation, which is important to ascertain.
- The distribution of correct answers should be balanced. If five options are being used, A, B, C, D, and E (or 1, 2, 3, 4, and 5) should each be the correct answer about 20% of the time.
- The content of one item should not give away the correct answer to another item. Such items are commonly called "enemies."

Sometimes several items are based on common stimulus materials. For example, a patient description may be followed by an item about laboratory evaluation, an item about the most likely diagnosis, and one focused on treatment. Within these item sets, the items should be independent, so that if examinees get one wrong they will not necessarily get the others wrong as well. Another caveat is to not oversample a topic by large item sets.

Matching items consist of a set of homogeneous options matched with a set of item stems. These are another MCQ variant that offer an efficient way to test some content areas. There should be a mismatch in the number of options and items so that examinees cannot get some items correct by the process of elimination. Again, oversampling of a content area is to be avoided.

> True/false items, which could be considered MCQs with two options, are not recommended. In the health professions it can be difficult to construct situations that are entirely true or entirely false, and this often leads to questions that focus on relatively trivial material. In addition, examinees have a 50% chance of getting these items correct by guessing.

Short-Answer Items

These are items in which the examinee supplies a short (usually a few words or sentences or numbers) answer. The items should be as clear and succinct as possible, and a scoring key should be developed before administration.

Essay Questions

Essay questions, which should only be used if no other format is suitable for a content area, usually require the examinee to write several paragraphs or pages in response to a question. Again, clarity and simplicity are desirable. Guidance for the examinee in terms of the general framework for responding as well as length of response should be provided. Developing a scoring key or scoring rubric is even more important than for short-answer items. For example, will the essays be graded holistically or will specific points need to be addressed?

Item Review

All items should be reviewed by knowledgeable subject matter experts before administration to ensure that the items are worth asking and expressed clearly. If illustrative materials (e.g., photographs, X-rays) are used, they should also be reviewed for interpretability. The reviewers may also suggest alternative or additional options. In addition to training item writers, this type of review is one of the most important things that can be done to ensure a quality examination, but it is often difficult to accomplish in educational settings with already overcommitted faculty members. Professional editing can also be very helpful, if available.

Administer the Test

Whether an examination is administered via paper-and-pencil or computer, the final version should be carefully proofread. Instructions to the examinee need to be written specifying at a minimum the number of items and amount of test time available. Procedures for breaks and handling examinee questions also need to be anticipated and specified in writing for the proctors.

Security issues need to be considered, including identification requirements, seating arrangements, and handling irregular behavior. If tests are in a paper-and-pencil format, procedures for distributing and collecting them should be followed to ensure that all test materials, including answer sheets, are collected at the end.

There may be some examinees who need special arrangements to take the examinations due to a disability. Procedures for applying for accommodations and evaluating these requests should be established.

Score the Test and Analyze the Results

Test scoring must be done with rigorous attention to detail so that all examinees receive accurate scores. For constructed-response items it is likely that the scoring rubric will have to be modified based on examinee responses. It is also desirable to have at least two judges score at least a subset of answers to establish inter-rater reliability.

For tests with selected-response items, computerized scoring programs are widely used to calculate item statistics. The two item statistics most widely used are difficulty and discrimination, and they can also be calculated by hand.

Difficulty is the percentage of examinees who got the item correct and can range in value between 0% and 100%. Items that are too easy or too difficult do not discriminate among the examinees. Test developers often strive for items with difficulty levels of 40%–80%. A low difficulty may indicate that a given topic was not taught resulting in a "guessing pattern" in which all options are selected about equally often. Sometimes a low difficulty will indicate an answer key error. If another answer is selected more often than the "correct" answer, the item should be reviewed carefully.

Discrimination is the correlation between performance on one item (right/wrong) and the total test score. Like any correlation it can range in value from -1.00 to $+1.00$. In general, we expect more knowledgeable examinees to perform better on any given item than those who are less knowledgeable. For classroom tests, discrimination indices >0.20 are generally considered acceptable. Items with negative discrimination indices should be reviewed to determine why the better examinees did less well on an item than the poorer examinees. There may have been something in the stem or options that misled the more able test takers.

Based on item statistics, test developers have two options for dealing with poorly performing items. In addition to correcting key errors and rescoring, items can be deleted from the final scoring (reduces the total number of items) or all examinees can get credit for the item. These item statistics should be stored with the items in the "item bank" so that they can be used to inform item selection for the next version of the examination, as well as revisions that would possibly strengthen the item.

The statistics typically used to summarize performance on a test are the mean, standard deviation, and range of examinee scores, and the mean and standard deviation of the item difficulties and discrimination indices.

In addition to these descriptive statistics, a measure of reliability is typically computed. Reliability is discussed in Chapters 2 (Criteria for a Good Assessment) and 4 (Research on Assessment Practices). For MCQ tests, the main indicator of reliability is internal consistency reliability calculated with Kuder-Richardson formula 20 or 21. Reliability can range from 0.00 to 1.00, and the higher the test stakes, the higher the reliability should be. For high-stakes examinations, reliabilities >0.90 are desirable. For classroom assessments, reliabilities within the range of 0.60–0.80 are acceptable. The reliability index is used to compute the standard error of measurement, which can be used to construct confidence intervals around examinee scores.

A number of factors can affect score reliability. One of the main factors is the number of test items. Longer tests generally produce more reliable scores than shorter tests. Hence, the primary method for improving score reliability is to increase the number of quality test items. The Spearman-Brown prophecy formula is used to estimate the reliability likely to result if a test is increased by a given factor. Composition of the examinee group can also affect reliability. A more homogeneous group will yield lower reliability indices than a more heterogeneous group.

Set Pass-Fail Standard
•••••••••••••••••••••••••

A pass-fail standard may not be needed for formative tests or for summative tests if combining with the results from other measures. When a pass-fail standard is needed, there are two broad approaches to setting one. Norm-referenced standards, also called relative standards, are based on performance of the group. For example, those scoring two standard deviations below the mean may fail or the bottom 10% may fail. In health professions education, criterion-referenced or absolute standards are generally preferred. The emphasis is on competence, and, theoretically, everyone can meet the standard and pass, or everyone can fail.

Several methods have been developed to set criterion-referenced standards, and they all involve systematic collection of data from subject matter experts. The most commonly used approach is the Angoff method, in which subject matter experts are asked to define the borderline examinee and specify how he or she should perform on each item. The results are then summarized across judges.

If the standard is set before the test is administered, actual performance will usually be considered before setting the final standard to ensure that it is "reasonable." For example, it is common for subject matter experts to overestimate examinees' ability, and hence the pass/fail score may need to be adjusted downward.

More detailed discussions of standard setting may be found in Norcini[8] and Yudkowsky et al.[9] As Yudkowsky et al.[9] remind us:

> There is no single correct or best method to set standards for an examination; nor is there a single correct or "true" cut score that must be discovered. All standards are, to some extent, arbitrary. Thus standard setting can best be viewed as "due process"—a procedure to be followed to ensure that the cut score is not capricious; that it is reasonable, defensible, and fair.

Report Results
•••••••••••••••••••

The test developer must decide what type of scores will be reported to examinees. Some options include raw scores (number correct), percentage scores (number correct divided by total number of items), and scaled scores (raw scores are converted to a scaled score based on means and standard deviations). The latter are typically not calculated for classroom tests.

In some situations it might be desirable to only report pass/fail status.

However, this is problematic for failing examinees because they need feedback about how close they were to the pass-fail standard.

Another issue is deciding whether to report a single total score or additional subtest scores. With computer administration it is also possible to provide key word feedback on all items answered incorrectly. While examinees typically want as much feedback as possible, scores from subtests with small numbers of items and keyword feedback can also be misleading because of limited sampling of a content area.

Item Banking

It is highly desirable to create a bank of previously used test questions with performance statistics, thus tests must be kept secure. There is often pressure from students to receive copies of questions and answers, and it may be school policy to provide them. Writing good test questions is a labor-intensive effort, and it is almost impossible to consistently give quality examinations if all new items are being constructed for each test. A better approach is to use a mix of new and pool questions on any given test. Pool questions can be modified if item statistics indicate there is room for improvement.

Future Directions

Computer administration of tests has not only facilitated the use of images (both static and moving) and sound, it has also permitted the development of new formats, although none of them are yet in widespread use. Some examples include multiple-response, drop-and-drag, and hot-spot items. Significant work has also been done on automated scoring systems for constructed response items and computer generation of test items.

Summary

This chapter began with the assertion that knowledge undergirds performance in the health professions and outlined a systematic approach to develop instruments to assess knowledge acquisition. The goal of giving any test is to yield scores that are usable for a specific purpose. The scores must be reliable and permit valid decisions about learner performance. The steps presented in this chapter increase the likelihood of accomplishing that objective.

References

1. Miller GE. The assessment of clinical skills/competence/performance. *Acad Med.* 1990; **65**(Suppl. 9): S63–7.
2. Bloom BS, Engelhart MD, Furst EJ, et al. *Taxonomy of Educational Objectives, Handbook I: cognitive domain.* New York, NY: David McKay; 1956.
3. Downing SM. Twelve steps for effective test development. In: Downing SM, Haladyna TM, editors. *Handbook of Test Development.* Mahwah, NJ: Lawrence Erlbaum Associates; 2006. pp. 3–25.
4. Rodriguez MC. Construct equivalence of multiple-choice and constructed-response items: a random effects synthesis of correlations. *J Educ Meas.* 2003; **40**(2): 163–84.
5. Clauser BE, Margolis MJ, Case SM. Testing for licensure and certification in the professions. In: Brennan RL, editor. *Educational Measurement.* 4th ed. Westport, CT: American Council on Education and Praeger Publishers; 2006. pp. 701–31.
6. Joorabchi B. How to . . . .: construct problem-solving MCQs. *Med Teach.* 1981; **3**(1): 9–13.
7. Case SM, Swanston D. *Constructing Written Test Questions for the Basic and Clinical Sciences.* Philadelphia, PA: National Board of Medical Examiners, 1998. Available at: www.nbme.org/publications/item-writing-manual.html (accessed July 7, 2011).
8. Norcini JJ. Setting standards on educational tests. *Med Educ.* 2003; **37**(5): 464–9.
9. Yudkowsky R, Downing SM, Tekian A. Standard setting. In: Downing SM, Yudkowsky R, editors. *Assessment in Health Professions Education.* New York, NY: Routledge; 2009. pp. 119–48.

Assessment of Professionalism

Brian David Hodges and Shiphra Ginsburg

Background: The Theme of Professionalism

This chapter represents a modified and expanded version of a previously published journal article:[1] Hodges BD, Ginsburg S, Cruess R, Cruess S, Delport R, Hafferty F, Ho M-J, Holmboe E, Holtman M, Ohbu S, Rees C, ten Cate O, Tsugawa Y, van Mook W, Wass V, Wilkinson T, Wade W. Assessment for professionalism: recommendations from the Ottawa 2010 Conference. *Med Teach.* 2011; **33**(5): 354–63.

Over the past 25 years, professionalism has emerged as a substantive and sustained theme within both clinical medicine and medical education. Featured in medical education conferences and journals, the definition, operationalization, and measurement of professionalism has become a major concern for those involved in the education and development of medical students, as well as residents (house officers, foundation year doctors, etc.), fellows, faculty, clinicians, and researchers. And yet it is a topic characterized by much ambiguity, confusion and at times controversy. The idea that the medical profession should attend to the professional behavior of students and practitioners is not in dispute. However, the process of establishing the elements that constitute *appropriate* professionalism is far more convoluted. Though myriad studies have addressed this topic, the question "What is professionalism?" remains complex, and defining best practices for its assessment even more so. Difficulty stems from the notion that professionalism stretches along a continuum from the individual (attributes, capacities, and behaviors) through the interpersonal domain (interactions with other individuals and with contexts) to the macro-societal level where notions such as social responsibility and morality but also political agendas and economic imperatives reside. Furthermore, there are interactions among these domains. For example, an individual's professional behavior may be influenced by context; similarly, the individuals within an institution may influence its collective professional values. While discussions and research about professionalism have appeared most prominently in English medical education literature in the past 2 decades, the globalization of medical education means increasing interest in the construct of professionalism in other languages, countries, and cultures. As professionalism is a complex and multidimensional construct, one should not look for one, simple, generalizable statement about what professionalism is and how to assess it. Rather, assessment of professionalism requires consideration of individual, interpersonal, and societal dimensions.

Method: The International Working Group

The International Ottawa Conference Working Group on the Assessment of Professionalism (IOC-PWG) was created by inviting individuals with a history of writing or speaking internationally about the assessment of professionalism. Attention was given to diversity of the group, which consisted of 18 individuals (7 women, 11 men) representing nine countries in North America, Europe, Asia, Oceania, and Africa. The group represented a mix of clinicians and PhD-level academics from different disciplines (sociology, psychology, education, medicine, etc.). Members of the group held a diverse set of views about the nature of professionalism and its assessment, something that the group both valued and recognized as a challenge for the creation of a consensus.

Discourses of Professionalism: Implications for Assessment

The working group chose to define the key issues related to the assessment of professionalism by undertaking a discourse analysis. The group began with a set of articles identified by the IOC-PWG as key to the consideration of the assessment of professionalism. A discourse analysis is quite different from a traditional review in that the goal is not simply to summarize and condense existing findings, as would be done in a meta-analysis or summary review paper, but rather to characterize different ways that language is used to talk about and create statements of truth about a given phenomenon. There are many approaches to discourse analysis. The approach used here is inspired by what is known as critical discourse analysis.[2] In this discourse analysis of literature on professionalism, it was not the purpose to identify all papers on the topic, or to try to reduce findings down to a single set of consensus statements. Rather, the objective was to identify several discourses that are currently used to frame what professionalism is, and to form guidelines for how professionalism might be assessed. While a discourse analyst tries to identify and classify samples of writing/text into a limited number of conceptual categories, it is important not to reduce or synthesize them to the point that paradigmatic nuances are blurred.

A discourse analysis is particularly well suited for something as complex and multifaceted as professionalism. Categorization helps to illustrate the diversity of active discourses related to professionalism. The terms *discourse* and *epistemology*, and other terms used in this analysis, are defined in a glossary in Appendix 1, at the end of this chapter. There is no assumption that these are the *only* categories or that they would be fixed over time or in different places. The purpose of this discourse analysis is to reveal different ways of thinking about professionalism so as to allow researchers, educators, and clinicians to preserve their core values, interests, and paradigmatic perspectives and at the same time to work collectively toward a multidimensional, multi-paradigmatic approach to assessing professionalism.

Discourse Analysis of Key Articles

The 18 members of the international working group each submitted two or three references (original research, theoretical article, review paper, etc.) that they considered key articles in assessment of professionalism. A few redundancies were eliminated and 50 articles were downloaded. Articles were then read in detail by the group lead (BH). Papers were coded for key words and concepts, and an anchoring/representative statement about the nature of professionalism for each of the articles was identified. Specific implications for assessment from each of the articles were extracted. Articles were sorted into groups according to similar discourses/statements about the nature of professionalism and its assessment. The preliminary classification was shared with working group members who provided feedback through an iterative approach of subsequent drafts refined and recirculated repeatedly over several months.

Implications for assessment were summarized from papers dealing with each level of discourse about professionalism. As well, potential limitations, weaknesses, and implications of thinking about professionalism using each discourse were considered. An anchoring concept of the work was that no one discourse would encompass every dimension of professionalism and that there was benefit in understanding what might be left out or obscured through using only one of the discourses. To paraphrase the words of Kenneth Burke, "Every way of seeing is also a way of not seeing."[3] Draft recommendations were created through an iterative process involving all members of the working group.

The draft recommendations were presented in multiple venues at the International Ottawa Conference in Miami in May 2010, the Association for Medical Education in Europe conference in Glasgow in August 2010, and Association of American Medical Colleges in Washington in November 2010. They were also posted on the website of the International Ottawa Conference for comment. All sources of feedback were used to make final refinements to the recommendations.[1] The data and recommendations presented in this chapter are based on those presented in the final working group publication, modified for clarity and adapted for the purposes of this chapter.

Results: Classification of Professionalism Discourses by Scope and Epistemology

During the analysis, which involved classification of articles and discussions among members of the working group, two overarching dimensions emerged in relation to professionalism: *scope* and *epistemology* (*see* Appendix 1 for definitions). Scope was also understood by the related terms *macro* and *micro*, and sometimes referred to as *level* reflecting that different authors and researchers were interested in different dimensions of professionalism. It was evident that trying to lump work related to individuals and their characteristics together with work examining institutions or societal constructions was a challenge. The group felt that both the terms *micro/macro* and *level* risked conveying a sense of hierarchical value of different approaches, so the term *scope* was employed. Epistemology, a term denoting notions about how knowledge itself comes to exist, was another important dimension in the sources examined. The most important branches are objectivist/positivist approaches, grounded in a belief that there is a fixed phenomenon called professionalism that transcends history and culture, and constructivist approaches grounded in a belief that professionalism is a social creation.

Articles about professionalism were classified according to the different discourses used by authors, underpinning their perspective on what professionalism is, how its nature can be discovered, and whether or not they believe it to be relatively constant across time and cultures or something that is highly changeable. Table 8.1 is an orientation matrix to the way in which the various professionalism discourses were grouped together. The organization follows the two dimensions: scope (individual, interpersonal, societal/institutional) and epistemology (objectivist/positivist or subjective/constructivist). It is important to note that these are not fixed, discrete categories; rather, they should be considered to represent continua. The levels of scope—individual, interpersonal, and societal/institutional—overlap and represent a continuum from the individual to the collective. The epistemological *positions* described in Table 8.1 can be thought of as *dominant* perspectives or *leanings* toward a certain view of how the world works. There were, in some instances, tensions or contradictions between positions and authors of papers (and members of the working group) often moved between perspectives.

TABLE 8.1 Classification of Professionalism Discourses by Scope and Epistemology

Epistemology		Scope		
		Individual	Interpersonal	Societal/Institutional
Positivist-objectivist	Generalizable	Professionalism is an objectively definable phenomenon to be found in individuals, generalizable across cultural contexts	Professionalism is an objectively definable phenomenon to be found in interpersonal interactions, generalizable across cultural contexts	Professionalism is an objectively definable phenomenon to be found in social groups, generalizable across cultural contexts
	Limited generalizability	Professionalism is an objectively definable phenomenon to be found in individuals, but shaped by context	Professionalism is an objectively definable phenomenon to be found in interpersonal interactions, shaped by context	Professionalism is an objectively definable phenomenon to be found in social groups, shaped by context
Subjectivist-constructivist orientation		Professionalism is subjectively constructed within individuals; arises from cultural context	Professionalism is an interpersonally constructed phenomenon; arises from cultural context	Professionalism is a socially constructed phenomenon; arises from cultural context

Having read and classified all of the key articles, and drawing on the collective expertise of the 18 members, the international working group created a set of general principles about the assessment of professionalism as well as three specific sets of recommendations for each "scope"—individual, interpersonal, and societal/institutional. The general principles are as follows:

- Professionalism is a concept that varies across historical time periods and across cultural contexts.
- The need to develop concrete and operational definitions, and from them effective teaching methods and defensible assessment approaches across the continuum of professional development, is strongly felt by many medical educators.
- Professionalism is intrinsically related to the social responsibility of the medical profession. Thus, developing an acceptable, clearly articulated and operational definition that is reviewed and refined regularly to reflect social and health care changes is an important responsibility of the profession and its educational institutions to the public.
- What professionalism is and how it will be taught and assessed should be clearly articulated through a dialogue between the profession and the public. Professionalism can be conceptualized and assessed using different "scopes": individual, interpersonal, and institutional/societal. A comprehensive understanding of professionalism requires attention to these multiple, and often interdependent, scopes.
- A culture that fosters continual improvement of all students and practitioners, and emphasizes personal and collective responsibility for that improvement is desirable. While summative assessment is important, formative methods should predominate including robust feedback supplemented where necessary by remediation.
- Professionalism, and the literature supporting it to date, has arisen predominantly from Anglophone countries. Caution should be used when transferring ideas to other contexts and cultures. Where assessment tools are to be used in new contexts, re-validation with attention to cultural relevance is imperative.
- Different perspectives lead to different statements about the nature of professionalism. They represent different lenses and focus attention on different aspects of education, assessment, and research in this domain. A diversity of approaches and perspectives (psychometrics, psychology, sociology, anthropology, etc.) should be embraced in professionalism assessment and research.
- Each perspective (and resulting assessment methods) will make some elements of professionalism visible, and each will deflect attention from other elements. Elements of professionalism are vast and include individual (attributes, characteristics, attitudes, behaviors and identities), interpersonal (relations, group dynamics, etc.) and social (economic, political, etc.).

Having defined some general recommendations about professionalism the group then turned to defining key issues for assessment for each of the three categories of discourse. These are presented here. In each section, we use examples of articles from the professionalism literature that illustrate the language and concepts associated with each particular discourse. We then review some of the strengths and limitations of viewing professionalism from the vantage point of each discourse, considering self-reflective critiques of insiders who use each discourse as well as critiques from others who hold different perspectives.

Three Discourses about Professionalism and Recommendations for Assessment

1. Professionalism as an Individual Characteristic, Trait, Behavior or Cognitive Process

In this discourse, professionalism is understood to exist or develop to varying degrees as a *characteristic* or *attribute* that is identifiable within individuals. Working within this discourse means focusing on the individual: attending to, and prioritizing, their attributes, whether believed to be inherent (essentialist) or mutable (developmental/learned). Significant attention is given to the measurement of these attributes, usually in the psychometric tradition. The context in which the attributes are expressed is less of a focus, and there is generally an assumption that the attributes are relatively stable and can be captured by tools that yield reliable data that permit valid inferences. The distinction between an essentialist perspective and a developmental perspective is not sharp, with some authors allowing for the presence of both elements. In addition, some attributes are considered to be more stable (traits) than others (states).

Authors working with an essentialist perspective view professionalism as a set of inherent personality traits apparent prior to admission to medical school (and therefore relatively fixed). They argue that diagnostic screening tools are necessary at the time of selection for admission to medical school.[4] They suggest that standardized instruments are needed to assess the personal qualities of medical school applicants that predict problematic performance; an improved system of evaluation to document deficiencies and that provides remediation, is also central.[5] However, one study reported that there were no consistent, significant correlations between any materials from the admissions packet and any of the outcomes of professional behavior by year 3 of medical school, although missing immunizations, missing evaluations, and self-assessment appeared to correlate with professionalism ratings.[6]

Another paper suggested there was a relationship between professionalism as estimated by medical students' peers and an index of "conscientiousness."[7] Principles distilled from such papers are that some component of professionalism may be related to inherent personality characteristics or traits. Assessment of traits (cognitive, personality, behavioral, etc.) prior to admission may be relevant to later professionalism, but this theory remains speculative. Links still need to be shown between preadmissions data, medical school performance, residency performance, and professionalism in practice. Cautions raised by authors working within this paradigm about this approach are that research has not yet identified specific characteristics or traits that robustly predict future behaviors from the premedical period. However, more evidence is available about the link between medical school performance and behavior in practice. Concerns associated with falsely identifying positive/negative characteristics are raised in relation to high stakes measurement, as well as hesitations about "homogenization" given the desire for a diverse student population that will serve different roles and purposes in practice.

Also using the individual discourse, but taking a somewhat more developmental/educational approach, is a variation on this discourse that conceptualizes professionalism as learned behaviors that develop *during* medical education. Some studies focused on the use of the "professionalism mini-evaluation exercise"—a four-factor, 24-item instrument with sufficient validity/reliability, with approximately eight raters.[8] Another measure of observable behavior reviewed was the Amsterdam Attitude and Communication Scale.[9] A third set of papers focused on deans' letters and their content about professional behavior.[10] Together, these papers argued for the need to clarify elements of professionalism and to develop better tools to assess behaviors (via psychometrics) by peers and teachers and during critical incidents.

Writing from this measurement perspective, one author suggested improving assessment by anchoring the assessed behaviors in real-world value conflicts.[11] Another underlined the need to create systems to foster peer feedback by emphasizing anonymity, immediacy, ubiquity, documentation, formative approaches (punishment/correction, "hold students responsible") for unprofessional behaviors, and to "reward" professional behaviors.[12] A challenge to these approaches is that measures of observed behaviors, self-reports, and single attributes are not considered adequate to assess professionalism by some authors who argue for the need to develop measures of values and attitudes and understand their relationship to behavior change.[13] It was argued that there are many existing assessment scales and ratings (one research group reported finding 88 of them) and that existing measures should be improved psychometrically, rather than continually creating new ones, and that assessment should involve multiple raters, more than one assessment method, and assessment in different settings using multisource feedback and patient questionnaires.[14]

Some authors taking an individualist approach focus on the postgraduate level. For example, it was shown that residency professionalism ratings and written examinations (American Board of Internal Medicine certification examinations) can predict some future problem behaviors.[15] At this level some have argued that most tools are designed to evaluate specific elements of professionalism but that few assess a comprehensive construct. One paper recommended that a one-shot assessment, even if gathered from multiple raters, should not be the sole measure of professional behaviors:

> A pragmatic approach is needed whereby multiple snapshots of an individual's professionalism can be taken and collated into a whole to develop a clear picture of that person's strengths and weaknesses and to provide a body of evidence on which to base summative decisions.[16]

Therefore, a complex, multi-tool blueprint is required. One study found that formal evaluation sessions (verbal discussions) actually contained more references to unprofessional behaviors than checklists or rating forms.[17] A final piece in relation to professionalism as an individual characteristic is that both student well-being and professional behaviors should be monitored continuously and rigorously, with a system of data collection, analysis, interpretation, and intervention. It seems to us that it is important to be clear whether the system is supportive or regulatory or whether it combines both elements.

Overarching principles distilled from the papers using an individualist discourse include the notion that professionalism may be understood as the observable, behavioral manifestations of the interaction of a complex set of cognitive, attitudinal, personality, and conative characteristics. This approach makes clear that the assessment of behaviors is a proxy measure, resting on the assumption that these behaviors are fully (or at least significantly) reflective of the underlying dimensions of professionalism. Thus, in order to be fair and defensible, the assessment of behaviors should be done using instruments that have demonstrable reliability and validity. Documenting behaviors alone, however, may be insufficient to capture a comprehensive construct of professionalism that also includes knowledge, attitudes, and the ability to employ professional behaviors in real practice settings. We have noted that in focusing on behaviors it is frequently forgotten that one can test a student's cognitive knowledge of professionalism. Professionalism has a knowledge base and including it in the subject matter to be tested will drive learning as it does in other areas. This understanding is rarely reflected in the literature on assessing professionalism, which concentrates on behaviors. Overall, the best assessments are part of a program that includes setting a safe climate, feedback, anonymity when appropriate, and follow-up of behavior change as documented by several measurements over multiple time periods. Finally, it appears that identification and documentation of *negative* behaviors may be distinct and, in the minds of some, less important than systems that recognize and document *positive* professionalism behaviors.

It is often cautioned that observable behaviors may have more to do with the exigencies of particular contexts than of deeply held values and attitudes. In other words, behaviors may be highly unstable across different contexts. There are aspects of professionalism that may be obscured by focusing on the individual. Students and teachers often struggle to define what professionalism means to them and note that what they consider "professional" in one setting may not be in another. By downplaying the importance of context, perfectly reasonable students can sometimes be demonized as "unprofessional" rather than just having "lapsed" because of time pressures, hierarchical pressures, and so forth. Further, if tools are created for specific contexts (institutions, specialties, cultures, countries), students and teachers may not value definitions or constructs of professionalism that feel "imported." For example, those writing about professionalism in Asian countries have noted a "buy-in" problem when definitions of professionalism and assessment tools are simply translated from North American versions. There are also generational issues that relate to the interpretation of behaviors, vis-à-vis such concepts as *altruism* and *lifestyle*. Trying to teach what Hafferty and Levinson[18] call *nostalgic professionalism* may result in simple rejection by the current generation.

The following recommendations were elaborated for assessment of professionalism as an individual phenomenon.

- Some component of professionalism may be related to inherent personality characteristics or traits. Assessment of traits (cognitive, personality, behavioral) prior to admissions may be relevant to later professionalism; however, use of such screening approaches requires that links between preadmissions data, medical school performance, residency performance, and professionalism in practice be demonstrated.
- Professionalism may be understood as the external, behavioral manifestations of the interaction of a complex set of cognitive and attitudinal elements and

personality characteristics with the environment. However, behavioral assessments are proxy measures, resting on the assumption that observed behaviors are reflective of underlying dimensions. Research shows that this assumption is not always accurate. For this reason, documenting behaviors alone may be insufficient to capture a comprehensive construct of professionalism, which should also include knowledge, values, attitudes, and the ability to employ professional behaviors in real practice settings.

- Where behavioral assessments are used, instruments should be employed that have demonstrable reliability and can be used to support valid inferences. Both quantitative measures (e.g., numeric scores derived from observation-based survey instruments) and qualitative measures (e.g., narrative data from deans' letters) have been studied and may be employed in a defensible manner. A combination of methods over a period of time is likely to be needed.

- Given the number of existing professionalism assessment tools, it may be more important to increase the depth and quality of the reliability and validity of a program's existing measures in various contexts than to continue developing new measures for single contexts.

- Triangulation of multiple kinds of measures, by multiple observers, synthesized over time with data gathered in multiple, complex, and challenging contexts is likely to be appropriate at all levels of analysis.

- Identification and documentation of *negative* behaviors is likely to require a distinct system from one in which there is recognition, documentation, and reinforcement of *positive* professionalism behaviors. Instrument design and validity research should be undertaken thoughtfully in such a way as to reflect this distinction.

- The overall assessment program is more important than the individual tools. The best programs use a variety of tools in a safe climate and provide rich feedback, anonymity (when appropriate), and follow-up of behavior change over time. Effective assessment and feedback programs also incorporate faculty development.

2. Professionalism as an Interpersonal Process or Effect

In this discourse, professionalism is understood to be something constructed (or suppressed) through interpersonal interaction. Working in this discourse means giving attention to interpersonal relationships, particularly that of student and teacher. While individual attributes are still a focus, these are understood to be cocreated between a student and another person (teacher, patient, etc.) and therefore more fluid. Context is given significant attention, as is the notion that the expression of professionalism is contextually determined. The detection and assessment of professional behaviors cannot take place without an analysis of the context in which they are expressed. Writers working with this discourse often express greater interest in formative assessment for teaching and learning, and somewhat less focus on summative assessment, but this need not be the case. The context, student-teacher, student-student, and student-health professional relationships and the learning climate itself may be targets for assessment as much, or more so, than individuals.

What this discourse makes visible/possible is the identification, documentation, and analysis of the impact of relationships on student and teacher perceptions of professionalism, and attention to context. On the other hand, this discourse can obscure macro-social forces acting on the teacher-student dyad and the institution in which learning occurs. It also gives less attention to personality attributes/traits and may not be as helpful in finding ways to address the rare but problematic individuals. Overly focusing on contextual dimensions might also diminish a sense of personal responsibility among students.

There are many variations on the interpersonal approach to professionalism. For example, studies have examined the idea that professionalism is a set of sociocognitive processes that an individual uses to interpret problems in the world and to select responses in relation to others. For example, Ginsburg and colleagues[19] set out to explore features of problem solving in the face of professional dilemmas that might shed light on the reasoning and rationales behind observed behaviors. They argued that, as no fixed list of traits could be defined, nor could raters be standardized, assessment should involve exposing students to dilemmas and having them produce a resolution, observing and scoring the process they use, the values and principles invoked, and the decisions made. They introduced the concept of "professionalism lapse" as more useful than the label "unprofessional."[19] Ginsburg et al.[20] wrote:

> Future efforts at evaluation need to look beyond the behaviors, and should incorporate the reasoning and motivations behind students' actions in challenging professional situations . . . sophisticated evaluation of professionalism requires an additional dimension, as behaviors alone do not give us all of the information we need to make accurate judgments.

Others have argued that there are definable stages that individuals pass through on the way from "proto" (rudimentary) professionalism to full professionalism in relation to learning environments. Evaluation involves the documentation of attainment (or attrition) of these characteristics.[21] To do this, reliable and valid ways to characterize the learning environment are needed. According to these authors, institutions should measure and maintain high professional standards of the learning environment. Initiatives to improve professionalism should be evaluated in terms of their impact on the environment.[22]

Taken together, principles distilled from these papers are that there are common features of unprofessional behavior/professionalism lapses that arise from particular kinds of social interactions and that these are generalizable across contexts. Assessment should include exploration of students' cognitive problem solving processes, monitoring learning environments as well as teacher-student relationships for interpersonal characteristics that could lead to unprofessional behaviors/professionalism lapses. Cautions voiced by authors working within this discourse include the idea that broadening the perspective to include teachers and the environment can be threatening to teachers. What using this discourse may obscure is that the nature of these interpersonal effects may be specific to cultures (by country, ethnicity, tradition, or even institutional).

Within the interpersonal scope, but taking a constructivist approach, is the notion that professionalism is a way of being that is entirely created in interpersonal interactions. According to this perspective, behavior results from the generation and negotiation of meaning through interaction with others. This view draws on social psychology, symbolic interactionism, and developmental psychology. For example, it is argued that professionalism is subtle and complex and does not reduce to numerical scales—that most assessment overemphasizes factors related to the person and underemphasizes factors related to the context. Some recommend exploring assessment that does not rely on scales at all.[23] As one author put it, the implication is that measurement of the student alone is only half of the equation.[24] The key point is that relying on behavioral assessment may lead to passing students with "professional behaviors" but unethical attitudes and failing students with "unprofessional behaviors" but ethical attitudes. Thus, assessment must include context-dependent nature of behaviors. Observation alone is not enough. Conversations about behavior, and behavioral explanations, are key. Thus it is necessary to collect data using multiple methods including observations and interviews, and focus on text and narrative.[25] A central idea here is that assessors have a role in constructing students' unprofessional behaviors.[26] The environment should therefore be monitored for conditions that lead to negative phenomena, such as the emotional detachment of students.[24]

A key principle distilled from these papers is that professionalism is a set of behaviors and responses to situational and contextual phenomena that arise much less from individual cognitive or personality dimensions and much more from context during learning and practice. The assessment of professionalism therefore involves assessing the thoughts, decisions, responses, and behaviors of all actors in each context, perhaps most importantly both teacher and student. Assessment of the learning/practice environment itself is also important. Inherent in this approach to assessment is feedback to improve the performance of individuals (teachers, other health professionals) and of the context/learning environment itself. The concept of "unprofessionalism" (a characteristic or trait) is less useful than "professionalism lapses" (situation).

There are cautions raised by authors working within this discourse especially over the fact that assessing characteristics and behaviors of students alone, without an assessment of other members of the system and of the context itself risks missing important forces that shape and determine behavior. It is important to make the connection between a necessarily reductionist set of observable behaviors and something more profound, and necessarily subjective. What may be obscured by a focus on this discourse of professionalism is how difficult it is to conceive of any program of evaluation of students' knowledge of professionalism and of professional behaviors that does not start with something fairly concrete. From this perspective, the need to define universal features of professionalism (e.g., *primum non nocere* or "patient interest above personal interest") may be strongly felt.

The following recommendations were elaborated for assessment of professionalism as an interpersonal phenomenon.

- In addition to its individual elements, professionalism also implies a set of behaviors and responses to situational and contextual phenomena that arise during learning and practice. The assessment of professionalism should therefore include assessment of the decisions, responses, and behaviors of all actors in each context (perhaps using multisource feedback), gathering longitudinal data from both teacher and student as well as from other key players such as health care professionals, administrators, patients, and so forth.
- Assessment of the learning/practice environment itself is also important. Inherent in this approach to assessment is feedback to improve the performance of teams (course faculty, clinical teaching teams, etc.) as well as to improve structural elements, be they organizational (e.g., policies that govern learning/work) or structural (in an architectural sense).
- Assessment of professionalism should include monitoring learning environments, student-student, teacher-student, student-health professional and student-patient relationships for problematic interpersonal phenomena. The

concept of situationally specific *professionalism challenges*, *dilemmas*, or *lapses* may be more useful than a global concept of *unprofessionalism* (characteristic or trait).

● While consensus on what are appropriate professional responses to complex problems and situations may not always be achieved, assessment and feedback should represent a collective perspective where possible.

3. Professionalism as a Societal/Institutional Phenomenon: A Socially Constructed Way of Acting or Being, Associated with Power

A key notion in this discourse is that professionalism emerges and is modified through the interaction of professional groups with society. Professionalism is something that serves a social purpose of some higher order. That is, professionalism has a function—be it in relation to the status of the profession, the organization of the health care system, or the cultural, social, or moral structure of institutions and societies of which medicine is a part. In this sense, professionalism is defined with and by society. Individual attributes and interpersonal processes are inseparable from consideration of these larger forces, but the emphasis is at the macro level.

There were two variations of this discourse in the papers reviewed. The first is an objective/positivist historical or utilitarian orientation. The second is a social constructivist view. The first perspective starts from the assumption that an objective professionalism exists and is relatively independent of context, generalizable, and therefore shaped by, but not wholly created by, social forces. Assessment means tying together attributes and behaviors of individuals, but also of teams and professional groups, to outcomes at organizational, systems, or social levels. Assessment is more likely to take the form of macro/social or institutional outcomes (patient outcomes) or processes (accreditation). What this discourse makes visible/possible is identification, documentation, and analysis of socio-organizational elements and functions of professionalism for evaluation of efficiency, productivity, relevance, or quality of medical professional practice and organization, and patient safety. What this discourse can obscure is the dynamics of power that construct particular definitions of what professionalism is in different times and places.

For example, it is argued that professionalism is an aspect of identity, status, and autonomy of the medical profession, drawing on systems theory and the study of professions. An implication is that medical schools, medical educators, and the profession in general must emphasize setting expectations, teaching, and assessing professionalism at a high level across the profession as a whole.[27] A related notion is that professionalism is a collective responsibility of the medical profession that arises from its social contract with society, with the implication that measurement should include the key elements outlined in the model. Both macro-dimensions (the contributions of each partner to the social contract— medical profession, but also government, society, etc.) and micro-dimensions (individual level comportment of physicians) need to be assessed. Cruess and Cruess,[28] for example, separate out the contextual/country-specific elements of the professional "social contract" and what they consider to be more universal dimensions of individual behavior associated with "the healer."

The related idea is that professionalism is a set of attitudes and behaviors linked to systems requirements of cost control, access to care, efficiency and quality (production imperative) of health care, notions that draw on politics, economics, and business management literatures. The implication is that attitudes and beliefs expressed should be measured against actual behaviors, recognizing the often large gap.[25] An example given is a conflict of interest scenario in which a doctor who owns a private clinic faces professional dilemmas about continuity of care that may challenge espoused beliefs because of a particular health care context.[29] An interesting argument in this literature is that attention to and assessment of professional values is necessary to ensure medicine does not become a "trade."[30] Assessment of professionalism would thus focus more on what individuals do in relation to the system in which they work rather than an individual's autonomy or self-determination.

Others taking this macro-societal perspective have argued that professionalism is a collective core set of values and approaches tied to morality and anchored in specific philosophical/ethical/religious traditions. The implications include a need to move beyond assessments targeted only at cognitive or behavioral competencies. There is a need for thick description to allow the interpretation of meaningful events from participants' perspectives, because, as several authors have written, social reaction and conduct are inseparable.[25,31] Finally, adding a contextual element are papers that suggest that professionalism is a set of definable and measurable behaviors that vary across cultures. For example, psychometric evaluation with the professionalism mini-evaluation exercise was reliable and acceptable in the Japanese context, but, nevertheless, new items were needed and the results obtained in Japan were different to those obtained in a Canadian setting.[32] Similarly, Taiwanese researchers proposed an approach to construct a professionalism framework that accounts for historical and socio-cultural context. The framework they built shared similarities with Western counterparts but differs in the centrality of self-integrity, harmonizing social roles, reflecting Confucian values.[33]

To summarize this first perspective, principles distilled from papers using this macro-societal discourse are that professionalism is an aspect of, and must be understood in the context of, the goals, aspirations, and exigencies placed upon the profession as a whole. Assessment involves characterizing those expectations and measuring the degree to which the profession (be it a subgroup such as students, a whole medical school, a professional practice group, or even the profession as a whole) meets those expectations. Assessment and research on assessment therefore may involve critiquing the dominance of certain ways in which those expectations are framed or enforced. Authors working with this discourse grapple to some extent with the profession as a whole and institutions as "actors" unto themselves. They start from the premise that what happens at the macro-level sets the stage for (and constrains) the ways in which individuals calibrate their own professional actions. Cautions raised by authors working within this paradigm are that the nature of the professionalism in the future will be strongly influenced by societal decisions relating to national health care systems and changes in self-regulation. What may be obscured by this discourse is that research has not yet established that the concept known as "professionalism" in the Anglo-Saxon countries/English literature exists or is fully understandable in other cultures and linguistic groups.

Also working at the macro-societal/institutional level, but taking more of a social constructivist/critical perspective, some authors start with the premise that there is no one fixed entity called professionalism in all places and historical periods. Rather it is a phenomenon created through discourse and power in certain places and times. For writers working from this perspective, the lack of cross-cultural validation of the concept raises concerns that perhaps professionalism as defined in the English literature might have a different nature, or possibly not even be understandable in a different language or culture. Working in this discourse means rejecting the notion that there are any fixed attributes or behaviors called professionalism that can be defined in the same way in all times and places. Rather, professionalism is something that has arisen in some places, cultures, or time periods together with specific social forces, discourses, or values. More focus is given to the processes that create different conceptions of professionalism (or make it possible to exist at all) than the actual attributes or behaviors of individuals or groups. Assessment, often qualitative, focuses on the meanings and attributions that individuals and groups give to their context and the ways in which their identity and certain behaviors are considered "professional" (or unprofessional) and how this determination is shaped by social forces, dynamics, and power (culture, gender, socioeconomic status, etc.). What this discourse makes visible or possible is the identification, documentation, and analysis of dynamics of power that lead to particular constructions of professionalism. It also highlights both the productive and repressive effects of power, hierarchy, and social organization and institutions. What this discourse can obscure is the sense of urgency felt by educators to classify positive/pro-social characteristics as well as problematic behaviors for the purposes of admission to medical school or pass, fail, and remediation decisions during medical training.

The key argument in such work is that professionalism is a social construction. This approach draws on sociology, political economy, historiography, and anthropology. Assessment of individual characteristics or behaviors is therefore seen as inadequate.[18] As a complex, adaptive system, assessment of professionalism should entail means of analyzing motivations and behaviors in context, at individual (the medical student/teacher), institutional (the medical school), and social (the medical profession) levels.[34] Authors working with this approach argue that professionalism is too complex and nuanced to be captured by checklists of individual characteristics or behaviors alone. Social-contextual factors shape the expression of behaviors, which may or may not reflect attitudes and values of individuals, or even small groups (e.g., teacher-student).[25] They argue that strategies for screening for character traits during admissions processes are not robustly predictive and may not even be desirable, given the need for diversity. As a "distributed" phenomenon, professionalism should be assessed in terms of the function of groups, settings, and institutions more than individuals.[35]

Principles distilled from this social-constructivist orientation include that assessment is a risky business because it is an act of power with the possibility to discriminate. Constructions of the definitions of what professionalism is are themselves subject to power relations, including the projects and agendas of social groups and institutions and may disguise problematic constructions. Assessment in this perspective is about gathering data to demonstrate equity and fairness in processes that discriminate between individuals and the accountability of professional groups and institutions as a whole. Cautions raised by authors working within this approach are that those accustomed to the objectivist/positivist orientation may find a social-constructivist perspective disorienting, and worry that constructivism means that all things are relative or of equal value. Those accustomed to a social-constructivist approach may find an objectivist-positivist orientation difficult, and worry that effects of power are hidden behind apparent objectivity. What may be obscured by this approach is that the "earnest search" for a measurable and teachable phenomenon articulated by frontline teachers and evaluators, seems difficult or impossible.

The following recommendations were developed for assessment of professionalism as institutional/societal phenomenon.

- Professionalism can be understood in the context of the goals, aspirations, and collective behaviors of health care and educational institutions and of the profession itself. Assessment involves characterizing social expectations, through dialogue and meaningful input from public stakeholders, and measuring the degree to which the profession (be it a subgroup such as students, a whole medical school, a professional practice group, or even the profession as a whole) meets these expectations. Accreditation requirements at every educational level require teaching and evaluating professionalism. Effectiveness should be measured in terms of clear institutional and social outcomes.

- Assessment may involve critiquing the dominance of certain ways that expectations and practices are framed or enforced (cultural, generational, gendered, hierarchical, etc.) and should lead to improved institutional and organizational climate and practice.

- Professional lapses may arise from particular kinds of social interactions and problematic organizational and institutional settings and politics. Examining and making explicit the *hidden curriculum* and tacit problematic organizational or institutional norms is important in assessing and contextualizing professional or unprofessional behaviors of students, teachers, and institutions.

Implications for Research on Professionalism Assessment

During the process of submitting and analyzing papers for the discourse analysis, it was widely recognized that further research in this area is warranted, especially in the two less well-developed perspectives (interpersonal process or effect and societal/institutional phenomenon). Further, during the public discussion sessions that were held at the Ottawa Conference (Miami, 2010) many audience participants made suggestions for future research. These areas will be briefly discussed here. As the purpose of the exercise was to focus on assessment of professionalism, we have limited this list to those relevant areas. We have also provided some elaborations and suggestions regarding the sort of research studies that may be effective for each.

Examine the concept of professionalism and its assessment across different linguistic and cultural contexts.

This exploration might be done by first researching the views of different stakeholder groups, as Ho et al.[33] did in Taiwan. Other groups have attempted to translate tools for use in different cultures (see Tsugawa et al.;[32] Ho et al.[36] in Taiwan are similarly studying the use of scenarios developed in Canada to explore perceptions of Taiwanese medical students). This sort of study is promising in that it may provide cross-cultural, comparative data to help us understand how professionalism is conceptualized between different groups.

Compare the definitions and conceptualizations of professionalism assessment in medicine to those held by other health care professions.

Interesting studies in nursing have suggested that nurses (and others) may view and evaluate professionalism differently than attending physicians.[37-39] These sorts of studies, done in the appropriate context and setting, can shed light on how others, including patients, view doctors' professionalism, and can be extremely useful for formative feedback to learners.

Characterize which elements of professional behavior are amenable to learning (and therefore remediation) and which may be more immutable and thus amenable to selection processes.

This suggestion was controversial because some participants were concerned that such tools might be ultimately used for "screening" for entry to medical school. Older research had suggested that this was not a profitable or even desirable approach. However, it may be productive to study the remediation of professionalism to guide educators on what sorts of professionalism issues are possible to remediate, what are the difficult versus the easier issues, and so forth. The literature in this area is sparse—even case studies or case series would be of great practical relevance.

Examine links between the assessment of professionalism and other assessment initiatives such as quality of patient care.

Research in this area could attempt to link measures of professionalism to indicators of quality or patient safety. It would be useful to determine, for example, which elements of professionalism may be responsible for better (or perhaps worse) outcomes for patients. These elements could then form a part of faculty development or remediation programs, if necessary.

Develop and evaluate means of incorporating patients' perspectives into the assessment of professionalism.

Patients' perspectives about the professionalism of their caregivers are not often sought. Research on patient satisfaction teaches that patients may be reluctant to evaluate health care professionals while they are still receiving care. Further, patients in hospital often cannot recall (or even name) their doctors after discharge. However, as in point 2, given earlier, patients may have critically different perspectives of their physicians, which could be very useful for formative feedback.[40] Interestingly, not only were patients in one study found to have different views than physicians when it comes to professionalism in general but also the authors found that some of the terminology physicians use in relation to professionalism did not resonate with patients and in some cases had negative connotations.[41] This finding stresses the need for further research in this area.

Explore professionalism assessment in complex clinical workplaces, including how individuals adapt to difficult or even dysfunctional systems and the gaps that arise between espoused values and actual practice.

Research in this area might begin by studying these complex systems in depth, determining who the actors are and how they interrelate, and also exploring the environment to determine its impact. Surveys have uncovered gaps between values and practice, but unfortunately could not explore why these gaps occur.[29,42] To address this issue, studies are ongoing at the American Board of Internal Medicine to explore in more depth why physicians might not always uphold the professional standards they agree are important.

Elaborate ways in which assessment data can be used to change the culture of education and practice, in particular the hidden curriculum.

The hidden curriculum, along with some of its more negative consequences, persists despite much research and writing in this area for many years. It seems that certain elements of the hidden curriculum may require further exploration to understand why they are replicated year after year. For example, one group is looking at how transitions in training (which may occur every 4 weeks) might cause dysfunctional adaptations—once this problem is recognized strategies can be developed to counteract its effects.[43,44] In other studies, researchers have developed instruments to measure the environment in which learning takes place. For example, the Postgraduate Hospital Educational Environment Measure has been used in several different settings (and, interestingly, required minor modifications between contexts).[45] It was able to be used to compare the environment across sites and identify areas for improvement. The present authors' own group (SG) is studying the clinical teaching units in depth, from multiple stakeholder viewpoints, to determine the environmental factors most affecting performance and evaluation. This research will be used to develop an instrument to measure and track change in relation to new initiatives (e.g., a change in call schedules, addition of new health care team members).

Consider what happens when expectations at an individual level conflict with those at the social/organizational/institutional level, and what the resolution means for professionalism assessment.

In some instances, it may be the case that behaviors that seem appropriate when viewed through one lens may seem inappropriate when viewed through another. As we discuss in the section on "sticking points" later in this chapter, further attention is needed to the issue of what happens when institutional or social demands conflict with those that physicians (or students) feel define their professional commitment.

Explore innovative ways to collect and analyze quantitative and qualitative assessment data from mixed-methods approaches, paying particular attention to threats to validity inherent in different assessment methods.

There are many methods available for studying the assessment of professionalism, and the choice of "best" method will depend on the purpose for which the study is being done. Studies trying to better understand different conceptualizations of professionalism, or that attempt to explore in depth how individuals might approach dilemmas, might be designed as qualitative studies with smaller numbers of participants. Studies attempting to determine opinions of broader groups might use surveys. Exploration of environmental impacts might require the opinions of many different stakeholder groups, or in-depth observations in practice. Studies should be designed to capitalize on the strengths of any number of these (or other) approaches. Further, more credible, generalizable conclusions might be drawn from studies (or programs of research) that are able to combine the best of each.

Conduct outcome studies to examine the impact of curriculum (formal, informal, and hidden) and other organizational interventions related to professionalism.

Studies looking at patient outcomes are scarce, and more research is certainly needed in this area. For example, which curricula or assessment methods are linked to better patient outcomes? It would also be important to look at institution-level outcomes, such as patient satisfaction scores, accreditation data, and so forth, to see which curricular or other elements are most effective in effecting change.

Sticking Points: Reflections on Controversies and Challenges for the Consensus Group

During the International Ottawa Conference in Miami in 2010 many of the participants on the consensus group came together and met in person, some for the first time. It was a great opportunity to discuss views and opinions, and to challenge each other's positions. In addition, there were two "open" forums where the consensus group presented the draft consensus document and solicited feedback from conference participants. These too led to stimulating discussion and debate regarding some of the recommendations. Subsequently, as lead authors (BH and SG) we have had opportunities to present the Consensus Recommendations to various audiences (e.g., at grand rounds, research presentations, working groups). We have often been asked, "What were the areas of disagreement?" or "Which areas were controversial?" This section provides a brief overview of our reflections on these questions.

One particular dimension that was troubling to some related to the issue of the medical profession's relation to society. Some members of the group felt strongly that the profession exists, and is able to function, only through its contract with society. The implication is that society should define what professionalism embodies. It was further noted that physicians alone do not always know what professionalism is or should be, and may not emphasize the same elements of professionalism as patients and other members of society. Further, argued some members of the group, when the profession is not seen to be accountable to society, certain privileges may be revoked, such as the capacity for self-regulation. On the other hand, we also heard from participants from non-Western countries representing non-Euroamerican cultures, that some individuals had significant concerns about entrusting such an important domain to others outside the profession. Examples were brought up of repressive political regimes that sometimes have governed what physicians are able or required to do. Some told stories about how physicians at various points in history have been required to comply with directives that go against their core beliefs or their role as healer. Some of these participants felt that physicians should be the ones to set the standards for the profession and that there is value in holding to these when societies or governments attempt to dictate things that run counter to professional values.

Related to this observation was the widely accepted recognition that professionalism may vary across cultures (see General Principle #1 listed earlier in this chapter), and that while we accept this statement as a general concept, we do not in fact know very much about the nature of these differences. Questions were raised about whether or not certain elements of professionalism should be considered universal or if all elements are potentially subject to local cultures and contexts. One often-cited example was that of respect for women and women's rights, something that is quite variable depending on society and culture. The question remained open as to whether or not the profession could or should set a standard, or at least attempt to develop common language, about professional behavior in relation to this and other sensitive cultural issues. Addressing this question was thought to be especially relevant for learners who train in cultures that are not their own and who return to practice in cultures different from those in which they undertook their studies.

Another related area of controversy was the issue of who gets to define a "lapse" in professionalism. One participant raised the example of a physician who speaks out against authority (e.g., their organization) and is, as a result, labeled as having displayed a lapse in professionalism. Acting against norms might reasonably be thought to be unprofessional by most people if, for example, a physician disclosed sensitive information or behaved in a hostile or violent manner. But what if a physician were questioning policies that could result in unfairly disadvantaging certain patient groups or that would interfere with the delivery of quality care? Concerns were raised that if organizations or authorities have too much power to define professionalism "lapses" that it might inhibit legitimate (and necessary) challenges to harmful policies and practices. Thus some participants felt it was important that health care workers themselves (including physicians or trainees) and patients have a role in evaluating questionable physician behaviors and cautioned about too much power of assessment residing with institutions.

There was much debate around the issue of how much of what we think of as professionalism or professional behavior is innate, and perhaps fixed, versus what might be malleable or remediable characteristics. If we knew more about these areas, some argued, we may be in a better position regarding selection for medical school. We learned that the older literature on admissions tended to discount strategies like personality testing at admissions, as research did not show an advantage to this approach and in fact may unfairly exclude reasonable candidates. It was clear that there has never been a particular test developed that can predict, for example, who might not be suitable as a physician, or who might have difficulties getting through medical training. However, some participants noted that newer models of understanding personality now exist, along with different sorts of personality tests, and that perhaps we should not yet close the book on this issue. Some suggested that further studies should be done taking these new models and theories into account. On the other hand, others were concerned about this approach in general, arguing that we do not know (and are unlikely to know in the foreseeable future) how much a person's attitudes and behaviors are subject to change, especially given the age at which most students begin medical training (early twenties), a time of important developmental change.

Finally, there were very interesting discussions regarding how professionalism has focused too much on behaviors and in so doing has gotten too far away from thinking of medicine as a moral profession. We no longer talk about *virtues*, *character*, or *calling*, which was concerning to some. For example, in one public session there was a spirited discussion about the notion of *courage*, which some felt was central to professionalism.

Clearly, the notion of *consensus* around professionalism was difficult to grapple with, as there were so many legitimate and nuanced points of view. We hope this short reflection around some of these controversial areas will continue to spark debate, new research, and greater understanding.

Conclusions

A common approach to developing consensus recommendations is to review a wide range of literature, consult with experts and work toward a shared set of guidelines or "best practices." In tackling the domain of professionalism, it was obvious from the outset that no unified consensus would be possible, or desirable, given the diversity of ways in which the phenomenon is understood. Rather than trying to force the paradigmatic richness that characterizes professionalism research into an overly simplistic list of recommendations, the International Working Group on the Assessment of Professionalism chose a discourse analysis approach. This allowed us to unearth, categorize, and represent three key discourses about professionalism—as an individual, interpersonal, or social-institutional phenomenon—discourses that are all in active use today. The strength of this approach is that we were able to create recommendations specific to each of the three identified discourses. The obvious corollary is that no unified "statements of truth" about what professionalism is or how it should be assessed are made.

The working group found the use of discourse analysis challenging but ultimately gratifying because the strength of this method is to retain and value diverse perspectives and at the same time emphasize that all approaches both illuminate and obscure what is "true" about professionalism. For those interested in the complex and important topic of professionalism, we hope that we have provided new insight as well as some helpful directions for both assessment and for future research.

Acknowledgments

The authors are very grateful to all members of the IOC-PWG for their contributions to the original paper on which this chapter is based, as well as their support for this chapter. The authors also extend their sincere thanks to Elisa Hollenberg for assistance in preparation of the manuscript.

Appendix 1: Glossary of Key Terms[1,46]

constructivism   A belief about knowledge (epistemology) that asserts that the reality we perceive is constructed by our social, historical, and individual contexts and so there can be no absolute shared truth.

discourse   A set of statements/logical system of thought that attempts to articulate the essence of what professionalism is as employed in a given article or body of work.

discourse analysis   A methodology that analyses language to enable an understanding of the role language has in construction of the social world. Critical discourse analysis focuses on the macro-level features of oral and written texts in their social contexts (as opposed to "linguistic discourse analysis," which includes the micro-level analysis of grammatical features).

epistemology   An underlying conception of how knowledge comes to exist; a theoretical approach to knowledge.

methodology   A method of data collection/analysis linked to an epistemological perspective.

objectivism   A belief about knowledge (epistemology) that asserts that there is an absolute truth or reality that can be discovered and that knowledge is objective and neutral.

positivism   A theoretical framework that is guided by the search for the objective truth that will contribute to the progress of humankind.

scope   Used here to denote the perspective or lens through which the phenomenon is being explored.

References

1. Hodges BD, Ginsburg S, Cruess R, et al. Assessment for professionalism: recommendations from the Ottawa 2010 conference. *Med Teach.* 2011; **33**(5): 354–63.
2. Hodges B, Kuper A, Reeves S. Qualitative research: discourse analysis. *BMJ.* 2008; **337**(879): 570–2.
3. Burke K. *Permanence and Change.* New York, NY: New Republic; 1935.
4. Knights JA, Kennedy BJ. Medical school selection: screening for dysfunctional tendencies. *Med Educ.* 2006; **40**(11): 1058–64.
5. Papadakis M, Teherani A, Banach M, et al. Disciplinary action by medical boards and prior behavior in medical school. *N Engl J Med.* 2005; **353**(25): 2673–82.
6. Stern DT, Frohna AZ, Gruppen LD. The prediction of professional behavior. *Med Educ.* 2005; **39**(1): 75–82.
7. Finn G, Sawdon M, Clipsham L, et al. Peer estimation of lack of professionalism correlates with low Conscientiousness Index scores. *Med Educ.* 2009; **43**(10): 960–7.
8. Cruess R, McIlroy J, Cruess S, et al. The professionalism mini-evaluation exercise: a preliminary investigation. *Acad Med.* 2006; **81**(Suppl. 10): S74–8.
9. Ten Cate TJ, de Haes J. Summative assessment of medical students in the affective domain. *Med Teach.* 2000; **22**: 40–3.
10. Shea JA, O'Grady E, Wagner BR, et al. Professionalism in clerkships: an analysis of MSPE Commentary. *Acad Med.* 2008; **83**(Suppl. 10): S1–4.
11. Arnold L. Assessing professional behavior: yesterday, today, and tomorrow. *Acad Med.* 2002; **77**(6): 502–15.
12. Arnold L, Shue CK, Kalishman S, et al. Can there be a single system for peer assessment of professionalism among medical students? A multi-institutional study. *Acad Med.* 2007; **82**(6): 578–86.
13. Jha V, Bekker HL, Duffy SR, et al. Perceptions of professionalism in medicine: a qualitative study. *Med Educ.* 2006; **40**(10): 1027–36.
14. Lynch D, Surdyk P, Eiser A. Assessing professionalism: a review of the literature. *Med Teach.* 2004; **26**(4): 366–73.
15. Papadakis MA, Arnold GK, Blank LL, et al. Performance during internal medicine residency training and subsequent disciplinary action by state licensing boards. *Ann Intern Med.* 2008; **148**(11): 869–76.
16. Wilkinson TJ, Wade WB, Knock LD. A blueprint to assess professionalism: results of a systematic review. *Acad Med.* 2009; **84**(5): 551–8.
17. Hemmer PA, Hawkins R, Jackson JL, et al. Assessing how well three evaluation methods detect deficiencies in medical students' professionalism in two settings of an internal medicine clerkship. *Acad Med.* 2000; **75**(2): 167–73.
18. Hafferty FW, Levinson D. Moving beyond nostalgia and motives: towards a

complexity science view of medical professionalism. *Perspect Biol Med*. 2008; **51**(4): 599–615.

19. Ginsburg S, Regehr G, Hatala R, et al. Context, conflict, and resolution: a new conceptual framework for evaluating professionalism. *Acad Med*. 2000; **75**(Suppl. 10): S6–11.

20. Ginsburg S, Regehr G, Lingard L. Basing evaluation of professionalism on observable behaviours: a cautionary tale. *Acad Med*. 2004; **79**(Suppl. 10): S1–4.

21. Hilton SR, Slotnick HB. Proto-professionalism: how professionalisation occurs across the continuum of medical education. *Med Educ*. 2005; **39**(1): 58–65.

22. Quaintance JL, Arnold L, Thompson GS. Development of an instrument to measure the climate of professionalism in a clinical teaching environment. *Acad Med*. 2008; **83**(Suppl. 10): S5–8.

23. Ginsburg S, Regehr G, Mylopoulos M. From behaviours to attributions: further concerns regarding the evaluation of professionalism. *Med Educ*. 2009; **43**(5): 414–25.

24. Haidet P, Kelly PA, Chou C. Characterizing the patient-centeredness of hidden curricula in medical schools: development and validation of a new measure. *Acad Med*. 2005; **80**(1): 44–50.

25. Rees CE, Knight LV. Viewpoint: the trouble with assessing students' professionalism: theoretical insights from sociocognitive psychology. *Acad Med*. 2007; **82**(1): 46–50.

26. Rees CE, Knight LV. Banning, detection, attribution and reaction: the role of assessors in constructing students' unprofessional behaviours. *Med Educ*. 2008; **42**(2): 125–7.

27. Stern D. *Measuring Medical Professionalism*. New York, NY: Oxford University Press; 2006.

28. Cruess R, Cruess S. Expectations and obligations: professionalism and medicine's social contract with society. *Perspect Biol Med*. 2008; **51**(4): 579–98.

29. Campbell EG, Regan S, Gruen RL, et al. Professionalism in medicine: results of a national survey of physicians. *Ann Int Med*. 2007; **147**(11): 795–802.

30. Walsh C, Abelson HT. Medical professionalism: crossing a generational divide. *Perspect Biol Med*. 2008; **51**(4): 554–64.

31. Holtman MC. A theoretical sketch of medical professionalism as a normative complex. *Adv Health Sci Educ Theory Pract*. 2008; **13**(2): 233–45.

32. Tsugawa Y, Tokuda Y, Ohbu S, et al. Professionalism mini-evaluation exercise for medical residents in Japan: a pilot study. *Med Educ*. 2009; **43**(10): 968–78.

33. Ho MJ, Yu KH, Hirsh D, et al. Does one size fit all? Building a framework for medical professionalism. *Acad Med*. 2011; **86**(11): 1407–14.

34. Hafferty FW, Castellani B. A sociological framing of medicine's modern-day professionalism movement. *Med Educ*. 2009; **43**(9): 826–8.

35. Martimianakis MA, Maniate JM, Hodges BD. Sociological interpretations of professionalism. *Med Educ*. 2009; **43**(9): 829–37.

36. Ho MJ, Lin CW, Chiu YT, et al. A cross-cultural study of students' approaches to professional dilemmas: sticks or ripples? *Med Educ*. 2012; **46**(3): 245–56.

37. Ogunyemi D, Gonzalez G, Fong A, et al. From the eye of the nurses: 360-degree evaluation of residents. *J Contin Educ Health Prof*. 2009; **29**(2): 105–110.

38. Brinkman WB, Geraghty SR, Lanphear BP, et al. Evaluation of resident communication skills and professionalism: a matter of perspective? *Pediatrics.* 2006; **118**(4): 1371–9.

39. Chandler N, Henderson G, Park B, et al. Use of a 360-degree evaluation in the outpatient setting: the usefulness of nurse, faculty, patient/family, and resident self-evaluation. *J Grad Med Educ.* 2010; **2**(3): 430–4.

40. Wiggins MN, Coker K, Hicks EK. Patient perceptions of professionalism: implications for residency education. *Med Educ.* 2009; **43**(1): 28–33.

41. Boudreau JD, Jagosh J, Slee R, et al. Patients' perspectives on physicians' roles: implications for curricular reform. *Acad Med.* 2008; **83**(8): 744–53.

42. Desroches CM, Rao SR, Fromson JA, et al. Physicians' perceptions, preparedness for reporting and experiences related to impaired and incompetent colleagues. *JAMA.* 2010; **304**(2): 187–93.

43. Holmboe ES, Ginsburg S, Bernabeo E. The rotational approach to medical education: time to confront our assumptions? *Med Educ.* 2011; **45**(1): 69–80.

44. Bernabeo E, Holtman MC, Ginsburg S, et al. Lost in transition: the experience and impact of frequent changes in the inpatient learning environment. *Acad Med.* 2011; **86**(5): 591–8.

45. Gough J, Bullen M, Donath S. PHEEM 'downunder.' *Med Teach.* 2010; **32**(2): 161–3.

46. Kuper A, Reeves S, Levinson W. Qualitative research: an introduction to reading and appraising qualitative research. *BMJ.* 2008; **337**:a288: 404–7.

9

Best Practices in Measuring Health Care Team Performance

Eduardo Salas, Michael A. Rosen, and Sallie J. Weaver

TEAMWORK IS CRITICAL TO SAFE AND EFFECTIVE HEALTH CARE delivery. This position has been repeated consistently over the past decade from both government[1] and industry regulating entities[2] and is being popularized in successful general audience books.[3-4] Health care teamwork represents a dramatic shift from traditional ideas about how health care is delivered, a shift made necessary by emerging evidence that the longstanding myth of the lone heroic provider does not work and is insufficient for managing the complexity of modern health care.

Communication and teamwork breakdowns are involved in approximately 50% of health care adverse events[5] and as many as 70% of all sentinel events.[2] Communication problems are the second most frequent contributing systems factor in surgical malpractice claims (43% of cases) behind only technical proficiency.[6] Observational studies suggest that approximately one-third of all communication acts in the surgical operating room include an error of some type.[7] Emergent data provides an increasingly detailed understanding of the nature, causes, and consequences of teamwork and communication failures. The big picture is clear: communication and teamwork failures are common, they adversely affect care delivery processes, and they contribute to numerous incidents of preventable patient harm.[8]

Consequently, there is a great need to systematically train, monitor, and sustain high levels of teamwork among health care providers through all phases of professional development. The educational continuum stretches from basic interpersonal communication skills development, to interprofessional education activities, multidisciplinary team training, and advanced coaching and leadership training in continuing education. Realizing this vision, however, requires the ability to measure team performance systematically and to obtain reliable data that permit valid decisions.

This chapter provides a summary of the team performance measurement literature and advances a series of best practices for the development of sound teamwork measurement systems. First, we define key concepts from the science of teams, training, and performance measurement methods to build common ground between the multiple disciplines involved in team performance measurement in health care. Second, we propose a set of 18 best practices for team performance measurement to illustrate how to develop, adapt, or adopt team performance measurement tools for specific contexts. These best practices are organized around a six-part design framework for team performance measurement systems previously introduced.[9] Third, we discuss future directions for team performance measurement systems in health care.

Key Definitions

There are many potential stakeholders in the development and implementation of team performance measurement systems including learners, educators and trainers, health care system administrators, and industry regulators. Measurement system development is ideally a multidisciplinary team effort, including clinicians, educators, team performance experts, and measurement experts. This diversity ensures a full range of perspectives is represented, but it also presents its own obstacles in terms of shared terminology. This section gives definitions from (a) the science of teams and (b) measurement science to create shared meaning about core concepts of team performance measurement.

Teams and Teamwork

Teams are defined as two or more individuals who see themselves and are seen by others as identifiable social entities working interdependently to achieve shared goals that require members to communicate, cooperate, and coordinate their efforts and resources.[10–12] Teams differ from groups because team members interact to complete a targeted task (task interdependency) and team members share the outcomes of these interdependent efforts (outcome interdependence).[13] Team members also have specific roles and responsibilities that contribute to achievement of overarching team goals.

Within health care, the National Library of Medicine first introduced the term *patient care team* to the Medical Subject Headings index in 1968, defining them as multidisciplinary entities in which each member "has specific responsibilities and the whole team contributes to patient care."[14] This was after the term *nursing team* was introduced in 1967 and defined as: "Coordination of various nursing care personnel under the leadership of a professional nurse. The team may consist of a professional nurse, nurses' aides, and the practical nurse."[15] This example demonstrates that care delivery teams have been defined based on professional identity (e.g., nursing teams), the type of patient population served (e.g., pediatric care teams), disease processes (e.g., cardiac care teams), clinical procedures (e.g., neurosurgical teams), care delivery settings (e.g., hospital, ambulatory care, long-term care), and by criticality in a crisis scenario (e.g., rapid response teams).[16,17] Clinical care teams have also been distinguished from management teams who focus on strategic visioning and policy setting, operations teams that focus on daily functions necessary to run a particular unit or function (e.g., central supply), and performance improvement teams that "conven[e] around organizational processes or systems problems."[18]

Teamwork refers specifically to the behaviors (e.g., backup behavior, communication, leadership), cognitive mechanisms (e.g., shared mental models), and affective states (e.g., collective efficacy, trust, cohesion) that enable team members to work effectively toward mutual goals.[19,20] More specifically, *teamwork* can be differentiated from *taskwork*—the technical components of a given task that can be completed by individual team members.[21] For example, cognitively calculating a dosage or reading an electrocardiograph output during a code can represent taskwork. Communicating one's interpretation of the output to other members of the team responding to the code illustrates teamwork. Teamwork refers to the mechanisms through which members leverage collective expertise and resources on the task at hand via individual team members.

Teamwork has processes and emergent states. Processes are team activities including behaviors and cognitions that change inputs into outputs. Emergent states are phenomena that come from social interaction. The process of teamwork is categorized as action processes, transition processes, or interpersonal processes based on their level of criticality at different task execution phases.[22] For example, mutual performance monitoring, information exchange, and providing backup behavior are action processes that teams fulfill as they get things done. Before and after actions, teams engage in transition processes related to planning (e.g., mission analysis, goal specification, strategy formation) and feedback (e.g., reflection). Finally, interpersonal processes such as conflict management, motivation and confidence building, and affect management support team performance in both action and transition.

Emergent states refer to phenomena that arise as a function of social interaction. They include intangible aspects of team functioning that both influence and are influenced by team processes. For example, engaging in such transition processes as goal specification and strategy formation during a pre-case briefing may help team members align their thinking about how the team will approach a new case. A shared mental model of the new case may emerge from these preplanning interactions. Similarly, if the team exchanges information during the case and members provide effective backup behavior to one another, this may trigger a shared belief about the team's collective ability to accomplish shared goals (i.e., collective efficacy) and breed team trust. These emergent properties can boost team coordination in future cases.

Teamwork competencies refer to the knowledge, skills, and attitudes (KSAs) underlying effective teamwork. They refer to what team members think, do, and feel to achieve mutual goals. Teamwork competencies are usually conceptualized as attributes that can be learned and developed, in contrast with personality traits or other dispositional factors.[23] Competencies are the foundations for team performance measurement. They define *what* we are measuring.

There are numerous teamwork competency models now available in the teams literature, and comprehensive reviews are available elsewhere.[19,24] However, health care reviews suggest that competencies underlying communication, situation awareness, leadership, and role clarity are some of the most commonly targeted in health care team training.[25,26] Table 9.1 defines some of the core teamwork competencies relevant for health care teams.

TABLE 9.1 Examples of the Knowledge, Skills, and Attitudinal Competencies Underlying Effective Teamwork[19]

Competency	Definition
Knowledge	
Accurate and shared mental models	Organized knowledge structures that capture cognitive representations of the patterns and relationships among the task, team members, and context in which they are functioning[27,28]
Cue-strategy associations	Compatible repertoire of performance strategies or courses of action associated with frequently occurring situations or problems shared among team members[22,29]

Competency	Definition
Skills	
Mission analysis	Formalizing an understanding of the team's core tasks, goals, and the conditions under which members will function as well as the resources available to the team[22,30]
Backup behavior	Shifting and balancing workload among team members during periods of high workload or high pressure[22,31]
Conflict management	Preemptively setting up conditions to prevent or control team conflict or reactively working through interpersonal disagreements between members[23,32,33]
Mutual performance monitoring	Team members' ability to track what others on the team are doing while continuing to carry out their own tasks[31,34]
Team leadership	Dynamic process of social problem solving involving information search and structuring, information use in problem solving, managing personnel resources, and managing material resources[35,36]
Standardized communication patterns (e.g., closed-loop communication, situation-background-assessment-recommendation protocol)	Patterned exchanges of information designed to ensure the passing of accurate information and confirmation of shared interpretation and understanding[31,37,38]
Team adaptation	Dynamic modification of strategy and/or reallocation of efforts and resources[27,39]
Attitudes	
Collective efficacy	The team members' sense of collective competence and their ability to achieve their goals[40–42]
Collective orientation	Team members' preference for working with others as opposed to working in isolation[43,44]
Mutual trust	The shared belief among team members that everyone will perform their roles and protect the interests of their fellow team members[43,45,46]
Psychological safety	The team members' shared belief that it is safe to take interpersonal risks[47,48]

Team Performance and Team Effectiveness

One point of clarification particularly important for team performance measurement is the distinction between team performance and team effectiveness. *Team performance* refers to the behavioral, cognitive, and affective processes teams use to achieve a collective outcome. *Team effectiveness* refers specifically to evaluative statements regarding the team outcome.[49,50] Team performance refers to the processes team members use to work toward shared goals. Team effectiveness refers to the outcomes that result from these processes.

Process versus Outcome Measures

Human performance measurement taxonomies mirror this differentiation by separating two primary types of performance measures: process and outcome.[27] *Process measures* are dedicated to providing information about why and how a particular outcome occurred. Specifically, process measures capture the specific procedures, steps, and interactions that happen during a team performance episode. Process measures are critical for formative feedback, development, and continuous improvement. *Outcome measures* are metrics that capture the end result of a team effort. Outcome measures gauge effectiveness and indicate where the end result falls on an evaluative continuum (e.g., effective versus ineffective, desirable versus undesirable). Outcomes have been conceptualized as three broad dimensions: (1) quality and quantity, (2) team member satisfaction, and (3) the degree to which the team's efforts strengthened or weakened the collective capacity and desire to work together in the future.[51,52]

Diagnostic approaches to team performance measurement should include measures of both processes and outcomes at both the team and individual level of analysis. Clear links between process measures and outcome measures are also important along with a way to distinguish individual versus team-level performance.[38] Table 9.2 outlines this framework for measurement in terms of type of measure (process/outcome) and level of analysis (individual/team).

TABLE 9.2 A Framework for Human Performance Measures[27]

		Level of Analysis	
		Individual	*Team*
Type of Measure	*Process*	Task relevant: knowledge procedural skills critical thinking	Backup behavior Information exchange Leadership/followership Mission analysis Mutual performance monitoring
	Outcome	Accuracy: precision of performance (e.g., correct interpretation of electrocardiogram) Time lines: how long (e.g., time to pass information to other team members)	Time lines: how long (e.g., time to incision) Productivity: how much (e.g., patient volume) Efficiency: ratio of resources required versus used (e.g., supplies opened versus used) Team effectiveness

Measurement, Evaluation, Assessment, and Performance Diagnosis

This also raises important differences between several terms used to describe team performance measurement.[53,54] Measurement captures the dimensions of a team performance episode.[55] Assessment takes measurement one step further, by telling if a performance feature met a standard or benchmark. Assessment, in its basic sense, provides a dichotomous index about whether or not a performance standard was met. Evaluation is one of the broadest terms used in the context of performance measurement. Evaluations are designed to provide information along a series of criteria that define the quality or value of a given performance.[56,57] Performance diagnosis can be an important component of evaluation. Performance diagnosis involves moving beyond "what" happened to "why" it happened, which is the underlying cause of observed performance.[58] This is critical for providing formative feedback about specific aspects of performance that can be used to improve future performance. Overall, (a) measurement captures what happened, (b) assessments indicate whether a given measurement achieved a standard or benchmark, (c) evaluation tells us where a given measurement would fall on the continuum of quality or value, and (d) performance diagnostics are formative information about what needs to be improved or maintained to reach high-quality evaluations.

Best Practices for Team Performance Measurement

As summarized in Table 9.3, this section provides a series of best practices for development and implementation of team performance measurement systems. These best practices are rooted in principles and methods of psychometric test development and the science of teams and team performance measurement. These best practices are also organized around a framework outlining six core components of a team performance measurement system: (1) purpose, (2) content, (3) location, (4) timing, (5) method, and (6) sources of data.[9]

TABLE 9.3 Summary of Best Practices for Team Performance Measurement Systems

Component of Team Performance Measurement System	Best Practices
Purpose: Why measure team performance?	*#1*: Develop a clearly articulated purpose statement, including who will be using the data and what types of decisions will be made using the performance measurement data
Content: What do you measure?	*#2*: Root measurement in theoretically based competency models of effective teamwork
	#3: Align content of measurement with training and development program objectives
	#4: Capture multiple levels of evaluation data
Location: Where do you measure?	*#5*: Measure teamwork across a variety of contexts to capture both typical and maximal performance
	#6: Measure teamwork in simulated environments to provide standardized opportunities to capture multiple aspects of teamwork and indicators of maximal team performance
	#7: Measure teamwork in the clinical environment to capture measures of typical performance, reinforce team learning, and to ensure transfer of teamwork competencies to the daily care environment
Timing: When should you measure?	*#8*: Measure team performance longitudinally
Method: How do you measure?	*#9*: Match the methods of measurement to the purposes of measurement
	#10: Use multiple measures from multiple sources to balance strengths and weaknesses of different measurement methods
	#11: Use observation for capturing observable aspects of teamwork (i.e., behaviors)
	#12: Use structured observational protocols and provide comprehensive rater training to ensure reliable and valid ratings
	#13: Use self-report methods for aspects of teamwork not directly observable (e.g., attitudes, beliefs)
Sources of data: Selecting, training, and supporting observers	*#14*: Select observers with clinical and teamwork expertise
	#15: Train observers to standards and monitor reliability over time
	#16: Support observers with job aids and continuing training
	#17: Train coaches to make use of the data collected
	#18: Train teams to use tools for self-assessments

Purpose: Why Measure Team Performance?

Defining the purpose for measuring performance and what will be done with the collected data is the cornerstone of effective team performance measurement. This means beginning with the end in mind to define (a) how the collected data will be used, (b) who has data access and use authority, and (c) what consequences (intended and unintended) may emerge as a result of measurement activities. There are multiple purposes for measuring team performance but they can be categorized broadly as formative or summative.[56,59] *Formative* measurement aims to facilitate team learning and development, while *summative* measurement intends to provide a final judgment about the proficiency or value of team outcomes or a performance feature. Box 9.1 lists some of the purposes for team performance measurement and builds on those identified by Epstein and Hundert[60] in their definition of professional competence.

Box 9.1 Examples of the Purposes of Team Performance Measurement[60]

For the Team
- Provide diagnostic feedback about team and individual team member strengths and weaknesses that guides future learning
- Foster habits of self-reflection and team self-correction
- Promote access to advanced team training

For the Institution
- Support strategic institutional decision making
- Promote workforce development by identifying candidates for further training opportunities
- Enhance selection processes by identifying candidates for leadership roles
- Express and reinforce institutional values and goals
- Provide data for evidence-based management and research

For the Patient
- Certify competence of interdisciplinary care teams
- Support patient safety through data-driven continuous improvement efforts
- Promote patient involvement

Identifying the purpose for measuring performance is critical because it drives other decisions, such as whether a single composite criterion or multiple criteria are most appropriate.[61-64] For example, the purpose may be to diagnose root causes of performance deficiencies to identify specific weaknesses or to provide team feedback about strengths and weakness. Such purposes demand a level of granularity that enables teams to identify specific aspects of their performance that went well and others that need improvement. Data are then used to define a development plan to remediate weaknesses and optimize future performance. Thus a measurement plan needs to be designed around multiple criteria that capture multiple teamwork processes. Conversely, if the goal is to provide an assessment of a team's level of proficiency or readiness, a single composite criterion that combines information from multiple sources or sub-criteria may be more useful for decision making and benchmarking.

> **Best Practice #1**: Develop a clearly articulated purpose statement, including who will be using the data and what types of decisions will be made using the performance measurement data.

Content: What Do You Measure?

All measurement systems can be defined broadly in terms of two fundamental components: content (i.e., *what* is being measured) and method (i.e., *how* data are collected).[65] For team performance measurement, there are at least two general categories of content that should be considered: teamwork competencies and multilevel evaluation frameworks. Issues of each method will be discussed in following sections.

Teamwork Competencies

As introduced previously and summarized in Table 9.1, teamwork competencies are the KSAs that team members must have to function effectively. Teamwork competencies are what team members must think, do, and feel to reach their shared and valued goals. Team goals include task performance outcomes, team learning, team member satisfaction, and viability—the ability of team members to work together in the future. Teamwork competencies can be categorized as either *team or task specific*—that is, teamwork KSAs that are unique to a given team type, set of team members, or task situation. Teamwork competencies can also be *team or task generic*—that is, apply across different teams, team members, or task situations.[29] This distinction becomes important when considering the development of teamwork throughout the career of a provider; for example, general competencies that can be developed at early phases of education and training, and advanced contextual competencies that can be developed at later stages.[25,26]

A large and expanding scientific literature documents teamwork KSAs and their relationship to team performance and task outcomes.[66] This literature is theoretically grounded, empirical, and has been summarized in recent reviews.[19,66,67] Its precepts address a broad variety of team types across wide-ranging application domains. Increasingly, there is high-quality empirical research available about specific health care contexts, primarily in graduate medical education.[68] Interdisciplinary and continuing education in the health professions are beginning to discuss the need for integrative teamwork competency models.[25,26] A recent comprehensive review of the team training literature in health care found that communication, situation awareness, leadership, and role clarity are currently the most commonly targeted teamwork competencies.[25]

Team performance measurement systems are usually developed in the context of a training, education, or quality and safety improvement initiative. In these cases, the content of the measurement tool must align with the objectives of the program or intervention.[27] Following the old adage "measure what you want to change" as well as the fundamentals of systematic educational, training, and instructional design,[69] the teamwork competencies targeted for acquisition should inform the content of the measurement system so that progress toward learning objectives can be gauged and decisions about feedback and remediation can be made systematically.

> **Best Practice #2**: Root measurement in theoretically based competency models of effective teamwork.

> **Best Practice #3**: Align content of measurement with training and development program objectives.

Multilevel Evaluation

Multilevel evaluation frameworks can guide development of a team performance measurement system. Diagnostic understanding of team performance requires performance data from several occasions. Multilevel frameworks outline several content sources that can be used to understand the broad set of factors that contribute to team performance. Multilevel frameworks also reveal how different team performance measures can be assembled to make sense of a situation. Several multilevel frameworks are used commonly in health care and other training and educational contexts for different purposes.

Kirkpatrick's multilevel training evaluation model[70] and its extensions[71] outline four hierarchical data levels to capture reactions, learning, behavior change, and results. Level 1, learner reactions to training, includes such variables as affective responses (e.g., do learners "like" the training?), utility judgments (e.g., do learners think the training content will be useful in their jobs?), and intent to transfer (e.g., do learners intend to use what was learned on the job?). Affective reactions do not correlate highly with learning outcomes, but utility judgments and learner self-efficacy (i.e., do the learners feel confident in their abilities to perform the acquired skills?) predict learning and behavior change.[72] Level 2, learning, involves assessing the acquisition and retention of targeted competencies. This can involve assessment of declarative (e.g., do learners know the basic concepts and terminology?) and procedural knowledge (e.g., do learners know how to apply the behaviors and skills?) as well as demonstrations of learned behaviors in controlled learning environments (e.g., simulations). Level 3, behavior change or transfer, involves assessing the degree to which acquired competencies are used in the work environment. This is a common deficit in educational and training initiatives including teamwork training in health care.[66] Level 4, results, includes the ultimate changes or impact on the organization (e.g., improved safety, quality, efficiency).

These levels of evaluation can be considered a series of effects that an intervention needs to produce to reach its intended goals. Collecting data at each of these levels helps answer questions about why an intervention is or is not effective. For example, if a teamwork intervention is introduced into a facility and the intended results are not achieved (e.g., improved staff satisfaction, a reduction in communication errors, improved efficiency), it could be due to one or more of the following: failure to transfer learned behaviors (a level 3 issue), failure to acquire the targeted skills (a level 2 issue), or a low level of perceived value or utility of the teamwork content (a level 1 issue affecting motivation to learn or transfer). Additional multilevel models can be used instead of or in addition to the levels outlined here, including the CIPP (Context, Input, Process, Product) model[73] used for program evaluation, and Bloom's taxonomy of learning outcomes.[74]

Best Practice #4: Capture multiple levels of evaluation data.

Location: Where Do You Measure?

Effective team performance measurement depends on the measurement tool used to capture performance (e.g., observational protocol and rater, survey instrument), the methods used to complete the measurement tool (e.g., the rater who is observing team performance), and the conditions under which performance occurs. Where (and when) team performance is measured can influence the type of captured performance. Specifically, the distinction between measures of typical and maximal performance is particularly relevant.[75,76] Maximal performance measures capture what a team or individual team member "can do." By contrast, typical performance measures capture what they "will do" in the context of normal, daily work.[77] Maximal performance measures are defined by three core characteristics: (1) team members are aware that their performance is being measured, (2) instructions say that the goal is to put forth maximal effort, and (3) the period of measurement is short enough that team members can maintain attention on the goal of maximizing their efforts.[78] For example, measures of team performance in simulated settings are often measures of maximum performance. Conversely, typical performance can be captured when it is not evident to team members that they are being watched or evaluated, when they are not consciously working to the highest level of their ability, and when performance is measured over an extended timespan. Observations of team performance in the clinical care environment can be measures of typical performance. Typical performance measures are important because they are vital to understanding the effects of efforts to boost team performance, such as team training, and are mechanisms for understanding barriers to team effectiveness that lie "outside" of the team, such as organizational, cultural, or other contextual factors.[79]

Simulated environments offer a mechanism for providing a standardized setting where team performance can be assessed. Whether in a dedicated simulation center or in situ, simulations allow multiple teams to experience the same tasks under the same environmental conditions with the same patient. This ensures that teams have the same opportunities to engage in and demonstrate targeted teamwork competencies. If the purpose of measurement is to compare teams, whether benchmarking them against a given standard or evaluating the effects of a team-training program, simulated environments can help ensure the construct validity of team performance measures by standardizing the contextual factors that can affect performance across teams. It is also important to connect measurement of simulated team performance with measures of performance in the clinical environment.

Best Practice #5: Measure teamwork across a variety of contexts to capture both typical and maximal performance.

Best Practice #6: Measure teamwork in simulated environments to provide standardized opportunities to capture multiple aspects of teamwork and indicators of maximal team performance.

Best Practice #7: Measure teamwork in the clinical environment to capture measures of typical performance, reinforce team learning, and to ensure transfer of teamwork competencies to the daily care environment.

Timing: When Should You Measure?

Determining the right frequency of team performance measurement and its specific timing (e.g., critical measurement time points) depends on other attributes of the performance measurement system including the purpose, content, and method. For example, some competencies change at different rates (e.g., attitudes change more slowly than behavioral skills).[80] Using performance measurement to facilitate corrective feedback may require more frequent data collection than summative assessments. However, most applications of team performance assessment require measurement at more than one point in time to accurately and reliably understand a team's performance.[58] Team performance is dynamic: it varies significantly over time and across contexts.[39] Consequently, a longitudinal approach that captures a team performance profile across multiple episodes will provide a more robust picture of team strengths and weaknesses. Longitudinal data also show change trajectories needed to diagnose and intervene, as needed, to advance team development.[27,58,81]

Best Practice #8: Measure team performance longitudinally.

Method: How Do You Measure?

Team performance can be measured using many methods including observational ratings, self-report surveys, and other techniques such as card sorts and communication analyses. Each approach differs in the facets of teamwork that can be captured. Each measurement method has strengths and weaknesses. The dynamic, multilevel nature of teamwork suggests that a single measurement tool is insufficient to capture all aspects of team performance. Thus it is critical to match measurement tools with measurement goals. For example, observational measures can capture behavioral aspects of team performance but are insufficient to capture cognitive and affective team components. The performance measurement literature emphasizes that performance ratings differ by source (e.g., external raters, team members, peers, managers, patients). To illustrate, external raters and managers tend to observe team members acting under maximal performance conditions for short, defined periods of time. Teammates and peers, by contrast, observe typical performance under a broader scope of conditions. Studies of multiple rating sources have found that self-ratings tend to agree least with managerial or peer ratings of performance while ratings from external sources agree more with managers and peers.[82] However, these differences are moderated by the aspect of performance being rated. Observable behaviors tend to be rated with greater agreement regardless of source. Ratings of implicit cognitive activities vary greatly due to their source. This is an important consideration for team performance measurement because external observers cannot see many of the tacit team processes that are the hallmark of highly effective teams, such as implicit coordination.

> **Best Practice #9**: Match the methods of measurement to the purposes of measurement.

> **Best Practice #10**: Use multiple measures from multiple sources to balance strengths and weaknesses of different measurement methods.

Multi-method team performance measurement is not always possible in practice. Team performance measures should at least strive to achieve several criteria such as capturing team processes that drive highly valued team outcomes, providing diagnosticity that enables constructive feedback, and producing assessments that are both reliable and valid indicators of team performance.[83] Box 9.2 summarizes the criteria that form the foundation for a comprehensive approach to team performance measurement. Examples of methods and instruments used to measure team performance are also described here.

Box 9.2 Criteria for Team Performance Measurement Tools[83]

Team Performance Measures Should . . .

1. Be designed or chosen based on the results of a team task analysis—a systematic method for identifying core team tasks, care process workflow, coordination requirements and communication flow among team members and with others outside of the core team, and individual, social, and organizational factors that can help or hinder team performance.
2. Identify processes linked to key team outcomes.
3. Distinguish between individual and team level performance deficiencies.
4. Describe interactions among team members in a way that captures or accounts for the moment-to-moment changes that occur throughout a given performance episode.
5. Produce information that can be used to deliver specific, diagnostic (i.e., process oriented) feedback.
6. Produce evaluations and assessments that are valid and reliable. This means ensuring that measures are indeed measuring what the instrument was designed to measure, predictive of meaningful team outcomes and consistent across both time and multiple raters.
7. Support operational use. This means ensuring measures are designed to be relatively intuitive and easy to use.

Observational Approaches

Observational measures of team performance are metrics where a trained expert observes a team over time and provides performance ratings based on the observations. Observational methods can involve live experience with teams during either simulated or real care scenarios or post hoc analyses using video recordings. Live observations are a core component of timely feedback. Observational methods usually involve a structured rating form such as a checklist, frequency count, behavioral observation scale (BOS), or behaviorally anchored rating scale (BARS).

Checklists have a long history as an assessment tool in health care given their use in medical education for objective structured clinical examinations.[84] Checklists contain item sets that list actions that raters assess using dichotomous categories (e.g., yes/no, performed/not performed, correct/incorrect). Checklists are best used for scripted simulation scenarios. This ensures that checklist items can be embedded as triggers into the simulated scenario. Each checklist item should represent a single action taken by an individual or team and the response categories should be labeled and defined. A rating guide that gives examples of legitimate responses (e.g., what responses qualify as a "yes" versus what behaviors are rated as a "no") should accompany checklists. The limited response range used in checklists usually boosts inter-rater reliability. However, checklists may not capture quality dimensions underlying team performance such as timeliness.

Frequency counts are check marks that indicate the quantity of specific team-work behaviors. They are generally better for measuring acts of commission (overt actions) rather than acts of omission (failure to demonstrate a given behavior). Frequency counts are useful when the purpose of measurement is to know how often specific teamwork behaviors (e.g., use of the standardized SBAR [situation-background-assessment-recommendation] protocol) are occurring. Frequency counts can also focus on a critical event that occurs during a team performance episode. For example, the number of times that critical patient information is called-out to the team during a code event can be captured as an indicator of effective team communication.

Behavioral observation scales, also known as graphic rating scales, are numerical Likert-type scales where observers rate either the frequency (e.g., 1 = never, 5 = always) or quality (e.g., 1 = low quality, 5 = high quality) of a team process. For example, raters may be asked to rate how often "team members used closed-loop communication" during a particular care episode using a numerical scale from 1 (never) to 5 (always). BOSs require observers to provide an assessment of average team behavior over time. These scales are not able to provide data about the dynamic nature of team performance as a particular scenario unfolds. Inter-rater reliability can be difficult to achieve with BOSs unless there is comprehensive rater training about each rating category.

BARSs are similar because they also use a Likert-type rating format. However, instead of using general ratings of frequency or quality, BARS anchor each rating point with specific examples of the behaviors that should be observed to achieve a particular rating. For example, a BARS assessing the use of check-backs during a trauma resuscitation could be anchored with:

1 = did not use check backs
2 = used a check back once to confirm care plans at beginning of care
3 = used check backs to confirm all medication orders
4 = used check backs to confirm critical orders during primary and secondary surveys
5 = used check backs to confirm all orders.

Overall, scale-based ratings are effective for assessing quality when it does not equate directly to quantity and for team tasks that are less procedural in nature. However, it is critical to clearly define each rating category and to increase inter-rater reliability.

Raters are a vital component of observational methods. Human raters are susceptible to both bias and use of heuristics that systematically color the lens they use to observe, interpret, and evaluate team and individual performance.[85] Box 9.3 lists and defines some of the most common rater errors.[86] Given this tendency, observational methods must incorporate rater training as a core component of measurement plans.[87]

Box 9.3 Rater Errors and Biases that can Affect Ratings of Team Performance

Central Tendency: Tendency for raters to primarily use performance ratings in the middle of a given rating scale (e.g., to give mostly 3s on a five-point rating scale), though team performance may warrant higher or lower ratings.

"Halo/Horns" Error: Rater error in which one really great (or really bad) behavior colors ratings of other behaviors.

Primacy/Recency Effect: Tendency for raters to most easily remember things observed early in a scenario and/or things observed at the end of the scenario and thus, weight them most heavily in their evaluations of performance.

Past Performance Error: Rater error in which ratings are implicitly influenced by previous team performance episodes, rather than only by the performance episode currently being observed.

High Potential Error: Rater error in which raters confuse future potential with current performance that often results in positively skewed ratings of performance.

Observation-based team performance measures within health care have included approaches that utilize BOSs and BARSs. Examples include the *Mayo High Performance Teamwork Scale*,[88] event-based checklists such as *SMARTER*,[89] and methods that combine frequency counts with indicators of performance quality like *ANTS*,[90] *OTAS*,[91] *CATS*,[63] and the *University of Texas Behavioral Marker Audit Form*.[92]

While we have focused on quantitative observational approaches to measurement it is also important to note that qualitative observational schemes have also been developed. Qualitative approaches that use direct observation of care teams in the clinical environment are important to understand the complex relationships underlying care processes and the individual, social, and organizational factors that influence team performance.[79] Qualitative measures are a critical component toward developing valid quantitative teamwork measurement tools.

> **Best Practice #11**: Use observation for capturing observable aspects of teamwork (i.e., behaviors).

> **Best Practice #12**: Use structured observational protocols and provide comprehensive rater training to ensure reliable and valid ratings.

Self-Report Approaches to Team Performance Measurement

Self-report measures of team performance refer to metrics completed by team members themselves that are often survey based. Such measures are the mechanisms through which attitude and knowledge-based aspects of team performance can be captured. While such measures have limits, they can provide data about team member perceptions of team processes such as communication and coordination of effort that are often implicit. There are numerous examples of self-report measures of teamwork in health care.[93] For example, one component of the *Operating Room Management Attitudes Questionnaire* developed by Sexton and colleagues[94] was specifically designed to capture individual team member perceptions about teamwork processes in their most recent surgical case. Similarly, the Agency for Healthcare Research and Quality's battery of surveys assessing patient safety climate including the *Hospital Survey on Patient Safety Culture*[95] includes scales dedicated to assessing perceptions of teamwork among one's usual team and across multiple teams.

> **Best Practice #13**: Use self-report methods for aspects of teamwork not directly observable (e.g., attitudes, beliefs).

Other Approaches to Team Performance Measurement

Other methods have also been developed to capture less-observable cognitive aspects of team performance. For example, card sorting and concept mapping are elicitation techniques that have been used to measure the accuracy and communality of team mental models.[28,96] Individual team members sort statements that describe various aspects of team performance into groups that represent their personal cognitive organization scheme about different aspects of teamwork. The data collected from individual team members can then be compared to assess if the data are organized in similar patterns and whether the data are organized in a way that is similar to recognized experts.

Communication analysis (CA) is another form of measurement that is emerging as a mechanism for assessing cognitive processes such as collaborative problem solving and the emergence of affective components of team performance such as cohesion and trust.[97] CA uses transcriptions of explicit team communications to examine the content (e.g., topics of conversation, frequency of specific words, standardized communication protocols) and flow of team communications (e.g., who speaks to whom, when particular team members speak, when new information is shared). Such analyses offer a unique view of team communication behaviors and can also offer insight into other aspects of performance such as backup behavior, problem solving, and psychological safety. While CA requires nothing more than audio or video data, it requires post hoc analyses that limit the timeliness of feedback. Thus, CA has mainly been used for research-focused assessments of team performance. Efforts to develop computer models that can interpret such data quickly may increase the feasibility of such methods for other measurement purposes.

Other methods have also examined the environmental artifacts used by team members to communicate and organize their cognitive schemas and situational awareness. For example, Xiao and colleagues[98] employed direct observation and photographs of whiteboards used by emergency department teams to examine team task management, communication, problem solving and negotiation, and situational awareness under dynamic conditions.

Sources of Data: Selecting, Training, and Supporting Observers

The "who" of team performance measurement refers to the source(s) of data. This is either team members themselves in self-report methods or an external observer. This section focuses on best practices for the selection and development of teamwork observational raters and best practices for using data for performance improvement (e.g., feedback during learning activities, real-time coaching).

Selecting observers is an important first step toward developing a reliable and valid observational measurement system. Both the type (i.e., clinical and teamwork knowledge and experience) and level of rater expertise are primary considerations for selection. Raters need to discriminate between different levels of team performance and understand the nature of the teamwork being rated and know the clinical rating environment. Expert raters can make fine-grained and accurate discriminations but their availability is low and they are difficult to train to an external criterion. Novices can be trained to expert standards but this is time-consuming. Tradeoffs made in selection must be addressed in training. If you cannot select raters with the needed expertise, you need to train them intensively. *Training observers* is a necessary second step to ensure that data generated across teams, from different raters, are reliable. There are three primary approaches to rater training: (1) rater error training, which seeks to minimize variation in ratings due to basic cognitive biases of raters;[99] (2) performance dimension training, which focuses on defining the rating dimensions for raters;[100] and (3) frame of reference training, which focuses on discriminating between different levels of proficiency.[101] Each of these approaches can be applied in isolation or together with team training measurement. A third step, *supporting observers* with job aids such as scoring guides and ongoing training, is necessary to prevent or detect and remediate rater drift over time.

Best Practice #14: Select observers with clinical and teamwork expertise.

Best Practice #15: Train observers to standards and monitor reliability over time.

Best Practice #16: Support observers with job aids and continuing training.

The preceding best practices focus on developing and maintaining high-quality data collection processes for an observational measurement system. However, team performance measurement on its own will not produce learning or change unless team members receive feedback about the results of measurement. Facilitated team debriefs are the preferred method for providing feedback to teams in learning environments. Here, a skilled facilitator guides the team members through a learning process including reflection on team performance, critique of that performance relative to standards, and generation of lessons learned and plans for improving future performance. The effectiveness of this method depends on facilitator skill. Consequently, developing skilled coaches who can use teamwork measures to drive learning is a key component of a program to improve teamwork. In addition, because a large portion of learning and development happens in the workplace (*see* Chapter 12) and access to instructors and coaches is limited, developing self-learning teams is necessary. These are teams that engage in a reflection and improvement without coaches. Team training programs such as *Team Dimensional Training* and *Guided Self-Correction* focus on developing such teams using standardized processes and tools for team self-analysis.[102]

Best Practice #17: Train coaches to make use of the data collected.

Best Practice #18: Train teams to use tools for self-assessments.

Future Directions

Standardized and systematic approaches to developing teamwork are relatively new to health care. Consequently, teamwork measurement is also new to health care. While progress has been made, much work remains to be done. This section discusses several key areas that need further development.

There is a great need for standards or consensus models for teamwork competencies. Health care providers in different clinical areas face a variety of teamwork demands. Teamwork competency models need to be sorted so that models applied in early education phases include generic team and task competencies. As learners move to advanced education levels, the teamwork competency models become increasingly specialized. This is similar to the broad Accreditation Council on Graduate Medical Education core competency model that applies across specialties with multiple specialty-specific features contextualized to meet the demands of provider subgroups. Further research is needed about the forms of teamwork competencies that are general or specific to clinical domains, teams, and situations.

Future work also needs to improve the practicality of data collection methods. Observation is still the "gold standard" for measuring team performance, especially for the purposes of feedback and development. However, measurement by observation is labor intensive but can be improved with technology and tools such as electronic data collection instruments that help to collect, process, and store team performance data. The use of "social sensors" to capture patterns of interaction among care providers is a new and promising approach to understand coordination and teamwork within units without the traditional burden of observation.[103]

Concluding Remarks

Teamwork matters. It is critical for delivering safe and efficient care. The bedrock of the health care system is skilled professionals, competent in their roles and technical skills. However, clinical skill alone is insufficient. Effective communication, coordination, and collaboration among professionals are essential. These competencies must be embedded within the educational, training, and certification processes of the health care professions and specialties. Achieving this type of integration requires reliable, valid, and practical forms of team performance measurement. This chapter offers a synthesis of the available methods and approaches and a starting point for further development and adaptation of existing techniques for the needs of the health care community.

References

1. Kohn LT, Corrigan JM, Donaldson MS, editors. *To Err is Human: building a safer health system.* Washington, DC: Institute of Medicine, National Academy of Sciences; 2000.
2. The Joint Commission. *Sentinel Event Data: root causes by event type.* Oakbrook Terrace, IL: The Joint Commission; 2011. Available at: www.jointcommission.org/Sentinel_Event_Statistics/ (accessed November 7, 2011).
3. Pronovost PJ, Vohr E. *Safe Patients, Smart Hospitals: how one doctor's checklist can help us change health care from the inside out.* New York, NY: Hudson Street Press; 2010.
4. Lee TH, Morgan JJ. *Chaos and Organization in Healthcare.* Cambridge, MA: MIT Press; 2009.
5. Rabøl LI, Andersen ML, Østergaard D, et al. Description of verbal communication errors between staff: an analysis of 84 root cause analysis reports from Danish hospitals. *BMJ Qual Saf.* 2011; **20**(3): 268–74.
6. Gawande AA, Zinner MJ, Studdert DM, et al. Analysis of errors reported by surgeons at three teaching hospitals. *Surgery.* 2003; **133**(6): 614–21.
7. Lingard L, Espin S, Whyte S, et al. Communication failures in the operating room: an observational classification of recurrent types and effects. *Qual Saf Health Care.* 2004; **13**(5): 330–4.
8. Nagpal K, Vats A, Lamb B, et al. Information transfer and communication in surgery: a systematic review. *Ann Surg.* 2010; **252**(2): 225–39.

9. Rosen MA, Schievel N, Salas E, et al. How can team performance be measured, assessed, and diagnosed? In: Salas E, Frush K, editors. *Improving Patient Safety through Teamwork and Team Training.* Oxford: Oxford University Press; 2012. pp. 59–79.

10. Cohen SG, Bailey DR. What makes teams work: group effectiveness research from the shop floor to the executive suite. *J Manage.* 1997; **23**(4): 238–90.

11. Kozlowski SWJ, Bell BS. Work groups and teams in organizations. In: Borman WC, Ilgen DR, Klimoski RJ, editors. *Handbook of Psychology, Vol. 12: industrial and organizational psychology.* New York, NY: Wiley; 2003. pp. 333–75.

12. Salas E, Dickinson TL, Converse SA, et al. Toward an understanding of team performance and training. In: Swezey RW, Salas E, editors. *Teams: their training and performance.* Norwood, NJ: Ablex; 1992. pp. 3–29.

13. Shea GP, Guzzo RA. Group effectiveness: what really matters. *Sloan Manage Rev.* 1987; **28**(3): 25–31.

14. National Library of Medicine. *Patient Care Team.* Available at: www.ncbi.nlm.nih.gov/mesh/68010348 (accessed September 19, 2011).

15. National Library of Medicine. Nursing, Team. Available at: www.ncbi.nlm.nih.gov/mesh/68009746 (accessed September 19, 2011).

16. Lemieux-Charles L, McGuire WL. What do we know about health care team effectiveness? A review of the literature. *Med Care Res Rev.* 2006; **63**(3): 263–300.

17. Manser T. Teamwork and patient safety in dynamic domains of healthcare: a review of the literature. *Acta Anaesthesiol Scand.* 2009; **53**(2): 143–51.

18. Heinemann GD. Teams in healthcare settings. In: Heinemann GD, Zeiss AM, editors. *Team Performance in Healthcare: assessment and development.* New York, NY: Kluwer Academic/Plenum Publishers; 2002. pp. 3–18.

19. Salas E, Rosen MA, Burke CS, et al. The wisdom of collectives in organizations: an update of the teamwork competencies. In: Salas E, Goodwin GF, Burke CS, editors. *Team Effectiveness in Complex Organizations: cross-disciplinary perspectives and approaches.* New York, NY: Psychology Press; 2009. pp. 39–79.

20. Salas E, Wilson KA, Murphy CE, et al. Communicating, coordinating, and cooperating when lives depend on it: tips for teamwork. *Jt Comm J Qual Patient Saf.* 2008; **34**(6): 333–41.

21. Morgan BB Jr., Glickman AS, Woodward EA, et al. *Measurement of Team Behaviors in a Navy Environment.* Technical Report No. 86-014. Orlando, FL: Naval Training Systems Center; 1986.

22. Marks MA, Mathieu JE, Zaccaro SJ. A temporally based framework and taxonomy of team processes. *Acad Manage Rev.* 2001; **26**(3): 355–76.

23. Stevens MJ, Campion MA. The knowledge, skill, and ability requirements for teamwork: implications for human resource management. *J Manage.* 1994; **20**(2): 503–30.

24. Weaver SJ, Feitosa J, Salas E, et al. The science of teams: the theoretical drivers, models and competencies of team performance for patient safety. In: Salas E, Frush K, editors. *Improving Patient Safety through Teamwork and Team Training.* Oxford: Oxford University Press; 2012. pp. 3–26.

25. Weaver SJ, Lyons R, Diaz Granados D, et al. The anatomy of health care team training and the state of practice: a critical review. *Acad Med.* 2010; **85**(11): 1746–60.

26. Weaver SJ, Rosen MA, Salas E, et al. Integrating the science of team training: guidelines for continuing education. *J Contin Educ Health Prof.* 2010; **30**(4): 208–20.

27. Cannon-Bowers JA, Salas E. A framework for developing team performance measures in training. In: Brannick MT, Salas E, Prince C, editors. *Team Performance Assessment and Measurement: theory, methods, and applications.* Mahwah, NJ: Lawrence Erlbaum Associates; 1997. pp. 45–62.

28. DeChurch LA, Mesmer-Magnus JR. Measuring shared team mental models: a meta-analysis. *Group Dyn-Theor Res.* 2010; **14**(1): 1–14.

29. Cannon-Bowers JA, Tannenbaum SI, Salas E, et al. Defining team competencies and establishing team training requirements. In: Guzzo R, Salas E, editors. *Team Effectiveness and Decision Making in Organizations.* San Francisco, CA: Jossey-Bass; 1995. pp. 117–51.

30. Mathieu JE, Schulze W. The influence of team knowledge and formal plans on episodic team process-performance relationships. *Acad Manag J.* 2006; **49**(3): 605–19.

31. McIntyre RM, Salas E. Measuring and managing for team performance: emerging principles from complex environments. In: Guzzo RA, Salas E, editors. *Team Effectiveness and Decision Making in Organizations.* San Francisco, CA: Jossey-Bass; 1995. pp. 9–45.

32. De Dreu CK, Weingart LR. Task versus relationship conflict, team performance, and team member satisfaction: a meta-analysis. *J Appl Psychol.* 2003; **88**(4): 741–9.

33. Jordan PJ, Troth AC. Managing emotions during team problem solving: emotional intelligence and conflict resolution. *Hum Perf.* 2004; **17**(2): 195–218.

34. Marks MA, Panzer FJ. The influence of team knowledge and formal plans on episodic team process-performance relationships. *Acad Manag J.* 2006; **49**(3): 605–19.

35. Burke CS, Stagl KC, Klein C, et al. What type of leadership behaviors are functional in teams? A meta-analysis. *Leadership Quart.* 2006; 17: 288–307.

36. Day DV, Gronn P, Salas E. Leadership capacity in teams. *Leadership Quart.* 2004; **15**(6): 857–80.

37. Bowers CA, Jentsch F, Salas E, et al. Analyzing communication sequences for team training needs assessment. *Hum Fact.* 1998; **40**(4): 672–9.

38. Smith-Jentsch KA, Johnston JA, Payne SC. Measuring team-related expertise in complex environments. In: Cannon-Bowers JA, Salas E, editors. *Making Decisions Under Stress: implications for individual and team training.* Washington, DC: American Psychological Association; 1998. pp. 67–87.

39. Burke CS, Stagl KC, Salas E, et al. Understanding team adaptation: a conceptual analysis and model. *J Appl Psychol.* 2006; **91**(6): 1189–207.

40. Bandura A. *Social Foundations of Thought and Action: a social cognitive theory.* Englewood Cliffs, NJ: Prentice-Hall; 1986.

41. Katz-Navon TY, Erez M. When collective and self-efficacy affect team performance: the role of task independence. *Small Group Res.* 2005; **36**(4): 437–65.

42. Zaccaro SJ, Blair V, Peterson C, et al. Collective efficacy. In: Maddux JE, editor.

Self-Efficacy, Adaptation, and Adjustment: theory, research, and application. New York, NY: Plenum; 1995. pp. 305–28.

43. Alavi SB, McCormick J. A cross-cultural analysis of the effectiveness of the learning organizational model in school contexts. *Int J Educ Manag.* 2004; **18**(7): 408–16.

44. Eby L, Dobbins G. Collectivistic orientation in teams: an individual and group-level analysis. *J Organ Behav.* 1997; **18**: 275–95.

45. Driskell JE, Salas E. Collective behavior and team performance. *Hum Factors.* 1992; **34**: 277–88.

46. Jackson CL, Colquitt JA, Wesson MJ, et al. Psychological collectivism: a measurement validation and linkage to group member performance. *J Appl Psychol.* 2006; **91**(4): 884–99.

47. Edmondson AC. Psychological safety and learning behavior in work teams. *Admin Sci Quart.* 1999; **44**(2): 350–83.

48. Nembard IM, Edmondson AC. Making it safe: the effects of leader inclusiveness and professional status on psychological safety and improvement efforts in health care teams. *J Organ Behav.* 2006; **27**: 941–66.

49. Campbell JP, McCloy RA, Oppler SH, et al. A theory of performance. In: Schmitt N, Borman WC, editors. *Personnel Selection in Organizations.* San Francisco, CA: Jossey-Bass; 1993. pp. 35–70.

50. Tannenbaum SI, Beard RL, Salas E. Team building and its influence on team effectiveness: an examination of conceptual and empirical developments. In: Kelley K, editor. *Issues, Theory, and Research in Industrial/Organizational Psychology.* Oxford: North-Holland; 1992. pp. 117–53.

51. Guzzo RA, Dickson MW. Teams in organizations: recent research on performance and effectiveness. *Annu Rev Psychol.* 1996; **47**: 307–38.

52. Hackman JR. The design of work teams. In: Lorsch J, editor. *Handbook of Organizational Behavior.* New York, NY: Prentice-Hall; 1987. pp. 315–42.

53. Brannick MT, Prince C. Overview of team performance measurement. In: Brannick MT, Salas E, Prince C, editors. *Team Performance Assessment and Measurement: theory, methods, and applications.* Mahwah, NJ: Erlbaum; 1997. pp. 3–16.

54. Salas E, Burke CS, Fowlkes JE, et al. On measuring teamwork skills. In: Thomas JC, editor. *Comprehensive Handbook on Psychological Assessment.* Vol. 4. New York, NY: John Wiley & Sons; 2003. pp. 427–42.

55. Wildman JL, Bedwell WL, Salas E, et al. Performance measurement at work: a multilevel perspective. In: Zedeck S, editor. *APA Handbook of Industrial and Organizational Psychology, Vol. 1: building and developing the organization.* Washington, DC: American Psychological Association; 2011. pp. 303–41.

56. Russ-Eft D, Preskill H. *Evaluation in Organizations.* 2nd ed. Philadelphia, PA: Basic Books; 2009.

57. Scriven M. The methodology of evaluation. In: Stake RE, editor. *Curriculum Evaluation: American Educational Research Association monograph series on evaluation.* Chicago, IL: Rand McNally; 1967. pp. 39–83.

58. Salas E, Rosen MA, Burke CS, et al. Markers for enhancing team cognition in com-

plex environments: the power of team performance diagnosis. *Aviat Space Environ Med.* 2007; **78**(Suppl. 5): B77–85.

59. Bloom BS, Hastings JT, Madaus GF. *Handbook on Formative and Summative Evaluation of Student Learning.* New York, NY: McGraw-Hill; 1971.

60. Epstein RM, Hundert EM. Defining and assessing professional competence. *JAMA.* 2002; **287**(2): 226–35.

61. Aram JD, Morgan CP, Esbeck ES. Relation of collaborative interpersonal relationships to individual satisfaction and organizational performance. *Admin Sci Quart.* 1971; **16**(3): 289–97.

62. Gaba DM, Howard SK, Flanagan B, et al. Assessment of clinical performance during simulated crises using both technical and behavioral ratings. *Anesthesiology.* 1998; **89**(1): 8–18.

63. Frankel A, Gardner R, Maynard L, et al. Using the communication and teamwork skills (CATS) assessment to measure healthcare team performance. *Jt Comm J Qual Patient Saf.* 2007; **33**(9): 549–58.

64. Yule S, Flin R, Maran N, et al. Surgeons' non-technical skills in the operating room: reliability testing of the NOTSS behavior rating system. *World J Surg.* 2008; **32**(4): 548–56.

65. Nunnally JC, Bernstein IH. *Psychometric Theory.* 3rd ed. New York, NY: McGraw-Hill; 1994.

66. Salas E, Almeida SA, Salisbury M, et al. What are the critical success factors for team training in health care? *Jt Comm J Qual Patient Saf.* 2009; **35**(8): 398–405.

67. Kozlowski SWJ, Ilgen D. Enhancing the effectiveness of work groups and teams. *Psych Sci Pub Int.* 2006; **7**(3): 77–124.

68. Fernandez R, Kozlowski SW, Shapiro MJ, et al. Toward a definition of teamwork in emergency medicine. *Acad Emerg Med.* 2008; **15**(11): 1104–12.

69. Goldstein IL, Ford K. *Training in Organizations: needs assessment, development, and evaluation.* 4th ed. Belmont, CA: Wadsworth; 2002.

70. Kirkpatrick DL, Kirkpatrick JD. *Evaluating Training Programs.* San Francisco, CA: Berrett-Koehler Publishers; 2006.

71. Kraiger K, Ford JK, Salas E. Application of cognitive, skill-based, and affective theories of learning outcomes to new methods of training evaluation. *J Appl Psychol.* 1993; **78**(2): 311–17.

72. Alliger GM, Tannenbaum SI, Bennet W, et al. A meta-analysis of the relations among training criteria. *Pers Psychol.* 1997; **50**(2): 341–7.

73. Farley DO, Battles JB. Evaluation of the AHRQ patient safety initiative: framework and approach. *Health Serv Res.* 2009; **44**(2 Pt. 2): 628–45.

74. Anderson LW, Krathwohl DR, Airasian PW, et al. *A Taxonomy for Learning, Teaching, and Assessing: a revision of Bloom's Taxonomy of Educational Objectives.* 2nd ed. Boston, MA: Allyn & Bacon; 2001.

75. Cronbach LJ. *Essentials of Psychological Testing.* 2nd ed. New York, NY: Harper & Row; 1960.

76. Sackett PR, Zedeck S, Fogli L. Relations between measures of typical and maximum job performance. *J Appl Psychol.* 1988; **73**(3): 482–6.

77. Dubois CLZ, Sackett PR, Zedeck S, et al. Further exploration of typical and maximum performance criteria: definitional issues, prediction, and white-black differences. *J Appl Psychol.* 1993; **78**(2): 205–11.

78. Sackett PR, Zedeck S, Fogli L. Relations between measures of typical and maximum job performance. *J Appl Psychol.* 1988; **73**(3): 482–6.

79. Jeffcott SA, Mackenzie CF. Measuring team performance in healthcare: review of research and implications for patient safety. *J Crit Care.* 2008; **23**(2): 188–96.

80. Mitchell TR, James LR. Building better theory: time and the specification of when things happen. *Acad Manage Rev.* 2001; **25**(4): 530–47.

81. Kendall DL, Salas E. Measuring team performance: review of current methods and considerations of future needs. In: Ness TJW, Ritzer D, editors. *The Science and Simulation of Human Performance.* Boston, MA: Elsevier; 2004. pp. 307–19.

82. Furnham A, Stringfield P. Congruence in job-performance ratings: a study of 360° feedback examining self, manager, peers, and consultant ratings. *Hum Relat.* 1998; **51**(4): 517–30.

83. Paris CR, Salas E, Cannon-Bowers JA. Teamwork in multi-person systems: a review and analysis. *Ergonomics.* 2000; **43**(8): 1052–75.

84. Frank C. Evidence based checklists for objective structured clinical examinations. *BMJ.* 2006; **333**(7576): 546–8.

85. Iramaneerat C, Yudkowsky R. Rater errors in clinical skills assessment of medical students. *Eval Health Prof.* 2007; **30**(3): 266–83.

86. Borman WC. Job behavior, performance, and effectiveness. In: Dunnette MD, Hough LM, editors. *Handbook of Industrial and Organizational Psychology.* Vol. 2. Palo Alto, CA: Consulting Psychologists Press; 1991. pp. 271–326.

87. Woehr DJ, Huffcutt AJ. Rater training for performance appraisal: a quantitative review. *J Occup Organ Psychol.* 1994; **67**: 189–205.

88. Malec JF, Torsher LC, Dunn WF, et al. The Mayo high performance teamwork scale: reliability and validity for evaluating key crew resource management skills. *Simul Healthc.* 2007; **2**(1): 4–10.

89. Rosen MA, Salas E, Wu T, et al. Promoting teamwork: an event-based approach to simulation-based teamwork training for emergency medicine residents. *Acad Emerg Med.* 2008; **15**(11): 1190–8.

90. Fletcher G, Flin R, McGeorge P, et al. Anaesthetists' non-technical skills (ANTS): evaluation of a behavioural marker system. *Br J Anaesth.* 2003; **90**(5): 580–8.

91. Healey AN, Undre S, Vincent CA. Developing observational measures of performance in surgical teams. *Qual Saf Health Care.* 2004; **13**(Suppl. 1): i33–40.

92. Thomas EJ, Sexton JB, Helmreich RL. Translating teamwork behaviors from aviation to healthcare: development of behavioral markers for neonatal resuscitation. *Qual Saf Health Care.* 2004; **13**(Suppl. 1): i57–64.

93. Heinemann GD, Zeiss AM, editors. *Team Performance in Health Care: assessment and development.* New York, NY: Kluwer Academic/Plenum Publishers; 2002.

94. Sexton JB, Helmreich RL, Glenn D, et al. *Operation Room Management Attitudes Questionnaire.* Technical report for The University of Texas at Austin Human Factors

Research Project; 2000. Available at: www.homepage.psy.utexas.edu/homepage/group/HelmreichLAB/Publications/595.doc (accessed March 26, 2011).

95. Sorra JS, Nieva VF. *Hospital Survey on Patient Safety Culture*. AHRQ Publication No. 04-0041. Rockville, MD: Agency for Healthcare Research and Quality; 2004.

96. Mohammed S, Klimoski R, Rentsch JR. The measurement of team mental models: we have no shared schema. *Org Res Meth.* 2000; **3**(2): 123–65.

97. Salas E, Milham LM, Bowers CA. Training evaluation in the military: misconceptions, opportunities, and challenges. *Mil Psychol.* 2003; **15**(1): 3–16.

98. Xiao Y, Schenkel S, Faraj S, et al. What whiteboards in a trauma center operating suite can teach us about emergency department communication. *Ann Emerg Med.* 2007; **50**(4): 387–95.

99. Stamoulis DT, Hauenstein NMA. Rater training and rating accuracy: training for dimensional accuracy versus training for rate differentiation. *J Appl Psychol.* 1993; **78**(6): 994–9.

100. Fay CH, Latham GP. Effects of training and rating scales on rating errors. *Pers Psychol.* 1982; **35**(1): 105–16.

101. Sulsky LM, Day DV. Frame-of-reference training and cognitive categorization: an empirical investigation of rater memory issues. *J Appl Psychol.* 1992; **77**(4): 501–10.

102. Smith-Jentsch KA, Cannon-Bowers JA, Tannenbaum SI, et al. Guided team self-correction: impacts on team mental models, processes, and effectiveness. *Small Gr Res.* 2008; **39**(3): 303–24.

103. Aggarwal CC, Abdelzaher T. Integrating sensors and social networks. In: Aggarwal CC, editor. *Social Network Data Analytics.* New York, NY: Springer; 2011. pp. 1–16.

10

Evaluating Outcomes in Continuing Education and Training

Paul E. Mazmanian, Moshe Feldman, Taylor E. Berens,
Angela P. Wetzel, and David A. Davis

WHAT HAPPENS TO PATIENTS ONCE CARE HAS BEEN DELIVERED IS AN outcome.[1] What happens to health care professionals once treated by an educational intervention is an outcome.[2] Many view outcomes as the only legitimate index for measuring whether education and health care systems are achieving their goals.[3] Current science to explain outcomes in education and in health care is incomplete and causal linkages from interventions to results are unclear.[2]

In health care, outcomes are the result of efforts to prevent, diagnose, and treat health problems encountered by a population. Clinical and functional health status and patient and provider experience are useful outcomes to assess the performance of a health system. Clinical status or measurements of the biological, physiological, and symptom-based aspects of health (including blood pressure, cholesterol, and mortality) are examples of outcomes of interest to physicians because such outcomes are amenable to treatment. Functional status includes physical, mental, role, and social effects. Functional status is important to patients because it represents how changes in clinical status affect their everyday lives.[3] Consumer satisfaction assesses whether experience in the health care system is consistent with expectations and acceptable to those receiving care.[1] Community health outcomes may be expressed as disease prevalence, calculated as the number of persons with a disease, divided by the number of persons examined in a select population.[4] Community outcomes may also be calculated as disease incidence, the number of new cases detected during a time period divided by the population size who are disease free.[4]

This chapter interprets original research and systematic reviews across disciplines including education, knowledge translation, implementation science, training, and organizational psychology. It presents a conceptual framework for measuring outcomes. The chapter also organizes educational interventions, stressing theories and linkages to evidence to assure the effectiveness of continuing education (CE) across a spectrum of desirable effects. Findings are discussed with implications for CE planners, evaluators, and physicians as learners. Continuing medical education (CME) emphasizes a physician's commitment to lifelong learning in practice. It refers to education after professional certification and licensure. CME is arguably the most complex but certainly the longest phase of medical education.[5,6] Evaluation of physician behavior change is featured in this chapter. The chapter reports how social research methods are used to study and improve the way CME is designed and implemented, including the measurement of its efficiency and outcomes.

Educational Outcomes and Planning for Instruction: A Conceptual Framework

Table 10.1 presents a conceptual framework for measuring outcomes in CME.[7] The framework represents variables aligned to guide practice and to set research agendas. It includes attendance as a method or data source for measuring *participation* at level 1. At level 2, participants' *satisfaction* with the setting and delivery of the CE activity is measured. A questionnaire completed by participants is the method typically used to collect such data. *Declarative knowledge* (level 3A) is the degree to which participants express the CME intentions. The data can be collected through pre- and post-tests of knowledge or through self-report of knowledge gain. *Procedural knowledge* (level 3B) is the degree to which participants report how to perform based on knowledge presented during a CME activity. Pre- and post-tests of knowledge and subjective self-reports of knowledge gain are key data sources. *Competence* is the outcome measured at level 4. Competence is defined as the degree to which participants show, in an educational setting, how to act as a result of CME experiences. Observation of behavior in controlled conditions and self-report of competence are central sources of data for measuring competence. At level 5, CME participants demonstrate *performance*. This is the degree to which they display the CME intentions in professional practice.

Observation in patient care settings, patient charts, administrative databases, and self-reports are data sources for performance measurement. Level 6 is *patient health*, the degree to which the health status of patients improves due to changes in practice behavior of CME participants. Reduced blood glucose and increased pulmonary function captured in medical records are examples of patient health outcome measures. Functional status measures recorded in patient charts, administrative databases, and patient self-reports of health status are major data sources at level 6. At level 7, *community health* is the degree to which the health status of a patient community changes due to adjustments in the practice behavior of CME participants. Disease prevalence and incidence derived from epidemiological data gauge changes in community health.

TABLE 10.1 Moore's Expanded Outcomes Framework for Planning and Assessing Continuing Medical Education (CME) Activities

Outcomes Framework	Miller's Framework	Description	Source of Data
Participation LEVEL 1		Number of learners who participate in the educational activity	Attendance records
Satisfaction LEVEL 2		Degree to which expectations of participants were met regarding the setting and delivery of the educational activity	Questionnaires/surveys completed by attendees after an educational activity, focus groups
Learning: Declarative Knowledge LEVEL 3A	Knows	The degree to which participants express the CME educational intentions	Objective: Pre- and post-tests of knowledge Subjective: Self-report of knowledge gain
Learning: Procedural Knowledge LEVEL 3B	Knows how	The degree to which participants report *how* to perform as a result of CME	Objective: Pre- and post-tests of knowledge Subjective: Self-reported gain in knowledge (e.g., reflective journal)
Competence LEVEL 4	Shows how	The degree to which participants *show* in an educational setting *how* to act as a result of CME experiences	Objective: Observation in educational setting (e.g., peer assessment and chart-stimulated recall) Subjective: Self-report of competence
Performance LEVEL 5	Does	The degree to which participants display CME intentions in professional practice	Objective: Observed performance in clinical setting; patient charts; administrative databases Subjective: Self-report of performance

(continued)

Outcomes Framework	Miller's Framework	Description	Source of Data
Patient health LEVEL 6		The degree to which the health status of patients improves as a result of changes in the practice behavior of CME participants	Objective: Health status measures recorded in patient charts or administrative databases Subjective: Patient self-report of health status
Community health LEVEL 7		The degree to which the health status of a patient community changes as a result of changes in the practice behavior of CME participants	Objective: Epidemiological data and reports Subjective: Community self-report

Moore et al.[7] compare features of the framework in Table 10.1 with elements of Miller's[8] well-known outcome pyramid. Miller's stages of clinical skill acquisition require that a physician *knows* what to do, *knows how* to do what is required and *shows how* expectations are met, before the physician actually *does* what is expected with patients in practice.

Moore et al.[7] recommend that CME planning should start with outcomes in mind. This is backward planning, starting with level 7 outcomes and working backward through levels 6, 5, 4, 3B, and 3A. The planner continuously analyzes gaps between current performance and desired results[9] at each level, until no gap is seen at level 7. Moore et al.[7] offer an example of how backward planning might work, using metabolic syndrome—high blood pressure, elevated insulin, excess midline body fat, high cholesterol levels—that together increase the risk of heart disease.

- Starting at the end of the outcomes framework, at level 7 (community health), data may show the health status of individuals with metabolic syndrome is suboptimal. Thus, at level 7, there is a gap between the current health status of these individuals and the desired health status, judged by a national standard.
- The next step for a CME planner is to determine if there is a gap at level 6, patient health, between the health status of patients with metabolic syndrome and what national and local guidelines report it should be.
- If a practice gap exists at level 6, a CME planner must decide whether a gap exists between what physicians in these practices currently do and what they should do at level 5, performance, to promote expected health status of patients with metabolic syndrome.
- If a gap is detected in the performance of certain physicians, the next step is to determine whether there is a gap at level 4, physician competence. This

shows what the physicians could do and what knowledge, attitudes, or skills (KSAs) they demonstrate in a controlled educational environment.

- Finally, if deficits are detected in the competence of physicians, the next step is to determine if there is a gap at level 3B, procedural knowledge. This reveals the discrepancy between the knowledge physicians should describe and what they actually describe.
- Most physicians can pass a test on procedural knowledge. Thus there is not likely to be a gap at level 3B for a CME planner to detect. Consequently, planning learning activities for physicians should focus on level 4, physician competence.

Backward planning using Moore's model presents challenges to CME planners. First, few CME planners have the time, money, and staff to devise such a roadmap. In addition, the transitions from knowledge at levels 3A and 3B to behavior at level 4, and from level 4, behavior, to level 5, performance in practice, are unclear. Few approaches exist to illuminate the processes and measures of change and to enable project replication. Tools to define, measure, and improve performance and outcomes must be identified, created, or improved.

Evidence for Measuring the Effectiveness of Continuing Education

The US Institute of Medicine (IOM) recently synthesized results from a literature search of more than 18 000 articles from fields including CE, knowledge translation, interprofessional learning and practice, and faculty development. The IOM report assessed study designs, methods, outcomes, and conclusions to disclose a range of issues informing a broadly defined research agenda for CE in the health professions. A final set of 62 studies and 20 systematic reviews and meta-analyses relevant to CE methods, cost-effectiveness, or educational theory formed the foundation of the report. The IOM research synthesis suggested a new scientific foundation is needed for CE to enhance health professional performance and patient outcomes. The new scientific foundation must include development of better measures to assure high-quality data collection, analysis, and dissemination of metrics. Continuing professional development (CPD) was defined not only to include components of CE but also to involve a broader focus. For example, the questions of how to identify problems and apply solutions and how to allow health professionals to tailor the learning process, setting, and curriculum to their needs are addressed in CPD. Principles of CPD are in place in Canada, New Zealand, the United Kingdom, and other member states of the European Union.[10,11]

Table 10.2 lists interventions and definitions taken from the Cochrane Library Database of Systematic Reviews.[12] The table includes references to studies in health professions CE and training, a designation of outcomes levels studied using Moore's expanded model, and examples of study findings. The list of interventions and studies is not exhaustive. It contains examples of outcomes studies where findings can inform best practices of education planners, learners, evaluators, and others interested in improving education and health care.

In 2007, Marinopoulos et al.[13] summarized the evidence from 136 studies and nine systematic reviews on the effectiveness of CME to boost knowledge and skills, change attitudes and practice behavior, and improve clinical outcomes. The investigators could not determine the effectiveness of all CME methods studied. However, CME was found generally effective for KSA acquisition; behavior change; and for improving clinical outcomes. There is additional evidence to support the overall effectiveness of CE in select instances,[10,14–16] but too little evidence exists to make a compelling case for the universal effectiveness of CE. For example, in 2009, print media was found ineffective, with exceptions such as brief messaging techniques.[17] Educational meetings alone or combined with other interventions can improve professional practice and health care outcomes for patients,[18] but education meetings do not alter complex behaviors. Mixed interactive and didactic education meetings are more effective than either didactic meetings or interactive meetings alone.[18] Outreach visits to practicing clinicians can improve patient care[19] when information is delivered by persons trained to help with practice changes.[6] On-screen, point-of-care reminders generally produce small to moderate improvements in provider behavior and patient health.[20] Opinion leaders alone or in combination with other interventions may successfully promote evidence-based practice, but effectiveness varies within and between studies.[21] Audit and feedback using clinical performance data can be effective, especially when delivered frequently and over long time periods.[22] Methods that include sequenced activities or multiple exposures to activities display mixed results, though tending to produce more positive results than one-time methods.[2,13,14,23–25]

TABLE 10.2 Educational Interventions, Definitions, References, Outcomes, and Findings on Health Professions Continuing Education (CE) Evaluations

Interventions	Definitions	References	Outcomes	Findings
Educational materials	Distribution of published or printed recommendations for clinical care, including clinical practice guidelines, audiovisual materials, and electronic publications	Prior et al.[66] Marinopoulos et al.[13] Rotter et al.[67] Farmer et al.[17] Taylor et al.[68,87] Machin and Fogarty[45]	Level 3: Examination scores Level 5: Improved documentation Level 6: Decreased complications, length of stay, mortality with clinical pathways	Passive dissemination strategies found ineffective at improving clinical processes Live media more effective than print; multimedia more effective than single-media interventions; multiple exposures more effective than a single exposure Providing behavioral video examples increases effectiveness on performance outcomes Content derived from a task analysis increases training effectiveness Higher similarity between training and work environment is more effective
Educational meetings	Participation in conferences, lectures, workshops, or traineeships outside the practice setting	Davis et al.[69] Forsetlund et al.[18] Keith and Frese[52]	Level 5: Practice performance Level 6: Changes in health outcomes on occasion	Interactive sessions provide opportunity to practice skills and can effect change in professional practice Didactic sessions did not appear to change performance Error-based training is more effective on performance outcomes than error-avoidant training when clear feedback is given
Outreach visits	Use of a trained person who meets with providers in their practice settings to provide information for improving the providers' performance	Van Eijk et al.[70] O'Brien et al.[19]	Level 5: Clinical behavior Level 3: Improved knowledge evaluated by a pre- and post-test Level 6: Patients more likely to receive drugs that were less anticholinergic	Improved propriety of clinical prescribing behavior Outreach visits alone or when combined with other interventions have effects on prescribing; most effects are relatively small, but potentially important
Local opinion leaders	Use of providers nominated by their colleagues as educationally influential	Goldberg et al.[71] Flodgren et al.[21]	Level 5: Change in prescription rate Level 6: Increased percentage of adequately controlled hypertensives	Continuous quality improvement teams and opinion leader effective at changing physician practice Opinion leaders alone or in combination with other interventions may successfully promote evidence-based practice.

(continued)

Interventions	Definitions	References	Outcomes	Findings
Audit and feedback	Any summary of clinical performance of health care over a specified period, with or without recommendations for clinical action; the information may have been obtained from medical records, computerized databases, patients, or by observation	Jamtvedt et al.[22] Lobach et al.[72] Kluger and DeNisi[56]	Level 5: Changes in professional practice Level 6: Changes in guidance compliance	Effects of audit and feedback greater when feedback is delivered more frequently and over longer periods of time Computer-generated, individualized feedback found to be effective at improving compliance Immediate feedback during training is more effective for competence but less effective for improving performance
Reminders	Any intervention (manual or computerized) that prompts the physician to perform a clinical action (e.g., concurrent or intervisit reminders to professionals about desired actions such as screening or other preventive services, enhanced laboratory reports, or administrative support like follow-up appointment systems or stickers on charts)	Demakis et al.[73] Gill and Saldarriaga[74] Hung et al.[75] Shojania et al.[20]	Level 6: Changes in compliance rates Level 6: Composite result of lipid-lowering therapy Level 5: Higher rate of complete documentation by physicians Level 7: Immunization rates increased in large sample	Computer-based reminders improved compliance screening and immunization rates Paper chart-based clinical reminder did not change lipid-lowering therapy subscription
Multifaceted/ sequenced interventions	Select combinations of the aforementioned seven interventions (e.g., outreach visits followed by clinical information collected directly from patients and a computer reminder to counsel certain patients regarding a specific disorder)	Davis et al.[14] Mansouri and Lockyer[25] Robertson et al.[15] Baker et al.[16]	Level 3: Physician knowledge as measured on ankle and knee examination Level 5: Prescribing behavior Level 6: Changes in guidance compliance	Multiple interventions using audit and feedback are less effective than interventions using clinical education alone Multifaceted interventions are more likely to be effective than one-method interventions; passive approaches generally ineffective; active approaches effective under some circumstances Effective CE is ongoing, interactive, contextually relevant, and based on needs assessment Interventions addressing prospectively identified barriers are more likely to improve practice than no intervention

Emerging Strategies
· ·

Simulation-based training is an increasingly visible approach to instruction for technical, clinical, and teamwork skills across health care specialties. Issenberg et al.[26] specified elements of effective design including feedback; repetitive practice; integration; scaffolding or increasing levels of difficulty; clinical variation; controlled environment to help isolate attention on targeted KSAs; individualized learning; and simulator fidelity.

Internet-based learning is associated with large positive effects, in comparison with no intervention.[27] Electronic communities of practice[28] show promise for internet-based informal networks among health professionals with common interests. Communities of practice can interact on an ongoing basis, sharing knowledge over a sustained time period. Evaluations of the effectiveness of internet-based interventions on health practitioner behavior are weak, which makes links to patient outcomes difficult to show.

Educational games that require learners to participate in competitive activities with preset rules have been used in nursing education.[29] While educational games have been used commonly with medical and nursing students, a recent review assessing the effect of educational games on qualified health professionals' performance, KSAs, satisfaction, and/or patient outcomes found only one study that met the inclusion criteria.[30] Workers in a hospital setting demonstrated increased retention of knowledge (level 3), but patient or process of care outcomes were not assessed.[31]

Interprofessional education (IPE) is any type of educational, training, teaching, or learning session in which two or more health or social care professions learn interactively. In a recent review by Reeves et al.,[32] four of six studies found IPE projects improved some ways that professionals worked together and improved the care they provided. Improvements include decreased errors in an emergency department and better management of care delivered to domestic violence victims. Additional studies are required to determine the relative value of component interventions on individual health professions and teams.

Zwarenstein et al.[33] recently reviewed studies of interprofessional collaboration, defined as practice-based interventions placed in health care settings to improve working behavior among two or more types of health care professions. The studies evaluated interprofessional rounds, meetings, and externally facilitated interprofessional audit. Three studies found patient care improvements such as use of pharmaceuticals, length of hospital stay, and total hospital charges. More research is needed to understand the effects of the various interventions, how they affect interprofessional collaboration, and how they lead to changes in health care including the circumstances where interventions are most useful.

Further research is necessary to determine whether simulation-based training, internet-based learning, educational games, IPE, and interprofessional collaboration improve outcomes at levels 5, 6, and 7.

Evidence for Outcomes Assessment and Instructional Design

Research findings show that multifaceted CE interventions are most effective at producing professional outcomes. However, research findings are inconsistent for changes in performance, patient health, and community health at levels 5, 6, and 7, respectively. This makes it difficult to (a) plan for the most effective CE activity, (b) estimate expected outcomes, and (c) determine the overall value of investing in CE in the health professions. One possible explanation for the inconsistent findings is that instructional strategies that underlie CE interventions vary within each intervention category.[34,35] For example, the amount of shared feedback, type of content, and degree of interactivity influence the effectiveness of an intervention on outcomes.[18,36] A more robust approach to research and planning is required to help explain the inconsistency within interventions and across variations in practitioners, settings, and behaviors. Measuring the unique effects of carefully specified instructional strategies should better inform education planners, learners, and evaluators about how interventions can be designed in an optimal fashion. A 2009 review of the effects of CE meetings and workshops on professional practice and health care outcomes identified only 17% of studies reporting the use of theory to design processes to create or support behavior change.[18] A more recent systematic review of interventions tailored to support transfer of training in health care showed that only six out of 26 studies (23%) reported use of theory to guide the instructional design of the tailored intervention.[16] Improved use of instructional theory and more treatment specificity are needed to strengthen educational interventions that yield powerful outcomes.[35,37,38]

Evidence for Training as a Mechanism of Change

Three major goals are served through health professions CE: (1) new knowledge, skills, or attitudes are learned; (2) knowledge, skills, or attitudes are maintained at a minimum level of competency; or (3) the level of proficiency for existing knowledge, skills, or attitudes is increased. CE interventions in the health professions aim to positively influence performance and patient outcomes[39] and studies suggest there is modest transfer of training to on-the-job performance (level 5).[13,14,16] The primary goal of training is to affect higher-level behavioral outcomes, but failure to detect the training impact on performance (level 5) is common in health care[16] and in other industries.[39,40] There are a couple of possible reasons for this limitation. First, those who plan or evaluate education and training of health professionals in organizations fail to evaluate outcomes at levels 5, 6, or 7. Second, workplace context effects prevent CE-acquired knowledge, skills, or attitudes to be manifest in the work environment.

The Cochrane Effective Practice and Organisation of Care Group[41] identified nine categories of barriers to change that prevent the effects of a CE intervention from reaching level 5, performance outcomes in the practice setting. The barriers include information management, clinical uncertainty, sense of competence, perceptions of liability, patient expectations, standards of practice, financial distinctiveness, administrative constraints, and others.[41] Baker et al.[16] investigated tailored interventions, defined as strategies planned to take account of prospectively identified barriers to change and to improve professional practice. The study found the effects of tailored interventions were inconsistent, and few studies collected outcomes data at levels 5 and 6. Out of 14 studies that met inclusion criteria for review, eight were found to be effective, two reported benefits for some outcomes, and four reported no benefits with outcomes measured at levels 5 and 6.

Training interventions can be manipulated to promote the degree to which training affects knowledge (level 3), competence (level 4), and performance (level 5) outcomes.[42,43] One example is the use of the theory of identical elements, which predicts that the more similar the learning environment is to the transfer environment, the more transfer will occur.[44] Machin and Fogarty[45] found that similarity of the training environment was positively related to self-reported performance (level 5) in a transfer task for advanced training of a computerized information system. Measuring across a variety of skills, Saks and Belcourt[46] found that using elements (e.g., training environment, setting, task characteristics) that were more similar to the work environment explained 20% of the variance in transfer of training on performance outcomes (level 5). Research has shown that increasing the similarity of training characteristics to the real-world task can increase the ability to detect training effectiveness on performance outcomes (level 5).[42,45,46]

Instruction is more deductive and focused when specific strategies, concepts, and rules for learning are provided explicitly. Studies show that instructional methods that maximize knowledge (level 3) and competence (level 4) may actually impair performance (level 5).[47–49] Alternative instructional approaches where trainees induce learning strategies and rules can be used to strengthen the effectiveness of training interventions on performance outcomes (level 5). Error-based training is a useful example. Error-based training is a strategy where learners are given minimal guidance and are encouraged to make errors during the training. Errors provide learning opportunities that lead to skills transfer on performance outcomes (level 5) compared with training where learners are told to avoid errors.[50] Other studies spanning a variety of tasks show that error-based training supports performance (level 5) on the job but impairs competence behavior (level 4) measured under controlled conditions.[51,52] Another instructional method, called guided discovery, organizes training so that learners are allowed to explore learning strategies with minimal guidance.[53] Such training provides information about appropriate strategies (e.g., advanced cardiac life support algorithms) but gives minimum feedback. Examples of guidance include providing leading questions or prompting without providing specific tactics and solutions.[54] Debowski et al.[55] found guided discovery to be most effective on complex, ill-structured tasks where there is less feedback received. Specific and immediate feedback may be important when evaluating learners for acquisition of new knowledge (level 3) and skills immediately after training (level 4), but less so for advanced skill development and transfer over time (level 5).[56] Less specific and immediate feedback is conducive to metacognitive processes that support training-appropriate processes that are needed when evaluating performance (level 5) in the transfer environment.[48] This is critical—for instance, when surgeons must adapt their strategies in response to complications in a surgery compared with no complications. Error-based training and guided discovery are two examples where instructional strategies may actually lead to lower levels of training effectiveness when measured on knowledge (level 3) and competence outcomes (level 4), yet yield higher levels of training effectiveness when measured on performance outcomes (level 5).[49,51–53]

Recent case studies of performance in primary care[57–59] suggest trained quality improvement coaches working on-site in primary care offices may use conference calls and performance feedback to increase office efficiency (level 5) and improve quality of care measures such as hemoglobin A1c and blood pressure (level 6). On-the-job training often occurs in surgical practice and has been shown to be effective in some instances. A study investigating how practicing surgeons trained for laparoscopic cholecystectomy procedures found that out of 1352 surgeons who used the procedure, 63.6% reported having had their first procedure supervised or assisted by a more experienced surgeon.[60] One study comparing patient outcomes 12 months after receiving endoscopic surgery showed no significant differences between patients treated by an expert surgeon and patients treated by a supervised trainee.[61] Other studies lend more support to the use of on-the-job training in surgical procedures. Yamashita et al.[62] investigated incidences of major complications during laparoscopic cholecystectomy procedures. They found surgeons who were supervised for their first 10 procedures demonstrated lower incidence of major complications in subsequent procedures than surgeons who were supervised for only their first two procedures. Liem et al.[63] suggested that supervision of a less experienced surgeon by an experienced surgeon during extraperitoneal laparoscopic hernia repair is vital when converting to a new technique, after finding a significant difference in patient complications.

A meta-analysis conducted by Winfred et al.[64] showed that the effects of various training strategies differed as a function of the targeted type of KSA and on the level of evaluation measured using Kirkpatrick's[65] four-level evaluation framework. In Kirkpatrick's framework, reactions (i.e., level 1) refers to the degree to which participants judge the training favorably and is similar to satisfaction (i.e., level 2) in the Moore et al.[7] framework. Learning, level 2 in the Kirkpatrick framework, refers to the degree to which learners acquire the targeted KSAs as a result of participating in the training and is comparable with declarative knowledge, procedural knowledge, and competence—levels 3a, 3b, and 4, respectively, within the Moore et al.[7] framework. Behavior, level 3 in the Kirkpatrick framework, refers to the degree to which the targeted KSAs are applied when the learner returns to the job environment and is comparable with level performance (i.e., level 5) within the Moore et al.[7] framework. Results, level 4 in the Kirkpatrick framework, refers to the impact training has on indirect outcomes the training is intended to improve; this is comparable with levels 6 and 7, respectively (patient and community health) within the Moore et al.[7] framework. A limitation of the Moore et al.[7] framework is that it explicitly addresses declarative knowledge, procedural knowledge, and skills but does not address the attitude measurement (e.g., patient safety attitudes) as an outcome. Given this limitation, the Moore et al.[7] framework is advantaged because it provides better sensitivity to detect training effects for knowledge and also addresses health care outcomes. Moore et al.'s[7] outcomes framework can be used as a guide to conceptualize which outcome level is most desired and realistic. This would be based ideally on a needs analysis that identifies KSA gaps. It is important to specify the targeted KSAs,

CE goal, and outcome level. Pre- and post-training activities may affect how well a particular CE intervention transfers to the workplace.[40] The effects of pre- and post-training activities will have the greatest effect on level 5, 6, and 7 outcomes, because of the context of measurement within an organization.[42,45,46]

Cost-Inclusive Evaluation

Those who plan CE and training in the health professions face steady pressures to control resource utilization and costs. Equivocal results about the effects of education and training on performance and patient health provide limited relief to planners and policy makers. This is especially the case as physicians respond to regulatory requirements that govern their free circulation to practice among various jurisdictions, medical institutions, or specialty certifications.[11,76–79] A more synchronized and aligned collection of medical registration or licensing boards, specialty boards, and organizations granting practice privileges is needed to inform the design of education and performance assessment. However, links of CE to practice and patient outcomes remain unclear. More data are required, not only to explain CE effectiveness but also to determine the costs and benefits of CE and training.[80]

Those responsible for leading the education and training of practicing health professionals must understand the economic relationships that sustain program budgets.[81] Cost-inclusive evaluation offers three main strategies for gaining knowledge of resource use.[81–83]

1. *Cost analysis* is the measured costs of program implementation—for example, an average of $200 per physician participating in a live, face-to-face, 4-hour workshop on incision and drainage of a skin abscess.

2. *Cost-effectiveness analysis* combines cost analysis with an assessment of the results of program implementation measured in nonmonetary units—for example, an internet-based program that costs $200 per physician and saves 4 hours of physician time spent learning incision skills relative to no training program at all. When comparing two programs (e.g., live, face-to-face and an internet-based program), a cost-effectiveness analysis might find that the internet-based program costs $200 more per physician but that it saves 4 hours of physician time spent learning incision skills.

3. *Cost-benefit analysis* combines cost analysis with an assessment of the value of resources gained through the program measured in the same units as costs (typically money)—for example, a cost of $1000 to teach five physicians

incision skills, which allows them to perform an additional 20 procedures annually, where each procedure can be billed at $85 per procedure generates a cost-benefit ratio of $20 \times 5 \times \$85 / \$1000 = 8.5$.

There are varied perspectives on cost-inclusive evaluation. For example, to a CME administrator the costs of an educational activity differ from its costs to an individual physician participant who is interested in knowledge acquisition. Cost perspectives also differ for a sponsoring institution concerned with changing physician performance or to a health care payer sensitive to the utilization of health care resources and patient outcomes. Cost-inclusive evaluation can take one or more of these perspectives. At the outset of a project, an evaluation design should include consensus measures articulated to determine relative progress toward project goals.[81,83]

Three Models to Guide Instructional Design in Health Care Continuing Education and Training

Leaders in education and health care are challenged to improve the quality of care, decrease the risk of adverse events, and reduce expenses. Current health care systems fail to use evidence optimally, which results in inefficient care and reduced quantity and quality of life.[84] Three popular models offer value in helping to resolve challenges of instruction and measurement in the application of learning from knowledge (level 3) to competence (level 4) and from competence (level 4) to performance (level 5). One model derives from education and the study of physicians as learners, a second model derives from organizational psychology and the study of transfer of training, and a third model derives from a multidisciplinary perspective on knowledge translation.

Figure 10.1 depicts the process of change and learning,[85] a model generated from analysis of 775 changes reported from interviews with 340 physicians located across North America. In this model, three interrelated sets of forces drive change. Personal forces include curiosity and the desire for personal well-being. Professional forces include career stage, desire for competence, and advances in the clinical environment. Social forces include family and community, regulation, and interaction with other health professionals. Change occurs as the clarity and importance of discrepancies between present performance and required performance grow more meaningful to the physician-learner. Effort spent in learning activities, such as reading and educational meetings, depends upon the size and

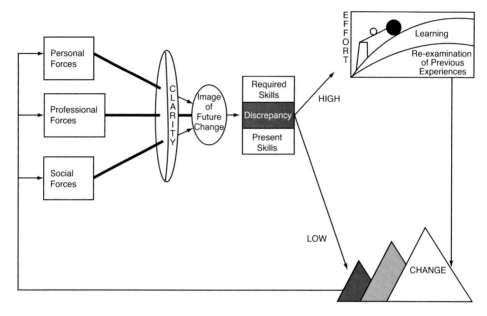

FIGURE 10.1 The process of change and learning

complexity of needed change. Accommodations are small, simple changes that are often attitudinal. Adjustments show incremental differences in an element of practice—for example, changing from use of a rigid sygmoidoscope to use of a flexible sygmoidoscope. Redirections and transformations are larger, more complex changes in the structure of lives or practices. Examples include dropping obstetrics from an obstetrics and gynecology practice or moving a clinic from one location of town to another. The role of the planner is to facilitate recognition of the gap between present and desired skills and to assure access to learning resources required to close the gap.

Figure 10.2, a model of training transfer,[37] emphasizes that much of what is being trained for knowledge acquisition (level 3) and competence (level 4) fails to be applied in the work setting. The model suggests six linkages among training inputs, training outputs, and the conditions of transfer. Three major sets of training inputs are described: (1) trainee characteristics, including ability, personality, and motivation; (2) training design, including principles of learning, the sequence of training of activities, and training content; and (3) the work environment, including support before and after training and opportunities to apply what was learned. The conditions of transfer require that the acquired knowledge and skills are generalized to the job and that learning is maintained over time. Training outcomes include the knowledge, skills, and affect acquired as a function of training and the retention of the training content.[37]

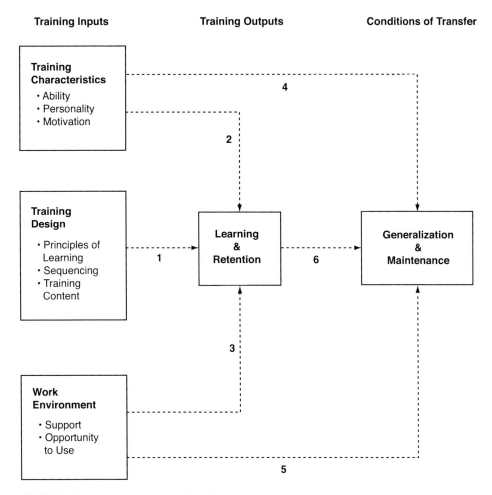

FIGURE 10.2 A model of transfer training

Source: Baldwin TT, Ford JK. Transfer of training: a review and directions for future research. *Pers Psychol*. 1988; **41**(1): 63–105. Reproduced with permission.

Figure 10.3 illustrates the knowledge-to-action framework,[86] a model deriving common elements from an assessment of 30 theories of planning action. A knowledge creation component involves three phases: (1) knowledge inquiry, (2) knowledge synthesis, and (3) knowledge tools and product creation. Knowledge creation (level 3) enables knowledge refinement for application by end users. Algorithms or practice guidelines form examples of knowledge tools shared in an action cycle of processes needed to implement knowledge in health care (level 5). The action cycle includes identification of a problem; identifying, reviewing, and selecting the knowledge to utilize; adapting or customizing knowledge to the local context; assessing knowledge use determinants; selecting,

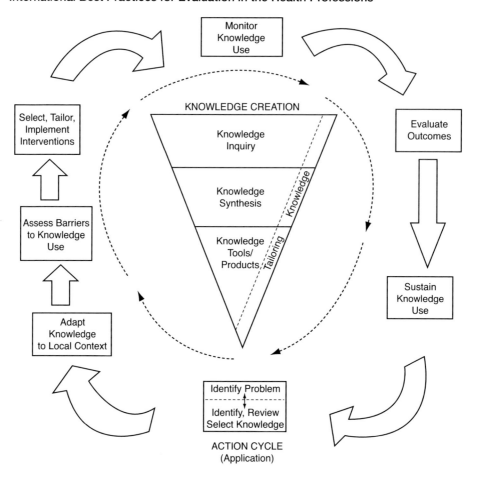

FIGURE 10.3 The knowledge-to-action framework

tailoring, implementing, and monitoring knowledge translation interventions (level 5); evaluating outcomes or impact of using the knowledge; and determining strategies for ensuring sustained use of the knowledge. Consideration of the end users is integral to the sensibility of the framework.

A positive aspect of the process of change and learning is its authenticity. It was generated from stories of successful changes made by practicing physicians. One strength of a model of training transfer is its emphasis on making improvements at the job site. A benefit of the knowledge-to-action framework is its unique focus on creation of knowledge tools to move evidence to practice in health care. A limitation of all the models is the lack of sound research testing hypotheses derived from their various theoretical constructs. The science must be improved to select and study the best models as planners and policy makers extend efforts and limited resources to improve the quality of education and health care.

Science in Continuing Education and Training in Health Care
• • • • • • • • • • • • • • • •

Taylor et al.[87] conducted a meta-analysis on the transfer of 107 management training interventions. They found performance ratings that linked training content derived from needs analysis were conducive to detecting effects of the intervention on performance, Moore's outcome level 5. Similarly, behaviorally anchored rating systems that narrowly define performance behaviors for each scale value can help align self-report of performance and supervisor expectations.[88] Self-report measures that are closely associated with training content and highly specified outcomes are more predictive of actual performance than using general statements.[89]

Many assessment methods fail to predict on-the-job performance.[48] Across the continuum of medical education, the educational planner's ability to make informed selection of outcomes measures is constrained by limited evidence for reliability and validity of data derived from assessment and evaluation instruments.[90–97] In a review of 115 instruments used for evaluation of evidence-based practice, of which 30 exclusively assessed physicians, Shaneyfelt and colleagues[94] found most studies reported at least one source of validity evidence but that only 10% used multiple types of validity evidence to support inferences made from the instrument scores. In a review of 32 CME evaluation studies, results indicate that of 10 studies that developed and applied a new instrument, none reported reliability or validity evidence.[95] Finally, Ratanawongsa and colleagues[93] reviewed CME evaluations limited to randomized control trial and historic/concurrent comparison designs, including only studies that reported either reliability or validity evidence. Of 62 instruments reviewed, only 16% reported both reliability and validity evidence. The majority of studies reported internal consistency reliability or inter-rater reliability; however, validity evidence was not reported for one-half of the instruments.

Table 10.3 reports four main findings of the current review: (1) effects are inconsistent across practitioners, settings, and behaviors, and gaps in performance present opportunities for improvement; (2) interactive learning and opportunities to practice skills can affect change; (3) sequenced and multifaceted activities can effect change in practice and patient outcomes; and (4) training content similar to the practice environment is more likely to affect change than training content that is dissimilar to practice, but providing varied cases and contexts is effective for transfer of training to multiple contexts.

Learners are advised to (a) set learning goals based on performance data and select educational activities that enable achievement of learning goals or identification of gaps in practice; (b) select educational activities that meet clinical performance needs individually and in teams, seeking educational activities with leaders who build on the learners' knowledge and skills and enable not only the observation but also testing of new skills in the practice setting; (c) participate in learning activities with clearly stated objectives that enable measured progress over a predetermined period of time; and (d) match the education or training environment to the practice contexts where performance will be demonstrated.

Planners are advised to (a) provide reliable data for learners to reflect upon present levels of performance compared with desired levels of performance; (b) offer consultation to help learners specify achievable and measurable goals while enabling comfortable communication and practice of what is learned among individuals or teams; (c) design activities with the goal of helping individuals or teams of learners adopt change incrementally, assuring compatibility with present systems and advantage over present behaviors and measuring results including clinical progress and costs; and (d) design education and training activities that provide more immersive and realistic contexts to practice or learn the intended KSAs.

Evaluators are encouraged to (a) develop consensus about an evaluation design that links evaluation to instructional objectives and includes an assessed need or gap in performance, a carefully delineated instructional strategy, evaluation tools, and costs; (b) select or develop observational tools to reliably evaluate knowledge, competence, and performance; (c) assess satisfaction and perceived value for each component of multifaceted interventions, including the overall impact of instruction on performance and patient health; and (d) evaluate demonstration of KSAs in variable contexts, including transfer of KSAs to practice.

TABLE 10.3 Findings and Implications for Learners, Planners, and Evaluators in Continuing Education and Training

Findings	What Learners Can Do	What Planners Can Do	What Evaluators Can Do
Need: Effects are inconsistent across practitioners, settings, and behaviors; gaps in current and desired performance present opportunities for improvement (Davis et al.,[14,24] Oxman et al.[98] Salas and Cannon-Bowers[99])	Set learning goals based on practice performance data Select educational activities needed to achieve goals or that help identify needs	Provide reliable data to enable learners to see present levels of performance compared with optimum performance Provide the learner with an opportunity to reflect upon present and desired levels of performance	Develop consensus about an evaluation design including assessed need or gap in performance, instructional strategies, evaluation tools, and costs Link evaluation items to educational objectives based on need

Findings	What Learners Can Do	What Planners Can Do	What Evaluators Can Do
Interactive: Interactive learning and opportunities to practice skills can effect change (O'Brien et al.,[100] Davis et al.,[14,69])	Select educational activities designed to meet your clinical performance needs and those of persons you may work with as members of a health care team Seek seminars, workshops, or other activities with leaders who build on your knowledge and skills as resources into the educational sessions Select activities that enable you and others to observe new knowledge and skills and to use them in your practice setting	Offer consultation to help learners specify goals that are achievable and measurable Enable comfortable communication among individuals or teams involved in the educational activity Enable physicians or teams to try in practice what is learned with limited fear of failure	Select or develop observational tools to reliably rate competence, knowledge, and performance
Multifaceted: Sequenced and multifaceted activities can effect change in practice and patient outcomes (Davis et al.,[14,69] Davis and Taylor-Vaisey[101])	Participate in learning activities with instructional objectives clearly stating what you will know or be able to do as you progress from one level of knowledge or skill to another Choose educational activities that enable you to progress incrementally (e.g., over a period of days or weeks in reading, seminars, or skills application sessions)	Design activities with the cumulative goal of helping physicians or teams of learners to adopt change incrementally, assuring there is compatibility with present systems and advantage over present behaviors Measure the results of educational activities intended to improve clinical care Assess the effects of educational and clinical improvements including budgetary performance	Assess satisfaction and perceived value of each component of multifaceted interventions Measure instructional strategies and sequence and evaluate impact on performance and patient health
Education and Training Content: Training content similar to practice environment is more effective (Saks and Belcourt,[40] Machin and Fogarty[45]) Providing varied cases and contexts is effective for transfer (Taylor et al.,[68] Schmidt and Bjork[48])	Match training environments, training content, and cases to the practice environment Provide variable contexts if learner is expected to perform skills in multiple contexts	Choose education and training activities that provide immersive and realistic contexts to practice or learn the intended knowledge, skills, and attitudes	Evaluate demonstration of knowledge, skills, and attitudes in variable contexts, including transfer of knowledge, skills, and attitudes in practice

An overarching concern for CE planners and evaluators involves the categorical approach to classifying and comparing the relative effectiveness of educational interventions. The approach may be helpful to understanding that some categories are more effective than others, but current approaches to categorization lack sensitivity and specificity to support an understanding of the causal mechanisms that undergird behavioral change.[35] A reliable method is required for specifying and reporting complex interventions. Michie et al.[35] suggest:

> The components involved in complex interventions include the techniques that facilitate behavior change that constitute the active ingredients of the intervention and procedures for delivery of those techniques. The techniques that target the behavior of individuals may be delivered in a variety of ways (e.g., prompts or patient reminders may be delivered by a telephone call from a health care professional or by a hand washing sign strategically located in an exam room). Techniques are the replicable components of an intervention designed to alter or redirect causal processes that regulate behavior; a technique proposed to be an "active ingredient" must have specified minimum criteria for implementation (e.g., feedback must involve providing the target audience with information about their behavior). The identification of behavior change techniques is critical to understanding how organizational change and policy changes, including policies around price and access, have their effects on individuals' health-related problems and physicians' capacity to help solve them through lifelong learning and self-assessment.

CE planners and evaluators must recognize that health care and education are delivered in highly complex and variable settings and must also recognize that results from uniform interventions are likely to vary and to be imperfect. Answering the question of what works in CE does not ask for a description of past performance of an intervention or for a prediction of future performance. It requires that the past and the future be addressed simultaneously; the former with evaluation results and the latter through a line of reasoning that connects past results to future actions.[102] This will be the case until a scientific substrate for change is more fully elaborated. As the processes and results of science advance theoretical understandings of instruction, learning, and change, evaluators must work together with researchers and practitioners to discover, apply, and measure results in practice.

References

1. Ganz PA, Litwin MS, Hayes RD, et al. Measuring outcomes in health-related quality of life. In: Anderson RM, Rice TH, Komnski GF, editors. *Changing the US Healthcare System.* San Francisco, CA: Jossey-Bass; 2007. pp. 185–211.

2. Mazmanian PE, Davis DA, Galbraith R. Continuing medical education effect on clinical outcomes: effectiveness of continuing medical education: American College of Chest Physicians Evidence-Based Educational Guidelines. *CHEST.* 2009; **135**(Suppl. 3): S49–55.

3. McGlynn EA. Evaluating the quality of care. In: Anderson RM, Rice TH, Komnski GF, editors. *Changing the US Healthcare System.* San Francisco, CA: Jossey-Bass; 2007. pp. 213–44.

4. Fletcher RH, Fletcher SW, Wagner EH. *Clinical Epidemiology: the essentials.* 2nd ed. Baltimore, MD: Williams & Wilkins; 1988.

5. Davis DA, Evans M, Jadad A, et al. The case for knowledge translation: shortening the journey from evidence to effect. *BMJ.* 2003; **327**(7405): 33–5.

6. Wentz DK, Jackson MJ, Raichle L, et al. Forces for change in the landscape of CME, CPD, and health-systems linked education. In: Davis D, Barnes BE, Fox R, editors. *The Continuing Professional Development of Physicians.* Chicago, IL: AMA Press; 2003. pp. 25–47.

7. Moore DE, Green JS, Gallis HA. Achieving the desired results and improved outcomes: integrating planning and assessment throughout learning activities. *J Contin Educ Health Prof.* 2009; **29**(1): 1–15.

8. Miller GE. The assessment of clinical skills/competence/performance. *Acad Med.* 1990; **65**(Suppl. 9): S63–7.

9. Moore DE Jr. Needs assessment in the new health care environment: combining discrepancy analysis and outcomes to create more effective CME. *J Contin Educ Health Prof.* 1998; **18**(3): 133–41.

10. Institute of Medicine. *Redesigning Continuing Education in the Health Professions.* Washington, DC: The National Academies Press; 2010.

11. Maisonneuve H, Matillon Y, Negri A, et al. Continuing medical education and professional revalidation in Europe: five case examples. *J Contin Educ Health Prof.* 2009; **29**(1): 58–62.

12. Cochrane Database of Systematic Reviews. *The Cochrane Collaboration.* Available at: www.thecochranelibrary.com/view/0/index.html (accessed July 13, 2011).

13. Marinopoulos SS, Dorman T, Ratanawongsa N, et al. *Effectiveness of Continuing Medical Education.* Evidence Report/Technology Assessment No. 149 (prepared by the Johns Hopkins Evidence-based Practice Center, under Contract No. 290-02-0018.) AHRQ Publication No. 07-E006. Rockville, MD: Agency for Healthcare Research and Quality; 2007.

14. Davis DA, Thomson MA, Oxman AD, et al. Changing physician performance. *JAMA.* 1995; **274**(9): 700–5.

15. Robertson MK, Umble KE, Cervero RM. Impact studies in continuing education for health professions: update. *J Contin Educ Health Prof.* 2003; **23**(3): 146–56.

16. Baker R, Camosso-Stefinovic J, Gillies C, et al. Tailored interventions to overcome identified barriers to change: effects on professional practice and health care outcomes. *Cochrane Database Syst Rev.* 2010; **3**: CD005470.

17. Farmer AP, Legare F, Turcot L, et al. Printed educational materials: effects on professional practice and health care outcomes. *Cochrane Database Syst Rev.* 2009; **3**: CD004398.

18. Forsetlund L, Bjorndal A, Rashidian A, et al. Continuing education meeting and workshops: effects on professional practice and health care outcomes. *Cochrane Database Syst Rev.* 2009; **2**: CD003030.

19. O'Brien MA, Rogers S, Jamtvedt G, et al. Educational outreach visits: effects on professional practice and health care outcomes. *Cochrane Database Syst Rev.* 2008; **4**: CD000409.

20. Shojania KG, Jennings A, Mayhew A, et al. The effects of on-screen, point of care computer reminders on processes and outcomes of care. *Cochrane Database Syst Rev.* 2009; **3**: CD001096.

21. Flodgren G, Parmelli E, Doumit G, et al. Local opinion leaders: effects on professional practice and health care outcomes. *Cochrane Database Syst Rev.* 2010; **1**: CD000125.

22. Jamtvedt G, Young JM, Kristoffersen DT, et al. Does telling people what they have been doing change what they do: a systematic review of the effects of audit and feedback. *Qual Saf Health Care.* 2006; **15**(6): 433–6.

23. Davis DA, Galbraith R. Continuing medical education effect on practice performance: effectiveness of continuing medical education: American College of Chest Physicians Evidence-Based Educational Guidelines. *Chest.* 2009; **135**(Suppl. 3): S425–85.

24. Davis DA, Thomson MA, Oxman AD, et al. Evidence for the effectiveness of CME: a review of 50 randomized controlled trials. *JAMA.* 1992; **268**(9): 1135–6.

25. Mansouri M, Lockyer J. A meta-analysis of continuing medical education effectiveness. *J Contin Educ Health Prof.* 2007; **27**(1): 6–15.

26. Issenberg SB, McGaghie WC, Petrusa ER, et al. Features and uses of high fidelity medical simulation that lead to effective learning: a BEME systematic review. *Med Teach.* 2005; **27**(1): 10–28.

27. Cook DA, Levinson AJ, Garside S, et al. Internet-based learning in the health professions: a meta-analysis. *JAMA.* 2008; **300**(10): 1181–96.

28. Ho K, Jarvis-Selinger S, Norman CD, et al. Electronic communities of practice: guidelines from a project. *J Contin Educ Health Prof.* 2010; **29**(3): 133–4.

29. Fitzgerald K. Instructional methods: selection, use, and evaluation. In: Bastable S, editor. *Nurse as Educator: principles of teaching and learning.* Sudbury MA: Jones & Bartlett; 1997, pp. 261–86.

30. Akl EA, Sackett KM, Pretorius R, et al. Educational games for health professionals. *Cochrane Database Syst Rev.* 2009; **1**: CD006411.

31. Burke CT. *The Influences of Teaching Strategies and Reinforcement Techniques on Health Care Workers' Learning and Retention* [dissertation]. Hattiesburg: The University of Southern Mississippi; 2001.

32. Reeves S, Zwarenstein M, Goldman J, et al. Interprofessional education: effects on professional practice and health care outcomes. *Cochrane Database Syst Rev.* 2009; **1**: CD002213.

33. Zwarenstein M, Goldman J, Reeves S. Interprofessional collaboration: effects of practice-based interventions on professional practice and healthcare outcomes. *Cochrane Database Syst Rev.* 2009; **3**: CD000072.

34. Bell BS, Kozlowski SWJ. Active learning: effects of core training design elements on self-regulatory processes, learning, and adaptability. *J Appl Psychol.* 2008; **93**(2): 296–316.

35. Michie S, Abraham C, Eccles MP, et al. Strengthening evaluation and implementation by specifying components of behavior change interventions: a study protocol. *Implement Sci.* 2011; **6**: 10.

36. Salas ES, Cannon-Bowers JA. The science of training: a decade of progress. *Annu Rev Psychol.* 2001; **52**: 471–99.

37. Ford JK, Weissbein DA. Transfer of training: an updated review and analysis. *Perf Imp Quart.* 1997; **10**(2): 22–41.

38. Winfred A Jr., Bennett W Jr., Edens PS, et al. Effectiveness of training in organizations. *J App Psychol.* 2003; **88**(2): 234–45.

39. Kozlowski SWJ, Brown K, Weissbein D, et al. A multi-level approach to training effectiveness: enhancing horizontal and vertical transfer. In: Klein K, Kozlowski SWJ, editors. *Multilevel Theory, Research and Methods in Organization.* San Francisco, CA: Jossey-Bass; 2000. pp. 157–210.

40. Saks AM, Belcourt M. An investigation of training activities and transfer of training in organizations. *Hum Res Manag.* 2006; **45**(4): 629–48.

41. Cochrane Effective Practice and Organisation of Care Review Group. *Data Collection Checklist.* EPOC resources for review authors, revised. 2002. Available at: www.epoc.cochrane.org/en/handsearchers.html (accessed July 13, 2011).

42. Brinkerhoff RO, Montesino MU. Partnership for training transfer: lessons from a corporate study. *Hum Res Dev Quart.* 1995; **6**(3): 263–74.

43. Kraiger K, Salas E, Cannon-Bowers JA. Measuring knowledge organization as a method for assessing learning during training. *Hum Factors.* 1995; **37**(4): 804–16.

44. Royer JM. Theories of the transfer of learning. *Educ Psychol.* 1979; **14**(1): 53–69.

45. Machin MA, Fogarty GJ. Perceptions of training-related factors and personal variables as predictors of transfer implementation intentions. *J Bus Psychol.* 2003; **18**(1): 51–71.

46. Saks AM, Belcourt M. An investigation of training activities and transfer of training in organizations. *Hum Res Manag.* 2006; **45**(4): 629–48.

47. Christina RW, Bjork RA. Optimizing long-term retention and transfer. In: Druckman D, Bjork RA, editors. *In the Mind's Eye: enhancing human performance.* Washington, DC: National Academy Press; 1991. pp. 23–55.

48. Schmidt RA, Bjork RA. New conceptualizations of practice: common principles in three paradigms suggest new concepts for training. *Psychol Sci.* 1992; **3**(4): 207–17.

49. Goodman, JS. The interactive effects of task and external feedback on practice performance and learning. *Organ Behav Hum Dec.* 1998; **76**(3): 232–52.

50. Keith N, Frese M. Self-regulation in error management training: emotion control and metacognition as mediators of performance effects. *J Appl Psychol.* 2005; **90**(4): 677–91.

51. Frese M, Brodbeck F, Heinbokel T, et al. Errors in training computer skills: on the positive function of error. *Hum-Comput Interact.* 1991; **6**(1): 77–93.

52. Keith N, Frese M. Effectiveness of error management training: a meta-analysis. *J Appl Psychol.* 2008; **93**(1): 56–69.

53. Bell BS, Kozlowski SWJ. Adaptive guidance: enhancing self-regulation, knowledge, and performance in technology-based training. *Pers Psychol.* 2002; **55**: 267–306.

54. Kamouri AL, Kamouri J, Smith KH. Training by exploration: facilitating the transfer of procedural knowledge through analogical reasoning. *Int J Man Mach Stud.* 1986; **24**(2): 171–92.

55. Debowski S, Wood RE, Bandura A. Impact of guided exploration and enactive exploration on self-regulatory mechanisms and information acquisition through electronic search. *J Appl Psychol.* 2001; **86**(6): 1129–41.

56. Kluger AN, DeNisi A. The effects of feedback interventions on performance: a historical review, a meta-analysis and a preliminary feedback intervention theory. *Psychol Bull.* 1996; **119**(2): 254–84.

57. Steiner RM, Walsworth DT. Using quality experts from manufacturing to transform primary care. *J Contin Educ Health Prof.* 2010; **30**(2): 95–105.

58. Newton WP, Lefebvre A, Donahue KE, et al. Infrastructure for large-scale quality improvement projects: early lessons from North Carolina improving performance in practice. *J Contin Educ Health Prof.* 2010; **30**(2): 106–13.

59. Bricker PL, Baron RJ, Scheirer JJ, et al. Collaboration in Pennsylvania: rapidly spreading improved chronic care for patients to practices. *J Contin Educ Health Prof.* 2010; **30**(2): 114–25.

60. Escarce JJ, Shea JA, Schwartz JS. How practicing surgeons trained for laparoscopic cholecystectomy. *Med Care.* 1997; **35**(3): 291–6.

61. Phillips JS, Vowler SL, Salam MA. Is training in endoscopic sinus surgery detrimental to patient outcome? *J Surg Educ.* 2007; **64**(5): 278–81.

62. Yamashita Y, Kurohiji T, Kakegawa T. Evaluation of two training programs for laparoscopic cholecystectomy: incidence of major complications. *World J Surg.* 1994; **18**(2): 279–85.

63. Liem MSL, van Steensel CJ, Boelhouwer RU, et al. The learning curve for totally extraperitoneal paparoscopic inguinal hernia repair. *Am J Surg.* 1996; **171**: 281–5.

64. Winfred A Jr., Bennett W Jr., Edens PS, et al. Effectiveness of training in organizations: a meta-analysis of design and evaluation features. *J Appl Psychol.* 2003; **88**(2): 234–45.

65. Kirkpatrick DL. *Evaluating Training Programs: the four levels.* San Francisco, CA: Berret-Koehler Publishers; 1994.

66. Prior M, Guerin M, Frimmer-Somers K. The effectiveness of clinical guideline implementation strategies—a synthesis of systematic review findings. *J Eval Clin Prac.* 2008; **14**(5): 888–97.

67. Rotter T, Kinsman L, James EL, et al. Clinical pathways: effects on professional

practice, patient outcomes, length of stay and hospital costs. *Cochrane Database Syst Rev.* 1999; **3**: CD006632.

68. Taylor PJ, Russ-Eft DF, Chan DWL. A meta-analytic review of behavior modeling training. *J Appl Psychol.* 2005; **90**(4): 692–709.

69. Davis DA, O'Brien MA, Freemantle N, et al. Do conferences, workshops, rounds, and other traditional continuing education activities change physician behavior or health care outcomes? *JAMA.* 1999; **282**(9): 867–74.

70. Van Eijk MEC, Avorn J, Porsius AJ, et al. Reducing prescribing of highly anticholinergic antidepressants for elderly people: randomized trial of group versus individual academic detailing. *BMJ.* 2001; **322**(7287): 654–7.

71. Goldberg HI, Wagner EH, Fihn SD, et al. A randomized controlled trial of CQI teams and academic detailing: can they alter compliance with guidelines? *Jt Comm J Qual Improv.* 1998; **24**(3): 130–42.

72. Lobach DF. Electronically distributed, computer-generated, individualized feedback enhances the use of a computerized practice guideline. *Proc AMIA Annu Fall Symp.* 1996; 493–7.

73. Demakis JG, Beauchamp C, Cull WL, et al. Improving residents' compliance with standards of ambulatory care: results from the VA cooperative study on computerized reminders. *JAMA.* 2000; **284**(11): 1411–16.

74. Gill JM, Saldarriaga AM. The impact of computerized physician reminder and a mailed patient reminder on influenza immunizations for older patients. *Del Med J.* 2000; **72**(10): 425–30.

75. Hung CS, Lin JW, Hwang JJ, et al. Using paper chart based clinical reminders to improve guideline adherence to lipid management. *J Eval Clin Pract.* 2008; **14**(5): 861–6.

76. Younies H, Berham B, Smith PC. Perceptions of continuing medical education, professional development, and organizational support in the United Arab Emirates. *J Contin Educ Health Prof.* 2010; **30**(4): 251–6.

77. Al Mosawi AJ. Medical education and the physician workforce of Iraq. *J Contin Educ Health Prof.* 2008; **28**(2): 103–5.

78. Van der Velden T, Van HN, Vu Quoc HN, et al. Continuing medical education in Vietnam: new legislation and new roles for medical schools. *J Contin Educ Health Prof.* 2010; **30**(2): 144–8.

79. Okoro CC, Okoro I. The use of medical information in Nigeria: the influence of gender and status. *J Contin Educ Health Prof.* 2009; **29**(4): 254–8.

80. Gold MR, Siegel JE, Russell LB, et al., editors. *Cost-Effectiveness in Health and Medicine.* New York, NY: Oxford University Press; 1996.

81. Mazmanian PE. Continuing education costs and benefits: lessons for competing in a changing health care economy. *J Contin Educ Health Prof.* 2009; **29**(3): 133–4.

82. Yates BT. Cost-inclusive evaluation: a banquet of approaches for including costs, benefits, and cost-effectiveness and cost-benefit analyses in your next evaluation. *Eval Program Plann.* 2009; **32**(1): 52–4.

83. Herman PM, Avery DJ, Schemp CS, et al. Are cost-intrusive evaluations worth the effort? *Eval Program Plann.* 2009; **32**(1): 55–61.

84. Straus SE, Tetroe J, Graham ID. Knowledge to action: what it is and what it isn't. In: Straus SE, Tetroe J, Graham ID, editors. *Knowledge Translation in Health Care.* West Sussex, UK: Blackwell Publishing; 2009. pp. 3–9.

85. Fox RD, Mazmanian PE, Putnam RW, editors. *Changing and Learning in the Lives of Physicians.* New York, NY: Praeger; 1989.

86. Graham ID, Logan J, Harrison MB, et al. Lost in knowledge translation: time for a map? *J Contin Educ Health Prof.* 2006; **26**(1): 13–24.

87. Taylor PJ, Russ-Eft DF, Taylor H. Transfer of management training from alternative perspectives. *J Appl Psychol.* 2009; **94**(1): 104–21.

88. Bushardt SC, Fowler AR Jr. Performance evaluation alternatives. *J Nurs Adm.* 1988; **18**(10): 40–4.

89. Tracey JB, Tannenbaum SI, Kavanagh MJ. Applying trained skills on the job: the importance of the work environment. *J Appl Psychol.* 1995; **80**(2): 239–52.

90. Beckman TJ, Ghosh AK, Cook DA, et al. How reliable are assessments of clinical teaching? A review of the published instruments. *J Gen Intern Med.* 2004; **19**(9): 971–7.

91. Hutchinson L, Aitken P, Hayes T. Are medical postgraduate certification processes valid? A systematic review of the published evidence. *Med Educ.* 2002; **36**(1): 73–91.

92. Jha V, Bekker HL, Duffy SRG, et al. A systematic review of studies assessing and facilitating attitudes towards professionalism in medicine. *Med Educ.* 2007; **41**(8): 822–9.

93. Ratanawongsa N, Thomas PA, Marinopoulos SS, et al. The reported validity and reliability of methods for evaluating continuing medical education: a systematic review. *Acad Med.* 2008. **83**(3): 274–83.

94. Shaneyfelt T, Baum KD, Bell D, et al. Instruments for evaluating education in evidence-based practice. *JAMA.* 2006; **296**(9): 1116–27.

95. Tian J, Atkinson NL, Portnoy B, et al. A systematic review of evaluation in formal continuing medical education. *J Contin Educ Health Prof.* 2007; **27**(1): 16–27.

96. Veloski JJ, Fields SK, Boex JR, et al. Measuring professionalism: a review of studies with instruments reported in the literature between 1982 and 2002. *Acad Med.* 2005; **80**(4): 366–70.

97. Thannhauser J, Russell-Mayhew S, Scott C. Measures of interprofessional education and collaboration. *J Interprof Care.* 2010; **24**(4): 336–49.

98. Oxman AD, Thomson MA, Davis DA, et al. No magic bullets: a systematic review of 102 trials of interventions to improve professional practice. *JAMA.* 1995; **153**(10): 1423–31.

99. Salas ES, Cannon-Bowers JA. The science of training: a decade of progress. *Annu Rev Psychol.* 2001; **52**: 471–99.

100. O'Brien MA, Freemantle N, Oxman AD, et al. Continuing education meetings and workshops: effects on professional practice and health care outcomes. *Cochrane Database Syst Rev.* 2001; **2**: CD003030.

101. Davis DA, Taylor-Vaisey A. Translating guidelines into practice: a systematic review

of theoretic concepts, practical experience and research evidence in the adoption of clinical practice guidelines. *CMAJ*. 1997; **157**(4): 408–16.

102. Gargani J, Donaldson SI. What works for whom, where, why, for what, and when? Using evaluation evidence to take action in local contexts. In: Chen HT, Donaldson SI, Mark MM, editors. *Advancing Validity in Outcome Evaluation: theory and practice*. San Francisco, CA: Jossey-Bass; 2011. pp. 17–29.

11

Culture, Medical Education, and Assessment

Stewart Mennin, Vanessa Burch, Enoch Kwizera, Luiz E. A. Troncon, Tejinder Singh, and Rita Sood

Introduction

Stewart Mennin

Knowing is grounded in culture. The *Oxford Dictionary* online describes the origin of the word "culture" as Middle English, denoting a cultivated piece of land.[1] Another origin stems from the French *culture* or directly from Latin *cultura*, "growing, cultivation." The verb form is from obsolete French *culture* or medieval Latin *culturare*, both derived from the Latin *colere*, meaning "tend or cultivate." In late Middle English the active idea was "cultivation of the soil." From this early sixteenth-century legacy arose cultivation of the mind, faculties, or manners.

Today the word culture is used in many different ways. The authors of this chapter use the term culture to indicate patterns of human knowledge, belief, and behavior arising from social learning. "Most commonly, we refer to a set of shared attitudes, values, goals, and practices that characterize an institution, organization or group."[2] Everyone comes from and lives in one or more cultures. Culture is co-embedded in society, politics, education, and health. Power and legitimacy emerge from their confluence.

In recent decades, the influence of North American and European cultures on medical education has been pervasive, perhaps neocolonial.[3,4] Some Western educators and scholars argue that science is "value free," that science is objective as are its data. We disagree. Our position is that value-free science and objective thinking is a myth, especially in medical education and clinical practice. We argue that the marginalization of culture, which is typical of the education of physicians in Western-influenced models of medical education, is detrimental to professional identity development among persons studying to become doctors. Cultural disregard in health professions education also weakens the health of society.[5] Culture is dynamic and holistic and cannot be separated into curriculum segments or parts of an assessment program.

Medical education aims to prepare and graduate physicians capable of working with patients and their families to optimize health. Physicians also must be able to work with problems of local society that are progressively becoming nested in a global network.

This chapter examines the affect and relationship between culture and medical education. The discussion is first expressed in general and then more specifically between assessment and culture via the practical experience of five professional medical educators and authors from South Africa (VB, EK), Brazil (LT), and India (TS, RS). The authors write about culture, assessment, and medical education using a set of six provocative questions as an organizing framework.

The framework questions are:

1. You live and work in a unique culture that has within it hundreds of subcultures. South Africa, Brazil, and India are vastly multicultural. How are the tensions and challenges of the legacy of colonialism expressed in the health system and in medical education in general and more specifically in assessment of learning?

2. What challenges, if any, do you have in adopting and adapting assessment methods from Europe and North America into the cultural context of your school?

3. How have you dealt with these challenges and what can others learn from your experience?

4. What, if anything, has been detrimental or harmful from imposing Western culture on medical education in your country? What, if anything, have been the benefits?

5. What does your culture and its approach to medical education have to offer North America and Europe?

6. What challenges and changes do you see in the near future about the evolving relationship between culture and assessment?

Not all of the questions are fully addressed in the following three sections. The authors write courageously about controversial, perhaps unpopular, ideas. Political correctness is not the standard here. Instead, political need is emphasized. The three sections that follow were written independently. However, similarities are evident and are highlighted in the chapter. Learning about South African, Brazilian, and Indian experiences advances comparative medical education.

From my individual experience living in Brazil for 8 years and working in health professions education in many countries for more than 30 years, I thought I knew something about culture. After preparing this chapter with my colleagues, it's clear that I still have a great deal to learn.

1. Into Africa

The first chapter section is about medical education in South Africa. Vanessa Burch and Enoch Kwizera write about the political and cultural legacy of apartheid. Having been denied basic civil liberties for generations, they describe the struggle to gain equity of access to education while the multicultural society configures its identity. Creative approaches to education emerge in response to severely limited human and infrastructure resources and to the challenges of multilingual, multicultural communication. Community-based innovations are particularly important because they serve public interests best.

Cross-Cultural Assessment: Africa
Vanessa Burch and Enoch Kwizera

> There is no place for [the Bantu] in the European community above the level of certain forms of labour . . . What is the use of teaching the Bantu child mathematics when it cannot use it in practice? That is quite absurd. Education must train people in accordance with their opportunities in life, according to the sphere in which they live.
> —Hendrik Verwoerd, former South African Minister of Native Affairs[6]

Medical education, including assessment, is significantly influenced by the socio-political and economic milieu within any given country.[7] A striking example of the overwhelming influence of political policies on education has been the impact of the Bantu Education Act of 1953[8] that enforced racially segregated primary, secondary, and tertiary education in South Africa until the first democratic election in 1994. The conservative South Africa National Party viewed education to be a key element in their plan to create a completely segregated society.

Politics and Medical Education in South Africa

Race was historically the main determinant for segregated schooling, health care, recreation, and even dating and marriage. Apartheid adversely affected all spheres of the marginalized peoples' lives. One of apartheid's most profound effects was on the education of black South Africans in general,[9,10] and on the training of black South African doctors in particular.[11,12]

Five of the eight medical schools in South Africa were reserved for white students. Indian students or students of mixed ancestry were only admitted subject to local government regulations.[9] Black African students were trained at three historically black medical schools, which were built more than 50 years after the first white South African medical school opened its doors in 1900.

Historically white universities started admitting black African students in the mid-1980s. These students were not, however, permitted to see or examine white patients in racially segregated hospitals, which were abolished after the first democratic election in 1994. The impact of these draconian measures on the ethnic profile of the South African health professions workforce has been profound.

Getting Into and Staying in Medical School

Another impact of racially segregated education in South Africa has been the inadequate preparation of prospective students aspiring to enter medical school after segregation laws were relaxed and eventually abolished. In the case of Walter Sisulu University, rural black schools targeted for medical student recruitment were severely marginalized in terms of human, financial, and infrastructure resources. The academic prerequisites for admission were deliberately made lower than was the case in the other medical schools in the country – something one could call ironically "a culturally sensitive admissions policy."[13] In the late 1980s, the performance of black African students at the University of Cape Town, a historically white university, was very poor. The academic expectations at black schools are still low.[14] In response to the need to improve graduate throughput, the university developed an Academic Development Program, which dramatically improved black African student achievement between 1991 and 2001.[15] The Academic Development Program was later replaced by an Intervention Program, also aimed at providing additional support for academically disadvantaged students.[16]

A number of medical schools in South Africa now offer additional academic input for educationally disadvantaged students to close the gap between poor-quality secondary education and university admission. In addition, the Council for Quality Assurance in General and Further Education and Training, known as "UMULASI" has a "5% language compensation" policy whereby National Senior Certificate candidates, whose home language is neither English nor Afrikaans, have their marks in non-language subjects adjusted upward by 5%.[17] This has, however, been a source of controversy, especially as seen by schools catering mainly to those who speak English or Afrikaans as their first language.[18,19] The impact of the upward adjustment on the predictably poor National Senior Certificate grades of its beneficiaries is also apparently questionable,[20] and evidence suggests that home language may have little or no influence on the performance of undergraduates at historically white and English-medium South African universities.[21]

At Walter Sisulu University, a historically black university, there is a compulsory first-year "Communication Skills" module, which includes information technology skills for all, "English for Academic Purposes" for those who speak English as a second language, and "IsiXhosa" for those who speak English or Afrikaans as their first language.[14] This aims to ensure that the students with English as a second language are primed for learning and assessment in English, and that those who speak English or Afrikaans as their first language are trained to communicate with patients and communities in the latter's mother tongue. Similar courses in Afrikaans and IsiXhosa are now also being offered at historically white universities for students who have limited preuniversity training in Afrikaans or IsiXhosa.[22,23]

In common with South Africa, poor-quality secondary schooling is an ongoing challenge in the rest of sub-Saharan Africa (SSA). Additional preparatory academic support for medical students has been implanted in other SSA countries including Mozambique, Malawi, and Tanzania.[24] Ongoing political strife continues to have an impact upon medical school graduation rates in many other SSA countries, but there is little documentation of the negative impact of political strife on the production of health care professionals in countries such as Uganda during the dictatorship of Idi Amin in the 1970s, and of subsequent regimes, the brutal tribal conflict in Rwanda that culminated in the genocide of 1994 and its aftermath, and ongoing political instability in Nigeria and the Democratic Republic of the Congo.[25]

Challenges Adopting and Adapting Assessment Practices in Africa

Major advances in assessment practices have been achieved internationally during the past 3 decades, including the use of online multiple-choice examinations, modified essay questions, objective structured clinical examinations (OSCEs), simulated patients, and directly observed mini-clinical examinations in the workplace. Many of these innovations have not been adopted in SSA because of a lack of human and infrastructure resources. A recent survey of 98 SSA medical schools showed that more than 50% of medical schools had fewer than 100 teaching staff—full-time, part-time, or volunteers—and that university infrastructure such as information technology, internet, libraries, laboratories, and clinical teaching sites were significantly related to the gross domestic product of the country concerned.[24] Thus it is no surprise that a model predicting assessment preferences in SSA medical schools identified noncomputerized assessments such as essay and short-answer written examinations and problem-based oral examinations rather than patient-based clinical examinations (traditional long case) or OSCEs as the most suitable examinations in the setting of severe resource constraints.[26]

Adapting modern assessment methods to settings with limited resources poses significant challenges as reflected by the lack of published data about assessment innovations in SSA medical schools. For example, OSCEs and patient-based clinical examinations require floor space to set up multiple stations, real or simulated patients, and multiple examiners at one sitting. Floor space in African medical schools is typically very limited, simulated patients are expensive to train and use, and busy clinicians are difficult to recruit all at one time without significantly compromising clinical services on examination days.

One example of adaptation to a resource-constrained environment is the use of structured oral interviews to assess portfolio-based learning.[27] The limited availability of examiners to thoroughly read and assess individual portfolios, as done in the United Kingdom,[28] or the availability of tutors who meet regularly with students to discuss and assess their portfolio, as done in the Netherlands,[29] prompted development of an alternative strategy. The University of Cape Town now requires students in some of their clinical rotations (e.g., internal medicine) to compile a series of patient case studies that include reflective learning tasks addressing self-identified learning topics, pharmacotherapeutic issues, and primary health care and bioethics issues relevant to the patients clerked and managed. At the end of the clerkship, examiners interview students using a structured approach based on six key questions that focus on specific aspects of the patient encounter—in particular, the clinical reasoning process followed to establish a diagnosis and treatment plan. The response to each question is scored using a nine-point rating scale (1–3 indicates poor, 4–6 indicates adequate, 6–9 indicates good). An average score is calculated for each case and an aggregate of the four scores is used for summative assessment purposes.[27] The two key reasons for selecting an interview rather than document review to assess portfolio-based learning in the workplace are the lack of academic staff to engage in detailed document review and the observation that black African students, making up more than 50% of classes at some South African universities, often have better spoken than written proficiency in English, their second or third language. A similar approach to portfolio-based learning and assessment has been introduced at two other South African universities and recently also at Makerere University in Uganda.[30] This strategy demonstrates a pragmatic approach to the implementation and assessment of a workplace-based learning strategy that is sustainable with limited faculty resources and that affords students' opportunities to demonstrate clinical understanding and insight in the presence of language difficulties typically encountered by students for whom English is a second or even a third language.

What Can the Western World Learn from the African Experience?

Over the past 2 decades African medical schools have increasingly provided opportunities for community-based education.[31] Since 63% of SSA people live in rural areas, many medical schools are located in close proximity to rural and underserved communities. In Burundi, for example, 90% of the population lives in rural areas, and even in a wealthy country like South Africa, at least 38% of the population is rural.[32] Walter Sisulu University Medical School in South Africa,[33,34] the Medical University of South Africa,[35] the Catholic University of Graben Medical School at Butembo in the Democratic Republic of the Congo,[36] and Makarere University in Uganda[37] all have shown that rural origin, rural location of a medical school, and community-based programs improve the retention of medical graduates in rural areas. These findings are in keeping with those of the Western world.[38] The important difference between the programs in the Western world and those in SSA is that funding in Australia, for example, has government-supported initiatives[39] while those in Africa are self-funded by individual universities. Consequently, African programs operate with considerably smaller budgets and may serve as more useful examples for less affluent countries in the Western world.

One of the most important strengths of medical education in SSA is the rich spectrum of ethnic diversity typically found in student populations across the continent. For example, South Africa has 11 official languages, and medical schools typically have students from five or more different ethnic backgrounds. The same holds true for Nigeria (32 languages) and Uganda (32 languages), where a large number of regional dialects are spoken.[40] These rich melting pots of ethnic and cultural diversity generate high levels of cross-cultural tolerance, sensitivity, and insight. Language concordance between patient and health care provider has been shown to be an important predictor of the quality of clinical encounters.[41] The removal of language barriers has been identified as essential to reducing ethnic and racial health care disparities.[42] For these reasons, language competency is increasingly being assessed as part of communication skills in African health sciences faculties.[14,22,23]

In conclusion, we return to the questions posed at the beginning of this section. First, colonialism and racial segregation have contributed significantly to the historical and ongoing discrepancy between students from affluent backgrounds compared with those from disadvantaged impoverished communities. A number of strategies have been put in place to improve access for educationally disadvantaged students and adequate support to ensure academic success. The strategies adopted in Africa may prove useful to Western countries increasingly faced with ethnically and educationally diverse medical students. Second, Africa is starting to develop and describe assessment strategies that are suitable for low-resource settings. These methods of assessment may be suitable for implementation in other developing countries. Third, ethnic diversity is greater on the African continent than any other world region. Ethnic sensitivity, tolerance and language skills concordant with the needs of these diverse communities is an essential part of health professions education in Africa and we have created educational strategies that could assist the Western world faced with increasing cultural diversity in previously relatively homogenous populations. Finally, Africans need to explore current assessment methods used in affluent societies and adapt and design strategies that will allow us to use modern methods in resource-constrained settings.

2. From Africa to Brazil

Stewart Mennin

Brazil and Africa drifted apart millions of years ago. Many similarities are evident in Brazil's struggle to address wide social and economic disparities in a highly multicultural society that, like South Africa, carries a burden of centuries of European colonial domination. Luiz Troncon describes issues of inequity of access to higher education and medicine, in particular. The recent increase in the number of private for-profit medical schools, similar to what is happening in India, presents challenges to the Brazilian national health system (SUS) and to medical education in general. The influence of the introduction of newer assessment concepts and methods from North America combined with a greater awareness of the importance of formative assessment has had similar effects as the experience in Africa. The juxtaposition of new education methods with outdated educational approaches and attitudes is disturbing in a familiar and constructive way. Powerful national movements in health care reform and health professions education, unique to Brazil, are discussed. A sophisticated national approach to community health and health education is a model for other schools in other countries. Troncon touches on the need for faculty development and national licensing examinations, something being discussed at the present time in both Brazil and India.

Influence of Cultural Aspects on Assessment of Learners in Brazil

Luiz E. A. Troncon

Introduction

Writing about the influence of culture on student assessment in Brazil is not easy. The diversity of aspects involved and the scarcity of published data on the subject present significant challenges. Nevertheless, perspectives on concepts and practices regarding assessment of learners in Brazilian medical education are described here, as well as comments about how progress from the Northern Hemisphere has been adapted to the Brazilian context.

Brazilian society is highly multicultural. There is much variation in habits and values because of country region and social class. At the same time, there are common denominators that pervade society and influence educational practices. For example, the current national education system and SUS have principles and working norms determined by federal laws that make institutions more, rather than less, uniform.

Brazil has approximately 190 medical schools graduating more than 20 000 students annually. One hundred and twenty of these schools are private and most of these were opened within the last 20 years. The increase in private medical schools was not motivated by a shortage of medical graduates in Brazil. Instead, the increase addresses the scarcity of places in higher education for large numbers of students finishing high school because the state university system was unable to expand financially. Medicine is still attractive to high school students and some private universities found the opening of medical schools to be an excellent commercial opportunity. Accordingly, more than two-thirds of the new private medical schools are located in the wealthier southeastern states of Brazil (São Paulo, Rio de Janeiro, and Minas Gerais).

Admissions and Access to Medical School

The inequality of access to medical school, with its implications in both ethnic and economic composition of student populations, has been tackled by national affirmative action policies. This is important because the proportion of African Brazilians in the general population reaches nearly 50% in some states and the percentage of black students in any individual medical school rarely exceeds 5%. Similarly, almost 80% of applicants to state universities, which are free, come from free government high schools and yet the proportion of black applicants who succeed in entering medical school is negligible. Nearly all government universities recently have adopted a policy of reserving places for black students or applicants from government high schools. The effects on medical school educational processes and the capability of graduates are still unknown.

Brazilian society in general, and the higher education system in particular, is highly bureaucratic. Inertia and a number of unnecessary yet compulsory official procedures together with little autonomy for individual faculty members create barriers to innovation and limit the introduction of new educational methods. For example, in some Brazilian universities, proposals regarding curriculum change or modification of student assessment require approval from so many committees at different administrative levels that the actual introduction of the proposed measures may take several years.

Assessment and Culture in Brazilian Medical Schools

Medical student assessment has been influenced worldwide by concepts and methods developed in the Northern Hemisphere.[43,44] Changes in assessment involved a shift in focus to competence and performance, with an increased appreciation of formative assessment and an explicit concern regarding validity and reliability.[44] Assessment of students and graduates has also become an important part of program evaluation. One assessment experiment carried out by the Educational Commission for Foreign Medical Graduates in six different countries showed that results from Brazil were similar to those from other

Northern Hemisphere countries.[45] This experiment consisted of a standardized assessment of clinical skills using simulated patients, portraying cases developed by the Educational Commission for Foreign Medical Graduates that were translated from English and were culturally adapted. The results indicated that there were no intrinsic difficulties for the local culture to adapt to the new approaches to learner assessment.[45] New concepts and methods of student assessment have been progressively introduced into Brazilian institutions with a variable degree of success.[46,47] Nevertheless, some features of Brazilian society, particularly Brazilian educational culture, make the progress slow, and sometimes these features hinder the full acceptance of proposed changes.[46,47]

Only recently has a positive "assessment culture" developed in Brazilian medical schools.[46–48] Still, in many parts of the Brazilian system of higher education, student assessment is regarded as a formal responsibility of the teachers who deliver lectures, without any external component. It is still seen as a bureaucratic set of procedures aimed only at fulfilling formal requirements and it is often neglected. Assessment of learners in many schools, following ancient Portuguese academic traditions, is still approached as an effective means of controlling student behavior and avoiding poor discipline. Punishing students who are not showing enough dedication to learning activities and inducing study habits seems to be the main functions of these outdated approaches to student assessment.[46,47] In this context, assessment is taken as a powerful determinant of "what" and "how" students learn and as an explicit way to point out the importance of topics, sometimes in a threatening way.[49] This approach to assessment has little concern regarding diagnostic and formative aspects of learning.[50]

Another cultural aspect of this distorted view of student assessment is the predominant focus on the cognitive domain. Admission into professional schools depends exclusively on achieving high marks on examinations. This usually involves only an extensive series of multiple-choice questions. Overvaluation of written knowledge to the detriment of skills, attitudes, and ethics, is evident from the observation that, in many Brazilian medical schools, not a single form of practical examination was routinely carried out, nor were performance tests applied to assess students in the clinical years, until the mid-1990s.[46–48]

The overvaluation of cognitive and technical aspects in the medical profession is an aspect of professional culture that influences teaching, learning, and assessment. Specialized procedures are seen as more important than primary care practices. Professionalism is still largely seen from a physician-centered perspective as the mastering of technical skills needed to diagnose and treat diseases. In addition, academic culture in the most prestigious Brazilian universities overvalues research, the training of PhD students and the search for more sophisticated diagnostic and therapeutic procedures compared to teaching and preparing future health professionals to serve the community. This has led to a delay in the incorporation of student-centered approaches and newer assessment methods, which require investment of faculty time and effort.[49,50]

These negative traces of the educational culture have influenced results from recent studies on assessment in different Brazilian centers. A high degree of student test-related stress was found in the first attempt to introduce an objective structured clinical examination in a traditional Brazilian medical school.[47] The medical students viewed the examination as a threatening experience because they had not experienced performance examinations.[47] One study exploring the differences between student and tutor assessment in problem-based tutorials showed that students tended to score themselves more generously than their tutors.[51] Students believe that achieving high marks is more important than collaborating to achieve a more accurate evaluation of learning activities. Another study aimed at identifying aspects of clinical competence valued by staff using global ratings to assess senior students in clerkships showed that staff tended to focus more on student technical skills than on humanistic qualities that reflect cultural traces prevailing in the medical profession.[52]

Movements in Medical Education

A powerful and broad movement for change has been developing throughout the Brazilian medical education system in the last 2 decades.[53] New National *Curriculum Guidelines* for undergraduate courses in medicine (DCN) were published, providing an essential framework for change.[54] These ambitious guidelines recommend a competence-based curriculum with active, student-centered learning. The aim is to graduate physicians capable of working as a general practitioner with critical, thoughtful, and humanistic characteristics. These doctors must be capable to diagnose and treat diseases and to interact with and assist communities to promote health and prevent disease.[54] It is noteworthy, however, that these *Guidelines* devote much more emphasis to teaching and program evaluation than to assessment of learners.

Even before this movement, interaction between a few Brazilian medical schools and North American and European institutions led to the introduction of community-oriented, problem-based curriculum and the adoption of newer approaches to medical education.[55] Student assessment began to be seen as a school responsibility, fostering the introduction of centralized and specialized assessment committees. Formative assessment has been gradually accepted as a major foundation of learning, although with some reluctance by both teachers unwilling to praise and students afraid of being criticized.[56]

Concomitantly, a broad health care reform led to the construction of a unified national health system (SUS) focused on comprehensive primary health care. A central tenet of SUS is that primary care is carried out through a family health program that works via multidisciplinary teams comprised of a doctor, nurses, and a number of health workers recruited from members of the community receiving assistance.[57] These teams are in close contact with the families who live within defined geographic areas and provide both health care and education for disease prevention and health promotion. The consolidation of SUS has been associated with remarkable progress concerning public health indicators.[58] However, there are still many barriers to overcome, including the shortage of physicians properly trained and committed to SUS as well as poor connections with secondary health care units and with tertiary care hospitals.

Convergence of the educational and health system reforms have been actively stimulated by both the education and the health ministries, working together to fund initiatives to reform the curriculum of all health professions schools nationwide. The strong forces propelling change in both Brazilian medical education and SUS have encountered resistance in some well-established features of Brazilian society. Economic and social inequality is the most prominent barrier. Access to higher education is limited to students from high-income families with resources to pay for preparation for the highly competitive admission tests. Nevertheless, these students will eventually learn in health care facilities that mainly assist low-income, uneducated people. Consequently, interaction and communication between patients and students is made difficult because of social inequalities, which also hold back the introduction of more humanistic, patient-centered approaches in education.

Further Developments in Assessment and Medical Education in Brazil

Increased interaction between Brazilian medical schools and North American and European institutions has led to an increased awareness of the importance of faculty development programs, which has helped to consolidate some important changes in medical education and in SUS. Progress into this direction has been slow, but steady, as shown by an evaluation initiative sponsored by the Brazilian Association of Medical Education.[53] Now, convinced about the need for change and informed about some ways to go, deans and teachers have engaged enthusiastically in the improvement of the assessment system. Many Brazilian medical schools have implemented centralized committees to address student assessment. Unified directions that emphasize formative assessment have been built collectively during recent national congresses of medical education.[59] Large-scale objective structured clinical examinations are now being carried out routinely in several medical schools and teaching hospitals during the clinical education years and as part of the selection of applicants to medical residency. This has prompted the use of standardized patients. Shortage of space in busy public hospitals has been overcome by running the performance examinations on Sundays. The unavailability of expensive mechanical or electronic models has been successfully overcome by the introduction of homemade devices.

A larger debate has begun about the introduction of national licensing examinations for medical graduates. This arose from concerns inside some state medical councils about poor performance and the weak demonstration of competence of graduates from some newly created schools. Starting in 2011, examinations for renewing specialist titles will be compulsory for those who have not acquired the minimum number of required credits of continuing medical education activities.

In conclusion, assessment of medical students and residents in Brazil is changing rapidly, together with improvements in medical education and the consolidation of the SUS (Unified National Health System). New concepts and methods originally developed in the Northern Hemisphere have been successfully introduced into Brazil with the necessary adaptations to the local culture, resources, and context. The dissemination of faculty development programs has been helpful in leaving behind practices from the authoritarian ancient Portuguese academic tradition. Nevertheless, there is still a long way to go toward increasing quality in assessment for selection to professional schools and admission to postgraduate programs, as well as improving assessment of graduate professionalism and teamwork.

3. India: Past, Present, Future

Stewart Mennin

Thousands of years of heritage, hundreds of years of colonial domination, and 60 years of independence contribute to India's unique cultures and their struggles with problems and issues in health and health professions education. The difficulties are similar to those in Africa and Brazil. Tejinder Singh and Rita Sood take us quickly through the evolution of India's values expressed in its approach to education in general and the British legacy of medical education in particular. The large and growing population of India, its economic disparities, and history of social divisions present unique problems. Like Brazil, there has been a rapid proliferation of for-profit medical schools that affects who becomes a physician. Whenever there is a rapid rise in the number of medical schools there is usually an issue of insufficient academic staff capable of delivering a quality program. Like South Africa but different from Brazil, India has problems concerning English as a second language. India's vast multicultural population features communication in many local languages. The issues of assessment in medical education and the role of the government control of medical education are similar to those in Brazil and South Africa, differing only in scale.

Indian Culture and Assessment in Medical Education
Tejinder Singh and Rita Sood

> Culture shapes mind, it provides us with the tool kit by which we construct not only our worlds but our very conceptions of ourselves and our powers . . . You cannot understand mental activity unless you take into account the cultural setting and its resources; the very things that give mind its shape and scope. Learning, remembering, talking, and imaging: all of them are made possible by participating in a culture.[60]

A Short History

The influence of culture on educational practices including assessment is very visible in the Indian subcontinent. Historically, Indian culture is based on a reverence for education that extends back thousands of years. In ancient times when the Gurukul system flourished, admissions were at the discretion of the Guru or sometimes a group of Gurus who assessed the student's background, aptitude, and suitability.[61] The Guru alone decided about the suitability of the student for certification, and unless the student attained a certain level of mastery, he continued with his studies. During the Aryan period, temporal seats of learning were established in universities like Takshila and Nalanda, to which learners traveled great distances to gain admission. Learning was prized for its own sake and the social status and intellectual freedom of teachers was great.[62]

The Moghul invasion saw a number of "madrasas" and "pathshalas" opened by the state, and those who were certified from these schools had a better chance of getting a job at the royal court. The teacher became a paid agent of the state. The state funded the cost of education with the objective of educating people to become a part of the court, thus maintaining an emphasis on quality.

The British changed the dynamics of education. While the basic objective of the state seemed to be producing people who could occupy the lower rungs of the administrative hierarchy, the prospect of social mobility attracted more and more people to education. As the number of people with basic qualifications grew, it became necessary to earn higher degrees in a competitive world. There was a mad rush for higher and higher degrees, not for higher learning but for certification. The quality of education took a backseat.

More Recently

The modern system of higher education began over 150 years ago, when the first three universities were established in affiliation with British institutions.[63] There was, over the next 90 years, a slow development of higher education, with a focus largely on Western arts education and much less focus on science education. Today, India's higher education system is the third largest in the world, after China and the United States.[61] Staff in various disciplines are expected both to teach postsecondary courses and to undertake original research in their specialty.

Every aspect of India's educational system has been based on the British colonial legacy: educational levels, curriculum frameworks, physical structure of schools and classrooms, and timing of examinations. The development of higher education has been rapid in the past 60 years. The number of higher education institutes has increased from 500 in 1947 to 5000 in 1980 and then to over 13 000 in 2000.[61] Prior to the liberalization of the economy in the late 1990s, the university system was funded largely from public funds.[62] Though private schools of medicine existed, the growth of the private system was blocked until about the year 2000.

More recently the expansion of the higher education system, including medicine, has been chaotic and largely unplanned. The initial growth of private medical colleges began with a drive to make the system socially inclusive. However, the rapid proliferation has been largely profit driven.[63] There has been a sudden and dramatic increase in the number of medical schools without a proportionate increase in funding or in intellectual resources.[64] Consequently, academic standards have suffered and there is a dilution in quality of medical graduates. India faces a similar situation today as the United States faced during the pre-Flexner era.[65]

India has the largest number (330) of medical schools in the world.[66] It has seen unprecedented growth in the private sector in the last few years, with the public sector being almost static. Many of these private medical schools have inadequate infrastructure and questionable (profit-making) motives. All public medical schools have caste-based reservations and a lower cutoff score is used for decisions about admission of social groups presumed to be disadvantaged.[67] Most private medical schools, on the other hand, make huge sums of money allowing rich people who can afford exorbitant fees to bypass the entrance examinations.[68] Still, many support privatization of medical education as a necessary consequence of caste-based reservations in government institutions.[69,70]

Language, Culture, and Education

The Medical Council of India (MCI) regulates almost all the medical schools, other than a few autonomous institutions.[67] Most of the 28 states and seven union territories in the country have different local cultures and values. English is almost the second national language in India, and it is the language in which medical courses are delivered throughout the country. The large majority of states have different languages and dialects that are used for communication at a local level. The proficiency in the English language among students and teachers varies drastically across different regions of the country beyond the metropolitan states. Outside the syllabus, the communication among students, teachers, and patients often occurs in their local language. Many students with poor English language skills remain at a disadvantage in terms of communication and, thereby, performance. While the issue of language seems to attract most attention, influences of culture, environment, and other factors (e.g., offensiveness of materials, level of a students' acculturation, behavioral issues, perspectives, and contexts) on a student's ability to do well on standardized tests are still poorly understood.[71] These factors must be accounted for in reaching a fair assessment of a student's cognitive abilities.[72] Teachers and educators should be aware of these and consider them when planning assessment.

There is a perception that the Indian education system produces people good at acquiring knowledge and certain skills but not necessarily efficient at applying the knowledge, problem solving, and "out of the box" lateral thinking. The entrance examinations for MBBS seats are based on multiple-choice questions (MCQs) of questionable utility, further encouraging rote learning among students. There are, with few exceptions, no aptitude tests or interviews for selection of medical students. Interviews recognized elsewhere as an important part of a selection process have not gained acceptance, perhaps because of a lack of transparency and public confidence.[69] Pursuit of objectivity without critical reflection takes its toll on validity and reliability with regard to the assessment for admissions.

Assessment

Almost all medical schools follow a curriculum based on guidelines from the MCI.[70] The MCI only gives guidelines on the expected outcomes and how students should be assessed. On paper the expected outcomes of medical graduates are the same across the country. However, individual and institutional variations in standards of undergraduate and postgraduate medical education are the rule rather than the exception. The only similarity that exists is in the weight given to various components of assessment, as it is dictated by the MCI.

Failure in examinations is considered highly negative by both parents and teachers in the Indian culture, is viewed negatively by society, and is often associated with lowered self-esteem. Thus, significant stress is paid to passing examinations and to the acquisition of degrees. One negative side effect of this cultural bias is that many of the undeserving students are passed by lowering the criteria. The pass mark across all medical schools is almost universally 50%, irrespective of the tools used for assessment. There are no formal mechanisms for standard setting for different attributes (e.g., theoretical knowledge, practical skills) and for using different assessment methods (e.g., essays or MCQs). Similarly, grades on different types of tests are often combined to produce an aggregate score with doubtful utility. Summative examinations are supposed to be criterion-referenced but they are more often norm-referenced, with poor generalizability of results.

What is ensured in the practical or clinical examinations are the following formalities:

- the number of examiners (external and internal)
- time allocated based on the total number of students appearing for examinations
- the number of cases—for example, one long and two short cases for examination of undergraduates in clinical disciplines
- oral viva voce (with not much structural uniformity).

There is an obsession with "objectivity," and anything that cannot be objectively measured is discarded. There is not much emphasis or focus on the assessment of attitudes, behaviors, communication skills, professionalism, or ethics. Most teachers claim they value these attributes as well as issues such as end-of-life care, palliative care, and care of the dying. However, these key issues are absent in the assessments practiced by the large majority of medical schools at the level of graduate and postgraduate medical education. Some examiners pay attention to these attributes, but no candidate ever fails because of a lack of these skills.

Adopting and Adapting Assessment Methods from Europe and the United States

The summative assessment of knowledge is tested using long and short essays and MCQs are used for most entrance examinations and a few in-course assessments. Most teachers recognize the educational limitation of MCQs focused predominantly on factual recall. Nevertheless, they are still used widely relying on objectivity and defensibility that reflect the loss of trust between the students and teachers and the lack of transparency and validity in the examination system. A very small proportion of faculty is trained and proficient in the construction of MCQs, particularly context-rich questions useful for assessment of clinical reasoning and decision-making abilities.

Well-defined and well-documented standards for preparation, editing, and improvement of questions are practiced at few universities. Poor-quality and ambiguous questions on high-stakes examinations often result in avoidable legal suits. Overdependence on questions eliciting factual recall reinforces poor learning habits among students. Ineffective faculty development in assessment results in MCQs for summative evaluations with inadequate attention to standard setting and minimum pass marks. Similarly, the objective structured clinical examination (OSCE) and its adaptation, the objective structured practical examination, used by some medical schools also lack stringent preparation with little to no evidence of validity and reliability. In addition, a major constraint is the lack of adequately trained faculty and infrastructure (e.g., videotaping of the OSCE or a protected space in which to conduct it). There is an acute shortage of faculty for the number of students.[73] Insufficient numbers of trained observers result in the use of OSCEs to elicit interpretative skills while performance and communication skills get little or no attention.

Insufficient regional educational research makes it more difficult to convince skeptics about the benefits of adapting different assessment methods, well established in the international community, to local contexts. The use of simulations and standardized patients for testing is almost nonexistent in most Indian medical schools. There are, however, motivated teachers at all levels who work hard to provide the benefits of newer methods and technology at individual levels. Unfortunately, they are few in number. The use of structured oral examinations, structured long case examinations, and mini-clinical examinations are good examples of adaptations in the resource constrained medical school settings.[74–76]

A recent advancement is that the MCI is considering introducing a national exit test similar to the United States Medical Licensing Examination.[77] The concern is that the modalities to be assessed are unclear. It is not known how the MCI proposes to introduce the test without a national group of well-prepared item writers, psychometricians, and assessment experts. There is a danger of further polarizing student learning toward factual recall by taking away the emphasis on in-course assessments.

A National Knowledge Commission[77] set up by the Government of India made the following observation about assessment at most institutions of higher education:

> The nature of annual examinations at universities in India often stifles the teaching-learning process because they reward selective and uncritical learning. There is an acute need to reform this examination system so that it tests understanding rather than memory. Analytical abilities and creative thinking should be at a premium. Learning by rote should be at a discount. Such reform would become more feasible with decentralized examination and smaller universities. But assessment cannot and should not be based on examinations alone. There is a clear need for continuous internal assessment which empowers teachers and students alike, just as it breathes life back into the teaching-learning process. Such internal assessment would also foster the analytical and creative abilities of students which are often a casualty in university administered annual examinations. To begin with, internal assessment could have weight of 25 percent in the total but this should be raised to 50 percent over time.[77]

These observations are, to a large extent, applicable to medical education.

The strength of medical education in India has been the knowledge base of students and the emphasis on clinical bedside teaching. There is extensive clinical exposure of students to patients during training and assessments with a focus on the skills of integration during examinations with real cases. Using real patients in examination settings brings assessment closer to life and thus is more authentic, but there is a trade-off in standardization and reliability. We believe there is a need to shed the dependence on simulated patients, dominant in the Western world, and explore further the possibility of working with real patients during high-stakes examinations. This is an important message to the West from countries like India with large populations, limited resources for health care and health professions education, and growing demands for authentic assessment in clinical settings.

In conclusion, we argue that assessment and instruction both influence and in turn are influenced by culture. It is not possible to design and interpret assessment and health professions education independent of culture. This becomes even more important in the wake of increased mobility of physicians and other health care workers. Multicultural societies can learn much from one another so that assessment and health professions education are viewed and understood through action in cultural contexts.

General Conclusions

Stewart Mennin

What appears obvious to us is understood only in relationships embedded in culture. The relationships are a complex series of webs nested in language, art, story, history, myth, ritual, gender, age, and beliefs that are essential for the interplay of communication from which learning and understanding continuously emerge. Across sub-Saharan Africa, Brazil, and India history combines with a colonial legacy to form and inform the sociopolitical infrastructures, institutional development, and higher education. These formations are especially influential concerning social well-being and health.

What is clear from these authors is that culture, health professions education, and assessment must be viewed as a continuously evolving sociopolitical, and economic environment. It is easy to lose this perspective in the rush to import and implement new educational tools, methods, and techniques from Europe and North America and in the challenges of seeking recognition from and parity with them. There still remains an ancient heritage about knowledge and its assessment that focuses mainly on memory-based tests. South Africa, Brazil, and India present a mix of first and third world institutions and values. The time scale of changes in assessment and educational practices is slow as old ways are culturally embedded individually, institutionally, and nationally. Only recently have more contemporary educational practices entered the medical education lexicon in these countries.

Another theme that emerges from these authors deals with equity of access to education, a reflection of the wide socioeconomic divide between rich and poor. Children from wealthy families have disproportionately greater opportunity to become physicians. They can afford the special private classes that prepare them for the entrance examinations and, in some instances, can buy their way into private for-profit medical schools. A rapid increase in the number of private medical schools is described in all three regions. It remains to be seen how these schools will contribute to the improvement of public health and to strengthen their respective national health systems. Inequity across the political, social, and economic landscape is often social class driven. Educational inequity in Brazil is mostly economic. India struggles with a lingering residue of the caste system, colonialism, and a growing divide in a rising economy. South Africa suffers from a legacy of centuries of colonialism and racial discrimination. An important role for government is to look out for and protect those who are excluded.

The authors discuss the political struggles that lead to improvements in health professions education. They acknowledge the importance of the role of government regulation and support while at the same time questioning the extent to which it is collaborative and responsive. They want to know who is watching and to what extent accountability and governance are functioning in the best interests of society. Numerous government initiatives in Brazil have been launched to improve family health, strengthen health professions education, and promote SUS, its Unique System of Health. Historically, the Medical Council of India has had a strong hand in controlling medical education and only in the last few years has it begun to loosen its grip. South Africa and sub-Saharan Africa continue to move forward in the midst of devastating HIV AIDS, infectious disease, and social upheaval.

What is remarkable about the stories of South Africa, Brazil, and India is their resolve in the struggle to strengthen the humanization of health professions education. Scholarly exploration, discovery, recognition, and understanding of local, regional, and national cultures central to health and education in society are achieving this.

The stories told by these authors reveal a culture of medical education embedded in a system of higher education, itself wrapped in an educational legacy deeply influenced by colonial and political history. These layers affect how we think about learning and assessment and how we organize and support education for tomorrow's health professionals. Bruffee[78] teaches that learning is a process of reacculturation, an extension over time of previous multicultural situations to include the new as a unified and purposeful whole. Common to each author in this chapter is recognition that the teaching-learning process is dominated by traditional methods while at the same time their institutions are adapting newer methods of assessment. Old and new approaches to assessment and medical education coexist and evolve together, moving toward a new entity adapted to the unique conditions of each region. A culture of collaboration and continuous exchange between the professoriate, university, community, and government is needed to nurture and sustain the vitality of this motion.

References

1. Oxford Dictionaries Online. *Culture*. Oxford: Oxford University Press. Available at: http://oxforddictionaries.com/definition/culture?region=us (accessed September 13, 2011).
2. *Oxford English Dictionary*. 2011. Available at: www.oed.com.turing.library.north western.edu/view/Entry/45746?rskey=yZ6f18&result=1&isAdvanced=false#eid (accessed May 31, 2011).
3. Bleakley A, Brice J, Bligh J. Thinking the post-colonial in medical education. *Med Educ*. 2008; **42**(3): 266–70.
4. Karle H, Christensen L, Gordon D, et al. Neo-colonialsim versus sound globalization policy in medical education. *Med Educ*. 2008; **42**(10): 956–8.
5. Bleakley A, Bligh J, Browne J. *Medical Education for the Future: identity, power and location*. Dordrecht, the Netherlands: Springer; 2011.
6. Clark NL, Worger WH. *South Africa: the rise and fall of apartheid*. Seminar Studies in History. Harlow, UK: Pearson Education; 2004.
7. Breier M, Wildschut A. *Doctors in a Divided Society: the profession and education of medical practitioners in South Africa*. Cape Town, South Africa: Human Sciences Research Council Press; 2006.
8. Bantu Education Act number 47 of 1953. Available at: www.sahistory.org.za/bantu-education-act-no-47-1953 (accessed October 23, 2012).
9. Colborn RP. Affirmative action and academic support: African medical student at the University of Cape Town. *Med Educ*. 1995; **29**(2): 110–18.
10. Treiman DJ. The legacy of apartheid: racial inequalities in the new South Africa. In: Heath A, Cheung SL, editors. *Unequal Chances: ethnic minorities in Western labour markets*. Oxford: Oxford University Press; 2007. pp. 403–49.
11. Kallaway P. An introduction to the study of education for blacks in South Africa. In: Kallaway P, editor. *Apartheid and Education: the education of black South Africans*. Johannesburg, SA: Raven Press; 1990. pp. 1–44.
12. Tobias PV. Apartheid and medical education: the training of black doctors in South Africa. *J Natl Med Assoc*. 1980; **72**(4): 395–410.
13. Faculty of Health Sciences, Walter Sisulu University. *Prospectus 2011*. Mthatha, South Africa: Walter Sisulu University; 2011. Available at: www.wsu.ac.za/study withus/images/resources/FHS prospectus.pdf (accessed September 13, 2011).
14. Van Niekerk JP. Missions of a medical school: an African perspective. *Acad Med*. 1999; **74**(Suppl. 8): S38–44.
15. Sikakana CN. Supporting student-doctors from under-resourced academic backgrounds: an academic development programme. *Med Educ*. 2010; **44**(9): 917–25.
16. Alexander R, Badenhorst E, Gibbs T. Intervention programme: a supported learning

programme for educationally disadvantaged students. *Med Teach*. 2005; **27**(1): 66–70.

17. UMULASI Council for Quality Assurance in General and Further Education and Training. *Quality Assurance of Assessment: policies, directives, guidelines and requirements*. Pretoria: UMULASI Council for Quality Assurance in General and Further Education and Training; 2006. Available at: www.nqf.org.za/download_files/nqf-support/8 Umalusi. Quality Assurance of Assessment. Policies, Directives, Guidelines and Requirements.pdf (accessed September 13, 2011).

18. Jones M. Top matrics robbed of As: teachers. *Cape Times*. January 11, 2011. Available at: www.iol.co.za/news/south-africa/western-cape/top-matrics-robbed-of-as-teachers-1.1010470#.UD1sSxzUT-l (accessed October 23, 2012).

19. Ngonyama S. ANC Statement on the 1998 Matric Results. Press Release. Marshalltown, South Africa: African National Congress; January 7, 1999. Available at: www.anc.org.za/show.php?id=7220 (accessed September 13, 2011).

20. Van der Berg S. Apartheid's enduring legacy: inequalities in education. *J Afr Econ*. 2007; **16**(5): 849–80.

21. Van Walbeek C. Does lecture attendance matter? Some observations from a first-year economics course at the University of Cape Town. *S Afr J Econ*. 2004; **72**(4): 861–83.

22. Faculty of Health Sciences, University of Cape Town. *Handbook 2011*. Cape Town, South Africa: University of Cape Town; 2011. Available at: www.uct.ac.za/downloads/uct.ac.za/apply/handbooks/fac_health_2011.pdf (accessed September 13, 2011).

23. Stellenbosch University, South Africa. *Review of the Language Policy*. Available at: www.sun.ac.za/university/taal/hersiening/woordvoerder_e.htm (accessed October 23, 2012).

24. Mullan F, Frehywot S, Omaswa F, et al. Medical schools in sub-Saharan Africa. *Lancet*. 2011; **377**(9771): 1113–21.

25. Longombe AO, Burch V, Luboga S, et al. Research on medical migration in sub-Saharan medical schools: usefulness of a feasibility process to define barriers to data collection and develop a practical study. *Educ Health (Abingdon)* [online serial]. 2007; **20**(1): 27. Available at: www.educationforhealth.net/publishedarticles/article_print_27.pdf.

26. Walubo A, Burch V, Parmar P, et al. A model for selecting assessment methods for evaluating medical students in African medical schools. *Acad Med*. 2003;**78**(9): 899–906.

27. Burch VC, Seggie JL. Use of a structured interview to assess portfolio-based learning. *Med Educ*. 2008; **42**(9): 894–900.

28. Davis MH, Friedman Ben-David M, Harden RM, et al. Portfolio assessment in medical students' final examinations. *Med Teach*. 2001; **23**(4): 357–66.

29. Driessen E, van Tartwijk J, Vermunt JD, et al. Use of portfolios in early undergraduate training. *Med Teach*. 2003; **25**(1): 18–23.

30. Mubuuke AG, Kiguli-Malwadde E, Kiguli S, et al. A student portfolio: the golden key to reflective, experiential, and evidence-based learning. *J Med Imag Radiat Sci*. 2010; **41**(2): 72–8.

31. Nazareth I, Mfenyana K. Medical education in the community: the UNITRA experience. *Med Educ*. 1999; **33**(10): 722–4.

32. United Nations Secretariat. *World Urbanization Prospects: the 2007 revision population database*. United Nations, Department of Economic and Social Affairs; 2007. Available at: http://esa.un.org/unup/ (accessed February 13, 2011).

33. Dambisaya YM. Career intentions of UNITRA medical students and their perceptions about the future. *Educ Health (Abingdon)*. 2003; **16**(3): 286–97.

34. Igumbor EU, Kwizera EN. The positive impact of rural medical schools on rural intern choices. *Rural Remote Health* [online serial]. 2005; **5**(2): 417. Available at: www.rrh.org.au/publishedarticles/article_print_417.pdf (accessed September 13, 2011).

35. De Vries E, Reid S. Do South African medical students of rural origin return to rural practice? *S Afr MEd J*. 2003; **93**(10): 789–93.

36. Longombe AO. Medical schools in rural areas: necessity or aberration? *Rural Remote Health* [online serial]. 2009; **9**(3): 1131. Available at: www.rrh.org.au/publishedarticles/article_print_1131.pdf (accessed September 13, 2011).

37. Kaye DK, Mwanika A, Sewankambo N. Influence of the training experience of Makarere University medical and nursing graduates on willingness and competence to work in rural health facilities. *Rural Remote Health* [online serial]. 2010; **10**(10): 1372. Available at: www.rrh.org.au/publishedarticles/article_print_1372.pdf (accessed September 13, 2011).

38. Dolea C, Stormont L, Braichet JM. Evaluated strategies to increase attraction and retention of health workers in remote and rural areas. In: World Health Organization (WHO), editor. *Bulletin WHO*. Geneva: World Health Organization; 2010. pp. 18–23.

39. Dunbabin J, Levitt L. Rural origin and rural medical exposure: their impact on the rural and remote medical workforce in Australia. *Rural Remote Health* [online serial]. 2003; **3**(1): 212. Available at: www.rrh.org.au/publishedarticles/article_print_212.pdf (accessed September 13, 2011).

40. www.britannica.com

41. Gonzalez HM, Vega WA, Tarraf W. Health care quality perceptions among foreign-born Latinos and the importance of speaking the same language. *J Am Board Fam Med*. 2010; **23**(6): 745–52.

42. Cooper LA, Roter DL. Patient-provider communication: the effect of race and ethnicity on process and outcomes of healthcare. In: Smedley BD, Stith AY, Nelson AR, editors. *Unequal Treatment: confronting racial and ethnic disparities in health care*. Washington, DC: National Academies Press; 2003. pp. 552–93. Available at: www.nap.edu/catalog.php?record_id=12875 (accessed September 14, 2011).

43. Epstein RM. Assessment in medical education. *N Engl J Med*. 2007; **356**(4): 387–96.

44. Wass V, van der Vleuten C, Shatzer J, et al. Assessment of clinical competence. *Lancet*. 2001; **357**(9260): 945–8.

45. Ziv A, Ben-David M, Sutnick A, et al. Lessons learned from six years of international administrations of the ECFMG's SP-based clinical skills assessment. *Acad Med*. 1998; **73**(1): 84–91.

46. Krasilchik M. Avaliação do ensino (Assessment of teaching). In: *Proceedings of the Assessment and Teaching Meeting, Faculty of Education, University of Sao Paulo, Sao Paulo, Brazil*. São Paulo, Brazil: Faculty of Education, University of São Paulo, Brazil; 1992. pp. 6–11.

47. Troncon LE. Clinical skills assessment: limitations to the introduction of an "OSCE" (objective structured clinical examination) in a traditional Brazilian medical school. *Sao Paulo Med J*. 2004; **122**(1): 12–17.

48. Aguiar A, Ribeiro E. Conceito e avaliação de habilidades e competência na educação médica: percepções atuais dos especialistas [The concept and evaluation of skills and competence in medical education: current expert perspectives]. *Rev Bras Educ Med*. 2001; **34**(3): 371–8.

49. Lowry S. Assessment of students. *BMJ*. 1993; **306**(6869): 51–4.

50. McManus IC. Examining the educated and the trained. *Lancet*. 1995; **345**(8958): 1151–3.

51. Machado JL, Pinheiro-Machado VM, Grec W, et al. Self- and peer assessment may not be an accurate measure of PBL tutorial process. *BMC Med Educ*. 2008; **8**: 55.

52. Domingues R, Amaral E, Zeferino A. Global overall rating for assessing clinical competence: what does it really show? *Med Educ*. 2009; **43**(9): 883–6.

53. Lampert J, Costa N, Perim G, et al. Change trends in a group of Brazilian medical schools. *Rev Bras Educ Med*. 2009; **33**(1 Suppl. 1): S19–34.

54. Ministry of Education B. *Diretrizes Curriculares Nacionais do curso de graduação em Medicina* [National Curriculum Guidelines for undergraduate courses in Medicine]. Resolução CNE/CES N° 4, 7 de novembro de 2001. Available at: http://portal.mec.gov.br/cne/arquivos/pdf/CES04.pdf (accessed September 13, 2011).

55. Feuerwerker L. *Além do discurso de mudança na educação médica: processos e resultados* [Beyond the discourse of changing medical education: processes and results]. Rio de Janeiro: Editora Hucitec; 2002.

56. Zeferino A, Domingues R, Amaral E. Feedback como Estratégia de Aprendizado no Ensino Médico [Feedback as a learning strategy in medical education]. *Rev Bras Educ Med*. 2007; **31**(2): 176–9.

57. Harris M, Haines A. Brazil's Family Health Program. *BMJ*. 2010; **341**: c4945.

58. Barros F, Matijasevich A, Requejo J, et al. Recent trends in maternal, newborn, and child health in Brazil: progress toward Millennium Development Goals 4 and 5. *Am J Public Health*. 2010; **100**(10): 1877–89.

59. Zeferino A, Troncon L, Hamamoto-Filho P, et al. Avaliação do Estudante de Medicina [Medical Student Assessment]. Cadernos da ABEM 2009; **5**: 30–3.

60. Bruner J. *The Culture of Education*. Cambridge, MA: Harvard University Press; 1996.

61. Dehaan R. National cultural influences on higher education. In: Dehaan R, Narayan K, editors. *Education for Innovation: implications for India, China and America*. Roterdam: Sense Publishers; 2008. pp. 133–65.

62. Government of India. *Compilation of 50 Years of Indian Education: 1947–97*. Available at: www.education.nic.in/cd50years/15/8P/84/8P840B01.htm (accessed September 13, 2011).

63. Kaul R. Whither equity? *Semin Mag.* 2000; **494**: 23–5.

64. Bansal R. Private medical education takes off in India. *Lancet.* 2003; **361**(9370): 1748–9.

65. Amin Z, Burdick WP, Supe A, et al. Relevance of the Flexner Report to the contemporary medical education in South Asia. *Acad Med.* 2010; **85**(2): 333–9.

66. Medical Council of India. *List of Colleges Teaching MBBS* [search tool]. Available at: http://mciindia.org/InformationDesk/MedicalCollegeHospitals/ListofColleges TeachingMBBS.aspx (accessed August 26, 2011).

67. Sood R. Medical education in India. *Med Teach.* 2008; **30**(6): 585–91.

68. Singh T. Commercialisation of medical education: a review of capitation fee colleges. *J Indian Med Assoc.* 1994; **92**(9): 301–3.

69. Bal AM. Medicine, merit, money and caste: the complexity of medical education in India. *Indian J Med Ethics.* 2010; **7**(1): 25–8.

70. Medical Council of India. *Salient Features of Regulations on Graduate Medical Education, 1997* [cited February 19, 2011]. Available at: http://mciindia.org/Rulesand Regulations/GraduateMedicalEducationRegulations1997.aspx (accessed August 26, 2011).

71. Geisinger KF, Carlson J. Assessing language minority students. *ERIC Clearinghouse on Tests and Measurement and Evaluation.* 1992; ED356232.

72. Demmert W G Jr. The influences of culture on learning and assessment among Native American students. *Learn Disabil Res Pract.* 2005; **20**(1): 16–23.

73. Ananthakrishnan N. Acute shortage of teachers in medical colleges: existing problems and possible solutions. *Nat Med J India.* 2007; **20**(1): 251–5.

74. Lobo J, et al. The viva-voce examination. In: Sood R, editor. *Assessment in Medical Education: trends and tools.* New Delhi: KL Wig Centre for Medical Education and Technology; 1995. pp. 169–78.

75. Singh T, Sharma M. Mini-CEX as a tool for formative assessment. *Natl Med J India.* 2010; **23**(2): 100–3.

76. Medical Council of India. *Vision 2015.* New Delhi, India: Medical Council of India; 2011 [cited May 30, 2011]. Available at: www.mciindia.org/tools/announcement/ MCI_booklet.pdf (accessed August 26, 2011).

77. National Knowledge Commission. *Report to the Nation.* National Knowledge Commission, Government of India; 2006 [cited 2008, 15 March]. Available at: http://knowledgecommission.gov.in/reports/report06.asp (accessed August 26, 2011).

78. Bruffee KA. *Collaborative Learning: higher education, interdependence, and authority of knowledge.* 2nd ed. Baltimore, MD: The Johns Hopkins University Press; 1999.

12

Workplace-Based Assessment

Tejinder Singh and John J. Norcini

THERE ARE MANY WAYS TO VIEW WORKPLACE-BASED ASSESSMENT (WPBA). The Postgraduate Medical Education and Training Board defines it as the assessment of working practices based on what doctors actually do in the clinical setting and predominantly carried out in the workplace itself.[1] This definition includes two attributes of WPBA: (1) it is a direct observation of performance and (2) it is conducted in the workplace.

WPBA is not a replacement for some other form of assessment;[2] rather, it is a vehicle for collecting quantitative and qualitative data about trainee performance from various sources and using it to provide feedback that fosters learning. Consequently, many WPBA programs assume a continuum based on a developmental model of competence such as the expertise model of Dreyfus and Dreyfus.[3] With this framework, WPBA is a good tool for providing feedback along the way while providing some assurance that there is ongoing growth in trainee competence.

In some settings, however, WPBA is used to provide summative as well as formative assessment. Additional work is needed before such use is recommended. Because most of the methods rely on clinical encounters and assessors that vary in difficulty across trainees and sites, final results are not necessarily equivalent.

This chapter reviews the state of the art in WPBA. Specifically, it provides the rationale for using WPBA in view of its ability to evaluate authentic tasks. The fact that WPBA occurs in real-life settings gives it certain advantages in terms of validity. We will also look at how learning happens in the workplace and the role that timely, effective, and specific feedback can play to improve that learning.

Rationale for Workplace-Based Assessment
• •

WPBA plays an important role in assessment for four reasons. First, it aims at clinical skills that are critical to diagnosis and treatment. Second, observation and feedback are lacking in clinical training and they are critical to learning. Third, traditional forms of assessment used in clinical education have several limitations. Fourth, there is a lack of alignment among learning objectives and assessment in the workplace.

Clinical Skills are Important

There are many reports that suggest a good history and physical examination can provide an accurate clinical diagnosis in the majority of cases. Hampton et al.[4] reported this figure to be as high as 80%, laboratory investigations adding only marginally to diagnostic accuracy. Peterson et al.[5] reported that patient history and physical examination are definitive on 76% of encounters in a primary care setting. This is a high figure compared with diagnostic imaging, which provided the correct diagnosis in only 35% of the cases.[6]

There are other aspects to clinical skill assessments than patient history and physical examination. Clinical skills assessments generally focus on "hard" competencies but there are many "softer" skills and competencies that are important for a physician. Medical practice involves both objective and subjective skills and knowledge. Physicians use both because tacit knowledge is the basis of mental schemas and pattern recognition is needed to reach diagnoses that are dependent on "noncognitive" factors.[7] A recent review summarizes the variety of noncognitive abilities that may be important in professional education.[8] WPBA can also promote a collaborative rather than a competitive environment. Lane[8] emphasizes that, "Competence in health care professions includes nontechnical skills that tap into diverse talents and 'intelligences.' Evidence is growing that such skills influence overall success in school and clinical settings."

Physicians' interpersonal and communication skills, for example, are important not only in gathering a useful history but also in building a meaningful doctor-patient relationship. There are a number of verbal and nonverbal cues that can help to develop such a relationship. However, these skills do not lend themselves easily to assessment except by direct observation. Standardized patients can provide data about these "soft" skills but cannot replace direct observation of medical trainees working with real patients. Context plays a major role in deciding the way physicians act.[9] Physicians are known to perform differently in the controlled setting of a clinical performance examination and the real work setting.[10]

Observation and Feedback are Lacking

A meta-analysis by Hattie[11] brings out the importance of feedback as a learning tool. Summarizing the results of over 1800 studies, Hattie[11] demonstrated a feedback effect size of 0.79 on student achievement compared with 0.40 for overall schooling. There was variability depending on the type of feedback, and largest effects were seen when information was provided about a specific task. In the field of medical education, a meta-analysis by Veloski et al.[12] demonstrated a beneficial effect of feedback in 74% of the 41 studies reviewed. The magnitude of these effects was increased further when feedback was combined with other educational interventions. Reports by Gipps[13] and Holmboe et al.[14] also suggest positive effects of feedback on learning behaviors.

Despite its importance as a learning tool, delivery of feedback based on observation of performance does not occur as frequently as one might expect.[14,15] Observed assessment of clinical performance was experienced by only 7.4%–21.3% of medical students during clinical clerkships in one study[15] and up to 33% of students were not observed performing a physical or mental health examination during clerkships in a national study reported by the Association of American Medical Colleges.[16] Other reports also suggest that less than one-third of the clinical encounters are actually observed during training.[17,18] This limits the number of opportunities where feedback could have been provided to the students.

The situation is no better at the postgraduate level, where there are fewer trainees. Day et al.[19] reported that up to 80% of postgraduate residents had only one observed clinical encounter during training. Isaacson et al.[20] reported that 80% of the trainees infrequently or never received feedback following direct observation. Even in situations where feedback was provided, less than a third elicited any reflection from the trainee.[21] Even when direct observation occurs, it is not being used as an opportunity to provide feedback. While assessors may not fully appreciate the role of feedback in creating learning, lack of training in providing quality feedback may be another important factor.

Concerns have also been raised regarding assessors missing student errors and thereby not being able to provide appropriate feedback.[22] The use of checklists may increase error detection but they do not seem to influence the accuracy of the assessors. Many assessors rate marginal performance of students as superior, which further limits the utility of feedback.[23,24]

Traditional Clinical Assessment is Flawed

Assessment of trainees in the clinical setting is not well developed. Problems that distort clinical assessment include small numbers of trainees, scattered resources, and the need to focus on clinical skills and performance when trainees are not responsible for patient care. The assessment focus is on the potential to practice rather than on actual practice.[25] The clinical training curriculum itself is unstructured because trainee experiences are dictated by the patients that appear in the clinic or on the ward.

Meaningful assessments must be longitudinal, sample multiple areas of work, and focus on the process of learning as much as on the product of learning. Assessment results should simultaneously provide timely and appropriate feedback to improve learning. Competency and performance should also be distinguished. In general, competence assessment in controlled settings is easier to administer than performance assessment in clinical environments. Patient and social expectations are that doctors should meet the assessment standards in workplace settings.[26]

Miller's pyramid is frequently used to design assessment at different levels.[27] While it is a good conceptual model for setting up curricula and learning experiences, its utility for assessment in practice settings is questionable.[10] Among other concerns, Miller's pyramid fails to take account of various factors that can influence practice. System influences like facilities and infrastructure or individual variables, such as trainee mental state during assessment, can have a major influence on practice. Assessment under examination conditions can meaningfully predict future performance only if factors such as efficiency and consultation time are taken into account.[26]

The major flaw with traditional assessment is its summative focus without equal attention to formative assessment to improve learning.

Lack of Alignment with Learning in the Workplace

Research suggests that learning in the workplace is triggered by specific problems in patient care that are solved by consulting directly available resources (colleagues, books, etc.).[28] In contrast, courses and independent study are useful for learning about general problems. This difference between on-the-spot learning and planned learning has been delineated by Hoffman and Donaldson.[29] On-the-spot learning is influenced by the type of patient cases encountered, the tension between work load and the time available for teaching and learning, and the learning climate. Differences of opinion, explaining things to others, and feedback and criteria for performance all seem to influence on-the-spot learning.

Activities that contribute to learning in medical practice are embedded in providing high-quality patient care.

These ideas are no surprise to practicing physicians. However, doctors do not engage as extensively in deliberate practice of essential skills as other professional groups.[30] This work implies that learning opportunities in the workplace could be better recognized and used more deliberately. The challenge for improving diagnosis and treatment is to increase experience with challenging cases that provide opportunities for deliberate practice during interactions between faculty and trainees.

Tools for Workplace-Based Assessment

Commonly used assessment tools for WPBA generally fit into one of four categories.[2]

1. Documentation of work experience through logs such as clinical encounter cards (CECs).
2. Observation of individual clinical encounters, such as the mini-clinical evaluation exercise (mini-CEX), direct observation of procedural skills (DOPS), and clinical work sampling (CWS).
3. Discussion of individual clinical cases, such as chart-stimulated recall (called case-based discussion, or CbD, in the United Kingdom).
4. Feedback on routine performance from peers, coworkers, and patients, collected by survey and usually called multisource feedback. Tools for gathering these data include the mini-peer assessment tool (mini-PAT), team assessment of behaviors, and the various patient satisfaction questionnaires. In addition, data from these tools and information from other sources are often combined into a portfolio, which serves as documentation of experiences and achievements.

Documentation of Work Experience: Clinical Encounter Cards

CECs originated as a means of documenting the learning experiences of medical students but they are applicable across the educational continuum. In general, CECs are packets of 5" × 8" cards that can be read by computers. The CECs are given to students at the beginning of rotations along with an instruction booklet. The CEC contents can be tailored to reflect the clinical material seen in a department.[31] A diagnosis list is provided in the booklet, along with a list of codes, which are used to record clinical conditions. The booklet also provides an example of disease staging (stage 1 indicates a disease with no complication, stage 2 is disease with local complications, and stage 3 is disease with systemic complications). Trainees complete a card each time they participate in patient care (e.g., taking a history or performing a physical examination). Multiple encounters with the same patient are recorded on the same card. Trainees record the age and sex of patient, location (outpatient or inpatient), level of involvement, and supervision and procedures seen or performed. The cards are scanned weekly. Reports generated twice a year are reviewed by program directors. Individual reports and peer group comparisons are made available to the students.[32]

Experience shows good agreement between the diagnoses entered on patient charts and those coded by trainees. When secondary diagnoses were considered, the agreement rate reached almost 97%.[32] Rattner et al.[31] also reported similar patterns of diagnostic reporting, indicating reliability of the method.

Analysis of the trends revealed via CECs can help identify disease patterns not seen by students during a particular year. This allows remedial action. Keely et al.[33] used CECs as a teaching encounter card where students provided feedback about the teaching skills of faculty. Kim et al.[34] modified CECs to record medical students' oral case presentation skills. They required students to have one card completed per week following a case presentation. The card was graded on nine competencies, using a nine-point scale. Medical students received feedback based on these ratings, which correlated with other performance on other tools. Greenberg[35] reported a qualitative study where CECs significantly improved the value of feedback. Students' perception of feedback was also positively influenced by using CECs.[36] Despite the different uses made of CECs, a common thread running through several studies is the value of observation and assessment of trainees followed by contextual feedback and remedial action. The quality of feedback improves after use of CECs and these cards can also serve as a means to help faculty improve their teaching.[37]

Observation of Single Clinical Encounters: the Mini-Clinical Evaluation Exercise

The mini-CEX is a snapshot observation of a trainee in an actual practice setting. The trainee engages in a patient care activity (e.g., data gathering, physical examination, counseling). The assessor observes the performance, scores it, and then provides educational feedback. Usually the encounter takes 10–15 minutes and another 5–10 minutes may be spent providing feedback to the trainee.

Many assessors can assess trainees many times during the course of their training. The mini-CEX assessment focuses on the core clinical skills that trainees demonstrate with real patients.[38] The mini-CEX can be easily implemented in a variety of clinical settings and can therefore be integrated into the normal work pattern.

A global rating is given for the mini-CEX rather than the checklist-based recording typical of the OSCE. Whereas checklists usually capture a nominal rating (right or wrong), global ratings capture ordinal information. Some subjectivity may be involved in the process. In fact, the assessor can use discretion and calibrate the ratings according to the performance expected depending on the level of the trainee, case setting (ambulatory, emergency, etc.), and complexity of the patient's problem(s). This makes the whole process more authentic.

The initial use of the mini-CEX was made in assessing trainees during postgraduate education in internal medicine. A structured format was used for ratings, which were made on a nine-point scale, with 1–3 being considered unsatisfactory and 6–9 considered as superior or excellent. The performance was assessed across a number of dimensions including interviewing skills, physical examination, clinical judgment, counseling, organization and efficiency, and overall competence. There was flexibility because not all domains were assessed during the encounters. Specific areas were assessed depending on location and context. Aggregation of ratings across domains and across cases was guided by the purpose of assessment.

There has been considerable experience with the use of the mini-CEX since its introduction. Norcini et al.[38] report a number of presenting complaints covering almost all systems and various contexts (outpatients, emergency, behavioral problems, etc.), which have been assessed using the mini-CEX. It has also been useful in assessing trainees when patients have multiple problems.

There is increasing realization that the mini-CEX shows acceptable correlation with other methods of assessing competence. Kogan et al.[39] report a modest correlation with examination scores, clerkship ratings, and final course grades. Similarly, Durning et al.[40] report correlations between individual components of the mini-CEX and corresponding evaluations by faculty as well as the results of an in-training examination. Boulet et al.[41] demonstrate a good predictive relationship between standardized patient (SP) checklists and global faculty ratings as well as with faculty ratings of communication. Holmboe et al.[14] demonstrate successful discrimination of videotaped performance into unsatisfactory, satisfactory, or superior using mini-CEX forms.

The mini-CEX demonstrates a small but modest correlation with overall future clinical performance judged by SPs, both in the short as well as in the long run.[42] However, it is possible that since the SP examinations were used for high-stakes purposes in the study, trainees may have had different degrees of motivation and this may have affected the correlations. A number of other studies have demonstrated the mini-CEX's ability to discriminate between different levels of performance.

A number of changes have been made in the mini-CEX process to make it more useful for different settings and in different countries. Its use has been extended to various settings in undergraduate as well as postgraduate training. However, the basic character of the tool is constant—that is, making judgments on the basis of an observed clinical encounter and following those judgments with feedback. As with all other methods, task specificity limits the generalizability of a single encounter, so multiple observations in different settings and with different faculty members are needed.

Direct Observation of Procedural Skills

DOPS was designed to provide formative assessment and feedback about trainee procedural skills. It is analogous to the mini-CEX with a focus on procedures rather than clinical skills. The assessors observe a procedure, rate it, and then provide developmental feedback. The observation typically lasts for 10–15 minutes with 5–10 minutes of feedback.

The procedures are generally selected from a list, which often includes those commonly used in practice. Understanding of the indications, techniques, asepsis, analgesia, and communication are assessed. Trainees may also be asked about their earlier experience of performing similar procedures.

Logistics and measurement characteristics of DOPS are similar to the mini-CEX. A trainee undergoes multiple assessments with different procedures and different assessors. Consultants, senior registrars, specialists, general practitioners, or nurses can act as assessors.

Global ratings of procedural skills have been shown to produce valid results and assessors are able to distinguish between various levels of performance.[43] Other studies have also shown that global ratings can distinguish between levels of performance.[44]

Clinical Work Sampling

CWS has been developed as a tool to capture in vivo assessment information without recourse to retrospective recall. Many opportunities occur in everyday contacts among health professionals but go largely unreported. Various forms are used to capture the essential points in trainees' interactions.[45] The forms include admission rating, ward rating, multidisciplinary rating, and patient rating with some local modifications. Supervisors rate the first two, while multidisciplinary teams and the patients rate the last two. One of each form is generally required per patient.

There has been a mixed experience with the use of CWS. While two-thirds of the forms were returned for others, the patients' rating forms were returned for only one-tenth of the situations. Admission and ward rating forms provide acceptable reliability with reasonable numbers of assessments.

Discussion of Individual Cases: Case-Based Discussion

CbD is a variation of what was called chart-stimulated recall. In CbD, trainees are required to select two or three cases they have seen recently and give the patient records to the assessor in advance of the evaluation. Since the discussion is case based, trainees are encouraged to select patients they have seen a number of times. The case should represent a patient problem for which the trainee is competent. The assessor selects one case (two if time permits) for discussion. A statement about why that case has been chosen and what competencies it represents guides the assessor's choice.

The discussion is generally focused on one aspect of the case—for example, the choice of lab tests or a particular therapeutic method. The assessor probes the reasoning behind the actions taken by the trainee. As a general rule, the discussion revolves around the case and does not extend to hypothetical situations. The trainee is rated on any one of several different scales such as the four-point scale developed by Mehay and Bradford[46] comprising: (1) insufficient evidence, (2) needs further development, (3) competent, and (4) excellent. A prerequisite for making such an assessment is to have a description of competencies in each of the assessed areas appropriate for the level of training.

CbD offers advantages in assessing clinical reasoning skills because it encourages a focus on knowledge application, decision making, and other issues. Evaluation of record keeping is also included due to its importance. Like other tools used for WPBA, CbD also uses single encounters for making judgments about the quality of clinical acumen, investigations, treatment, referrals, and ethical issues.

CbD has many similarities with other tools of WPBA. The patient problems can be selected from a core list. CbDs are intended to address multiple encounters, each lasting 10–15 minutes with 5–10 minutes of feedback. Consultants, senior registrars, specialists, or general practitioners can act as assessors. The feedback after the encounter focuses on strengths, suggestions for development, and an action plan.

There are some subtle differences between CbD and what is known as a "case presentation." During a case presentation, "What would you do next?" is the usual question, while CbD looks at what the trainees have actually done. Hence, CbD is not a replacement for a case presentation because they focus on different aspects of competence. CbD is not intended as a knowledge test or as an oral or clinical examination. It is intended to assess the clinical decision-making process and the way in which trainees use medical knowledge when managing a single case.

CbD aims to explore professional judgment exercised in clinical cases. Recognizing uncertainty, application of medical knowledge, application of ethical frameworks, and the ability to prioritize options are some of the components addressed during a CbD. The question-answer portion of the encounter is meant primarily to help the assessors gather evidence rather than to teach.

There have been reports on the validity of CbD from North America. The score distribution and pass rates were consistent with other methods including oral examinations and record audit.[47] CbD also correlated well with an SP examination and was able to discriminate between levels of performance. Solomon et al.[48] also found positive correlations among CbD and an oral examination and positive correlations with written and oral examinations conducted 10 years earlier.

Feedback on Routine Performance: Mini-Peer Assessment Tool

Peers are a good source of information about one's clinical performance and have been used in assessment for many years. Recently, there has been renewed interest in peer assessment and in making collection of this information more systematic. The mini-PAT is a tool that has been modified from the Sheffield peer review assessment tool, an established multisource feedback instrument to assess senior doctors.[49] Mini-PAT has been content-validated against the Foundation Program curriculum in the United Kingdom.[50] Mini-PAT requires trainees to receive anonymous feedback (collected centrally) from their coworkers about a range of competencies. The trainee completes a self-rating and later receives aggregated information from peers and is compared to national norms. The focus is on assessing professional competence within a teamwork environment. Verbatim comments from assessors are also included anonymously. These are reviewed by the trainee and supervisor together to assess strengths, identify areas for improvement, and devise an action plan. This process is undertaken twice per year. Like most other tools for WPBA, the mini-PAT is intended to provide formative feedback to the trainee and is not intended for summative purposes.

Peer assessments have a long history of use in a number of programs. Their value has been mixed. At some places, most of the negative reports about trainee behaviors have emanated from peers, while at others, peer assessment has been used to recognize trainees with outstanding professionalism.

The validity of the mini-PAT has been established in a number of publications. Ramsey et al.[51] found higher mini-PAT scores among certified physicians compared to noncertified doctors. The Sheffield peer review assessment tool, the predecessor of the mini-PAT, has also been shown to be feasible, reliable, and not susceptible to extraneous influence.[50]

Portfolios

A portfolio is a tool for collecting, storing, and presenting evidence about learning and competence development at all levels of training. A portfolio has been defined as "a collection of evidence that is gathered together to show a person's learning journey over time and to demonstrate their abilities."[52] Portfolio is a general term because it can include many different types of content depending on its intended purpose. It can contain educational experiences (procedures, continuing medical education, conferences, etc.), reflections on those experiences, publications, critical incidents, performance on WPBA methods, or multiple-choice question (MCQ) tests.[25] The information may pertain to a single encounter or it may cover an extended period of time. Portfolio data may be evaluated either as representative samples or in total. Portfolios can be paper based or electronic.

Assessors evaluate portfolios to make judgments. These judgments may relate to the frequency, quality, or value of a trainee's educational experiences and outcomes. The power of a portfolio lies in its reflective potential. Reflection separates portfolios from logbooks or dossiers because it allows learning from actions.[53]

Portfolios are a response to the belief that assessment should enhance and support learning as well as measure performance.[54] Portfolios can counteract the reductionist approach to assessment by facilitating a broad view of complex and integrated abilities while also accounting for level and context of learning. Portfolios provide evidence for learning and progress toward desirable educational outcomes.

Portfolios have high face validity because they reflect what is actually done in the workplace. Their validity and reliability depends entirely on the quality of their contents. At our present level of understanding, portfolios are best used for formative purposes. It is possible to increase their quality by making them standardized, developing acceptable scoring criteria, and training both learners and assessors. Driessen and colleagues[55] suggest that qualitative methodologies like triangulation, member checking, and prolonged engagement can be used to increase portfolio dependability.

Feedback

Based on direct observation, feedback is the backbone of WPBA. Timely and quality feedback is crucial to learning, especially in areas related to patient care. An observer who compares trainee performance with an expected standard usually provides feedback. The expected performance standards may be either stated explicitly or derive from the observer's professional judgment. The trainee is expected to reflect on this information and use it to improve behavior. The effect of feedback on physician performance has been well researched. A Best Evidence Medical Education review published in 2006 identified 683 studies on feedback and physician clinical performance between 1966 and 2003.[12]

Feedback must be given in an acceptable and actionable form to be useful by trainees. Some evaluators believe that feedback should be nonjudgmental. However, judgment is always involved if feedback is to be useful. The person providing feedback must present it constructively. If feedback is too negative, trainees may become defensive, dismiss the evidence, or attempt to justify their actions. Learners generally welcome constructive feedback.[56]

Various models of giving feedback have been described. The simplest one is the "sandwich model," where an observer tries to provide critical feedback between layers of praise. While this has the appeal of simplicity, it is now recognized that following a line of praise, the trainee generally recognizes what is coming next and may not attend to the positives. This removes the reinforcing utility of feedback. Pendleton et al.'s[57] framework is another model commonly used for this purpose. In this framework, the trainee first identifies what went well. The trainee then indicates what could have been done better and how the performance could be improved. The trainer also provides suggestions for improvement. The trainer and trainee conclude by formulating an action plan that specifies areas for improvement.

There is an analogy between doctor-patient communications and educational feedback. In a clinical communication, the first step is to build a therapeutic relationship through empathy and rapport. In educational feedback, one needs to build a climate of trust and comfort for the learner by being objective and reducing emotionally charged situations.[58] The rapport building skills used in a clinical situation can also be used in the educational setting. The "PEARLS" mnemonic

(**P**artnership for joint problem solving; **E**mpathetic understanding; **A**pology for barriers to learners' success; **R**espect for learners' values; **L**egitimation of feelings; and **S**upport for efforts at correction) is a useful framework for building rapport.[59]

Whatever feedback model the observer chooses, it is important to own the feedback (use of "I" statements). Equally important is being clear by avoiding general statements. Using current observations as the basis of feedback avoids inferential comments. Being descriptive rather than evaluative (*you did not make eye contact with the patient* rather than *you were not interested in the patient*), avoiding interpretation (*I think you meant*) and advice giving (*I think you should*), and focusing on behavior that can be changed are some other attributes of constructive feedback.

Quality Assurance

Unlike paper-and-pencil tests, WPBAs are more prone to measurement errors, which can compromise their reliability and validity. The problem is further compounded by relatively small sample sizes. While a number of psychometric methods can be applied to improve the reliability of such assessments,[41] some believe the approach to WPBA should take a constructivist, social-psychological perspective and integrate elements of theories of cognition, motivation, and decision making.[60] A central assumption in this proposition is that performance assessment is a judgment and decision-making process in which rating outcomes are influenced by interactions between individuals and the social context of assessment.

Research has shown many problems related to the reliability and accuracy of performance ratings.[61,62] Assessors tend to give above-average ratings, which fail to distinguish between students despite obvious differences in performance.[63] Raters appear to use a one- or two-dimensional concept of performance and do not tend to distinguish between more detailed performances dimensions.[64] Leniency, halo effects, and range restriction are other rater errors that contribute to the low reliability of performance ratings. There are reports to suggest a lack of rating consistency between raters and within raters, across different occasions, with reliability coefficients approaching zero.[65] Even the validity of the interpretations could be doubted because of content specificity and small sample sizes.

Govaerts et al.[60] argue that many of these issues stem from the quantitative psychometric framework, which aims at getting a "true" score reflecting "true" performance. Trainee ability is assumed to be fixed, permanent, and acontextual and any changes due to context or rater interactions are considered as unwanted sources of bias. Efforts to improve in-training assessments have been made from this perspective and include development of precise rating formats and rater training to improve consistency.

Studies on expertise provide some interesting insights to the design of WPBA systems. Task-specific expertise is a key variable in information processing. Experts demonstrate rapid automatic pattern recognition and are likely to take more time to gather and analyze information, when confronted with unfamiliar problems.[61] Studies on teacher supervision have shown that inexperienced supervisors provided literal description while analyzing verbal protocols whereas experienced ones interpreted their findings and made evaluative comments.[62] Experts focused on learning; nonexperts focused on discrete teaching. Experts spent time monitoring, gathering and analyzing information; nonexperts focused on providing the correct solution. Experts had more elaborate and well-structured mental models, replete with contextual information.

More enriched processing and better incorporation of contextual cues by experienced raters can result in qualitatively different, more holistic feedback to trainees, focusing on a variety of issues. Thanks to more elaborate performance scripts, expert raters may rely more often on top-down information processing or pattern recognition when observing and judging performance, especially when time constraints or competing responsibilities play a role.[63] Optimization of WPBA may therefore require rating procedures and formats that force raters to elaborate their judgments and substantiate their ratings with concrete and specific examples of observed behaviors.

Assessment of competence under examination circumstances can have a higher predictive value for performance in actual practice when factors such as efficiency and consultation time are taken into account. Substandard performance of physicians does not necessarily reflect a lack of competence. Performance and competence are two distinct constructs.[26] This has important implications for assessment design. The competence of physicians is a necessary but insufficient condition for performance in actual practice. Therefore, assessments in real settings are likely to reflect and predict future performance better than standardized assessments.

In essence, WPBA requires (a) specification of standards, criteria, and scoring guides; (b) training and calibration of assessors and moderators; (c) use in the context of a system of assessment; and (d) ongoing audit of the results.[64] Triangulation of results with other assessments external to workplace should also help to improve the utility of the process. Adding a knowledge test component (e.g., MCQs) or skills test (e.g., the objective structured clinical examination) should be part of an overarching assessment and learning system.

Faculty development remains an important strategy for maintaining quality of WPBA. Two areas that need to be developed are assessment and providing feedback. Some good examples of focused training programs are available, which target behavioral observation with minimum obtrusiveness, performance dimensions, and frame of reference training.[21] Such training has been reported to positively affect the process of WPBA. Provision of educational feedback is a vital component of many of the tools used for WPBA, and efforts to improve the quality of feedback will help in making WPBA more effective. While it stands to reason, there are conflicting reports about the effect of rater training on accuracy or reliability of assessments.[65]

Several other issues also warrant attention. Many of the concerns related to scoring under Kane's framework, discussed in an earlier chapter, may relate to seeing WPBA as yet another "examination" by the trainees. This may limit the utility of the entire exercise as trainees may view low scores as failures rather than as an opportunity to learn.[66] The competitive nature of trainees may override the philosophy of WPBA as a developmental tool. There are also concerns that early success in WPBA may decrease the motivation to learn more. It is imperative to project WPBA as an intergral part of teaching-learning at the workplace rather than as an end itself. From this perspective, it may be important to pay as much attention to student development as to faculty development.

Advantages of Workplace-Based Assessment

Assessment is most commonly associated with "having to prove," where the assessor tries to prove a hypothesis about the knowledge and skills of the trainee. However, there is an equally important function of assessment and that is to improve learning. Even though there may not yet be enough evidence about the better predictive utility of WPBA, it makes sense—at least theoretically—to use this form of assessment as a tool for better learning.

An advantage of the workplace-based methods is that they fulfill the three basic requirements for assessment techniques that facilitate learning.[67–70] First, the content of the training program, the competencies expected as outcomes, and the assessment practices are aligned. Second, trainee feedback is provided during and after assessment events. Third, assessment events are used to steer trainee learning toward the desired outcomes. The potential to foster and shape learning is WPBA's greatest strength.

WPBA has generally been seen from an assessment perspective as analogous to classroom tests. In this role, it exhibits much strength, especially as a tool to foster learning. However, this also puts WPBA at a disadvantage because ensuring equivalence among institutions or even among different assessors may be problematic.

Reliability

While it is true that most of the tools used for WPBA are unstandardized, they are not low in terms of utility. WPBA reliability can be improved by sensible and expert use. In addition, sufficient and representative sampling of competencies will improve reliability just as it does for objective structured clinical examinations and MCQ examinations. Triangulating the results with those obtained from other instruments and out of workplace assessments also helps in building confidence.

Reports on reliability of these instruments are interesting.[71] They often require eight to twelve encounters to reach an acceptable level of reliability, which compares very well in terms of testing time with standardized and objective instruments. Picking up information that is generalizable across encounters is responsible for this; broad sampling of assessors may balance out any inter-rater differences.

A recent publication reviewing the research in an effort to build validity arguments for the mini-CEX made some interesting observations.[65] It used Kane's conceptualization of validity—that is, building a structured argument involving scoring, generalization, extrapolation, and interpretation. This is necessary because on one hand, observation of a single encounter by a single observer raised issues of reproducibility and validity; on the other hand, the unit of analysis (i.e., history taking and physical examination) may not be representative of the typical work pattern of physicians. Some of the points that emerge from review of research on the mini-CEX include the use of a "shrunken" scale (i.e., not using the extremes), ratings skewed positively, leniency, and awarding high scores to professionalism and humanism. It has also been reported that there is a high correlation between various competencies assessed by the rating form. This could either be a true effect (i.e., a candidate who is good in one area is also good in another area) or a halo effect, or that raters are not able to distinguish between different constructs using the rating form.

While it may be possible to recreate a clinical situation using simulations and then test it using standardized tools, there are concerns that this encourages introduction of indirect or surrogate measures.[72] However, low reliability by traditional standards can be considered as an impediment for less reliance being placed on WPBA. Reliability of work-based assessments remains an issue because "they depend on subjective judgement of unstandardized material."[73] Reliability of "subjective" assessments can be improved by a number of interventions.[74] Increasing the size and representativeness of samples, increasing the number of assessors, using subject experts as assessors, training assessors, and calibration can all improve reliability. It may also be time to revisit the issue of reliability as "comparability" or "dependability," especially when dealing with performance testing.[75]

WPBA has the appeal of being able to directly, relevantly, and holistically measure the elements that comprise clinical competence. The challenge, however, is how to make this form of assessment more acceptable and dependable. The silver lining has been the turn of methodology full circle—from real patient-based examinations to simulations to real patients.[76]

Strategies to improve WPBA have typically followed the psychometric approach, focusing on precision of measurement and trying to limit uncontrolled variables. Low inter-rater reliability, halo effects, leniency, and range restriction have been reported for WPBA.[64,77,78] Attempts to improve objectivity and standardization through various means has met with only limited success.[62]

Another important issue may be related to trainees who are rated unsatisfactory during WPBA. For them, alternative methods of assessment may be needed, especially to provide remediation and diagnostic feedback. Traditional tests of knowledge and skills, and perhaps SP examinations may be required.

Trust and acceptance of WPBA by raters and trainees is a crucial factor in making it more useful. Authenticity, fairness, honesty, transparency, and quality feedback have been cited as some of the factors that promote trust.[79,80] The concept of trust is embedded in consequential validity.

Performance assessment in the workplace is a complex task because it is affected by a number of factors and is highly contextual. Doctors work in their own environments and their performance depends increasingly on how well they function in teams and how well the health care system around them functions. Rater behavior and rating outcomes are influenced by contextual factors. From this perspective, WPBA is not really a measurement issue but a decision-making issue. Govaerts et al.[60] argue that WPBA may benefit from better understanding of raters' reasons and cognitive processes that they engage in while assessing than that from quantitative properties of scores.

WPBA has the advantage of assessing performance under actual work conditions, climbing to the third and fourth levels of Miller's pyramid. It also allows a tight fit between curriculum, instruction, and assessment. The feedback loop makes early and appropriate remedial action possible.

The utility of any assessment—either an individual tool or an entire program—can be conceptualized as a product of its validity, reliability, feasibility, acceptability, and educational impact.[81] There are inevitable trade-offs between these components. Attempts to increase reliability by tightly structuring the assessments may reduce their educational impact. What WPBA loses in terms of standardization, it gains in terms of its educational impact by providing developmental feedback to trainees. Contrasted to standardized externally administered tests at the end of the program, WPBA integrates teaching, learning, and assessment. It has been rightly pointed out that WPBA *is "built-in" the program rather than being a "bolt-on."*[2]

There has been a renewed interest in using assessment as a tool of improvement. Typically, formative assessment is low stakes and opportunistic and is intended to stimulate learning. It provides specific actionable feedback in an ongoing and timely manner. If this is the purpose of formative assessment, then the need for high reliability is less than the need for educational impact. This conceptualization of the criteria for good assessment is addressed in Chapter 2 of this volume.

We conclude that WPBA is growing in popularity and utility across the health professions. Continuous, rigorous research on the processes, outcomes, and tradeoffs involved in WPBA schemes is needed to insure its quality, fairness, and validity for personnel decision making.

References

1. General Medical Council. *Workplace Based Assessment: a guide for implementation.* London; 2010. Available at: www.gmc-uk.org/Workplace_Based_Assessment__A_guide_for_implementation_0410.pdf_48905168.pdf (accessed October 22, 2012).
2. Swanwick T, Chana N. Workplace-based assessment. *Br J Hosp Med (Lond).* 2009; **70**(5): 290–3.
3. Dreyfus H, Dreyfus S. *Mind Over Machine: the power of human intuition and expertise in the era of computers.* Oxford: Basil Blackwell; 1986.
4. Hampton JR, Harrison MJG, Mitchell JRA, et al. Relative contributions of history-taking, physical examination, and laboratory investigation to diagnosis and management of medical outpatients. *Br Med J.* 1975; **2**(5969): 486–9.
5. Peterson MC, Holbrook JH, Hales DV, et al. Contributions of the history, physical

examination and laboratory investigation in making medical diagnoses. *West J Med.* 1992; **156**(2): 163–5.

6. Kirch W, Schafii C. Misdiagnosis at a university hospital in four medical eras. *Medicine (Baltimore).* 1996; **75**(1): 29–40.

7. Norman GR. Non-cognitive factors in health sciences education: from the clinic floor to the cutting room floor. *Adv Health Sci Educ.* 2010; **15**(1): 1–8.

8. Lane IF. Professional competencies in health sciences education: from multiple intelligences to the clinic floor. *Adv Health Sci Educ Theory Pract.* 2010; **15**(1): 129–46.

9. Regehr G. The persistent myth of stability: on the chronic underestimation of the role of context in behavior. *J Gen Intern Med.* 2006; **21**(5): 544–5.

10. Rethans JJ, Norcini JJ, Maldonado MB, et al. The relationship between competence and performance: implications for assessing practice performance. *Med Educ.* 2002; **36**(10): 901–9.

11. Hattie JA. *Influences on Student Learning.* Inaugural professional address, University of Auckland, August 2, 1999. Available at: www.education.auckland.ac.nz/webdav/site/education/shared/hattie/docs/influences-on-student-learning.pdf (accessed August 23, 2011).

12. Veloski J, Boex JR, Grasberger MJ, et al. Systematic review of the literature on assessment, feedback and physicians' clinical performance. BEME Guide No. 7. *Med Teach.* 2006; **28**(2): 117–28.

13. Gipps C. Socio-cultural aspect of assessment. *Rev Res Educ.* 1999; **24**: 355–92.

14. Holmboe E, Yepes M, Williams F, et al. Feedback and the mini clinical evaluation exercise. *J Gen Intern Med.* 2004; **19**(5): 558–61.

15. Kassebaum DG, Eaglen RH. Shortcomings in the evaluation of students' clinical skills and behaviors in medical school. *Acad Med.* 1999; **74**(7): 842–9.

16. Association of American Medical Colleges (AAMC). *Medical School Graduation Questionnaire: all schools report.* Washington, DC: AAMC; 2011. Available at: www.aamc.org/data/gq/allschoolsreport/2004.pdf https://www.aamc.org/download/256776/data/gq-2011-rm.pdf (accessed October 22, 2012).

17. Kogan JR, Hauer KE. Brief report: use of the mini-clinical evaluation exercise in internal medicine core clerkships. *J Gen Intern Med.* 2006; **21**(5): 501–2.

18. Daelmans HE, Hoogenboom RJ, Donker AJ, et al. Effectiveness of clinical rotations as a learning environment for achieving competencies. *Med Teach.* 2004; **26**(4): 305–12.

19. Day SC, Grosso LG, Norcini JJ, et al. Residents' perceptions of evaluation procedures used by their training program. *J Gen Intern Med.* 1990; **5**(5): 421–6.

20. Isaacson JH, Posk LK, Litaker DG, et al. Residents' perceptions of the evaluation process. *J Gen Intern Med.* 1995; **10**(Suppl.): 89.

21. Holmboe ES, Hawkins RE, Huot SJ. Effects of training in direct observation of medical residents' clinical competence: a randomized trial. *Ann Intern Med.* 2004; **140**(11): 874–81.

22. Noel GL, Herbers JE, Caplow MP, et al. How well do internal medicine faculty

members evaluate the clinical skills of residents? *J Gen Intern Med.* 1992; **117**(9): 757–65.

23. Herbers JE, Noel GL, Cooper GS, et al. How accurate are faculty evaluations of clinical competence? *J Gen Intern Med.* 1989; **4**(3): 202–8.

24. Kalet A, Earp JA, Kowlowitz V. How well do faculty evaluate the interviewing skills of medical students? *J Gen Intern Med.* 1992; **7**(5): 499–505.

25. Norcini JJ. Workplace based assessment. In: Swanwick T, editors. *Understanding Medical Education: evidence theory and practice.* West Sussex, UK: Wiley Blackwell; 2010. pp. 232–45.

26. Rethans J, Sturmans F, Drop R, et al. Does competence of general practitioners predict their performance? Comparison between examination setting and actual practice. *BMJ.* 1991; **303**(6814): 1377–80.

27. Miller GE. The assessment of skills/competence/performance. *Acad Med.* 1990; **65**(Suppl. 9): S63–7.

28. Van de Weil MW, van den Bossche P, Janssen S, et al. Exploring deliberate practice in medicine: how do physicians learn in the workplace? *Adv Health Sci Educ.* 2011; **16**(1): 81–95.

29. Hoffman KG, Donaldson JF. Contextual tensions of the clinical environment and their influence on teaching and learning. *Med Educ.* 2004; **38**(4): 448–54.

30. Ericsson KA. Deliberate practice and the acquisition and maintenance of expert performance in medicine and related domains. *Acad Med.* 2004; **79**(Suppl. 10): S70–81.

31. Rattner SL, Louis DZ, Rabinowitz C, et al. Documenting and comparing medical students' clinical experiences. *JAMA.* 2001; **286**(9): 1035–40.

32. Richards ML, Paukert JL, Downing SM, et al. Reliability and usefulness of clinical encounter cards for a third-year surgical clerkship. *J Surg Res.* 2007; **140**(1): 139–48.

33. Keeley E, Oppenheimer L, Woods T, et al. A teaching encounter card to evaluate clinical supervisors across clerkship rotations. *Med Teach.* 2010; **32**(2): e96–100.

34. Kim S, Kogan JR, Bellini LM, et al. A randomized-controlled study of encounter cards to improve oral case presentation skills of medical students. *J Gen Intern Med.* 2005; **20**(8): 743–7.

35. Greenberg LW. Medical students' perceptions of feedback in a busy ambulatory setting; a descriptive study using a clinical encounter card. *South Med J.* 2004; **97**(12): 1174–8.

36. Ozuah PO, Reznik M, Greenberg L. Improving medical student feedback with a clinical encounter card. *Ambul Pediatr.* 2007; **7**(6): 449–52.

37. Paukert JL, Richards ML, Olney C. An encounter card system for increasing feedback to students. *Am J Surg.* 2002; **183**(3): 300–4.

38. Norcini J, Blank L, Duffy F, et al. The mini-CEX: a method for assessing clinical skills. *Ann Intern Med.* 2003; **138**(6): 476–81.

39. Kogan JR, Bellini LM, Shea JA. Feasibility, validity and reliability of the mini clinical evaluation exercise in a medicine core clerkship. *Acad Med.* 2003; **78**(Suppl. 10): S33–5.

40. Durning SJ, Cation LJ, Markert RJ, et al. Assessing the validity and reliability of mini clinical evaluation exercise (mCEX) for internal medicine residency training. *Acad Med.* 2002; **77**(9): 900–4.

41. Boulet JR, McKinley DW, Whelan GP, et al. Quality assurance methods for performance-based assessments. *Adv Health Sci Educ Theory Pract.* 2003; **8**(1): 27–47.

42. Ney EM, Shea JA, Kogan JR. Predictive validity of the mini-clinical evaluation exercise (mCEX): do medical students' mCEX ratings correlate with future clinical exam performance? *Acad Med.* 2009; **84**(Suppl. 10): S17–20.

43. Larson JL, Williams RG, Ketchum J, et al. Feasibility, reliability and validity of an operative performance rating system for evaluating surgery residents. *Surgery.* 2005; **138**(4): 640–7.

44. Goff BA, Nielsen PE, Lentz GM, et al. Surgical skills assessment: a blinded examination of obstetrics and gynecology residents. *Am J Obstet Gynecol.* 2002; **186**(4): 613–17.

45. Turnbull J, MacFadyen J, Barneveld CV, et al. Clinical work sampling: a new approach to the problem of intraining evaluation. *J Gen Intern Med.* 2000; **15**(8): 556–61.

46. Mehay R, editor. *The Essential Handbook for GP Training & Education.* Available at: www.essentialgptrainingbook.com/ (accessed October 22, 2012).

47. Norman GR, Davis D, Painvin A, et al. Comprehensive assessment of clinical competence of family physicians using multiple measures. In: Bender W, Hiemstra R, Scherpbier A, et al., editors. *Teaching and Assessing Clinical Competence.* Groningen, NL: Boekwork Publications; 1990. pp. 357–64.

48. Solomon DJ, Reinhart MA, Bridgham RG, et al. An assessment of an oral examination format for evaluating clinical competence in emergency medicine. *Acad Med.* 1990; **65**(Suppl. 9): S43–4.

49. Davies HA, Archer JC. Multi source feedback using Sheffield Peer Review Assessment Tool (SPRAT): development and practical aspects. *Clin Teach.* 2005; **2**: 77–81.

50. Archer JC, Norcini JJ, Davies HA. Peer review of pediatricians in training using SPRAT. *BMJ.* 2005; **330**(7502): 1251–3.

51. Ramsey PG, Wenrich MD, Carline JD, et al. Use of peer ratings to evaluate physician performance. *JAMA.* 1993; **269**(13): 1655–60.

52. Rees C. The use (and abuse) of the term "portfolio." *Med Educ.* 2005; **39**(11): 436–7.

53. Izzat S. Portfolios: the next assessment tool in medical education? *Neo Rev.* 2007; **8**(10): e405–8.

54. Friedman MB, David MH, Harden RM, et al. Portfolios as a method of student assessment: AMEE Guide No. 24. *Med Teach.* 2001; **23**(6): 535–51.

55. Driessen E, van der Vleuten CP, Schuwirth L, et al. The use of qualitative research criteria for portfolio assessment as an alternative to reliability evaluation: a case study. *Med Educ.* 2005; **39**(2): 214–20.

56. Gordon J. ABC of learning and teaching in medicine: one to one teaching and feedback. *BMJ.* 2003; **326**(7388): 543–6.
57. Pendleton D, Schofield T, Tate P, et al. *The Consultation: an approach to teaching and learning.* Oxford: Oxford University Press; 1984.
58. Kaprielian VS, Gradison M. Effective use of feedback. *Fam Med.* 1998; **30**(6): 406–7.
59. Prochaska JO, DeClimente CC, Norcross JC. In search of how people change: applications to addictive behaviors. *Am Psychol.* 1992; **47**(9): 1102–14.
60. Govaerts MJB, van der Vleuten CPM, Schuwirth L, et al. Broadening perspectives on clinical performance assessment: rethinking the nature of in-training assessment. *Adv Health Sci Educ Theory Pract.* 2007; **12**(2): 239–60.
61. Van der Vleuten CP, Scherpbier AJ, Dolmans DH, et al. Clerkship assessment assessed. *Med Teach.* 2000; **22**(6): 592–600.
62. Williams RG, Klamen DA, McGaghie WC. Cognitive, social and environmental sources of bias in clinical performance ratings. *Teach Learn Med.* 2003; **15**(4): 270–92.
63. Nahum GG. Evaluating medical student obstetrics and gynecology clerkship performance: which assessment tools are most reliable? *Am J Obstet Gynecol.* 2004; **191**(5): 1762–71.
64. Silber CG, Nasca TJ, Paskin DL, et al. Do global rating forms enable program directors to assess the ACGME competencies? *Acad Med.* 2004; **79**(6): 549–56.
65. Littlefield JH, DaRosa DA, Anderson KD, et al. Assessing performance in clerkships: accuracy of surgery clerkship performance raters. *Acad Med.* 1991; **66**(Suppl. 9): S16–18.
66. General Medical Council. *Workplace Based Assessment: a guide for implementation.* London: General Medical Council; 2010.
67. Frederiksen N. The real test bias: influences of testing on teaching and learning. *Am Psychol.* 1984; **39**(3): 193–202.
68. Crooks TJ. The impact of classroom evaluation practices on students. *Rev Educ Res.* 1988; **58**(4): 438–81.
69. Swanson DB, Norman GR, Linn RL. Performance-based assessment: lessons from the health professions. *Educ Res.* 1995; **24**(5): 5–11.
70. Shepard LA. The role of assessment in a learning culture. *Educ Res.* 2000; **29**(7): 4–14.
71. Pelgrim EAM, Kramer AWM, Mokkink HGA, et al. In-training assessment using direct observation of single-patient encounters: a literature review. *Adv Health Sci Educ Theory Pract.* 2011; **16**(1): 131–42.
72. Sadler DR. Specifying and promulgating achievement standards. *Oxford Rev Educ.* 1987; **13**(2): 191–209.
73. Southgate L, Campbell M, Cox J, et al. The General Medical Council's performance procedures: peer review of performance in the workplace. *Med Educ.* 2001; **35**(Suppl. 1): 20–28.
74. Wass V, O'Neill P. What the educators are saying. *BMJ.* 2004; **328**(7433): 210.
75. Gipps C. *Beyond Testing.* London: Falmer Press; 1994.

76. Schuwirth LW, van der Vleuten CPM. The use of clinical simulation in assessment. *Med Educ.* 2003; **37**(Suppl. 1): 65–71.

77. Kreiter CD, Ferguson KJ. Examining the generalizability of ratings across clerkships using a clinical evaluation form. *Eval Health Prof.* 2001; **24**(1): 36–46.

78. Gray JD. Global rating scales in residency education. *Acad Med.* 1996; **71**(1 Suppl): S65–3.

79. Messick S. The interplay of evidence and consequences in the validation of performance assessments. *Educ Res.* 1994; **23**(2): 13–23.

80. Piggot-Irvine E. Key features of appraisal effectiveness. *Int J Educ Manag.* 2003; **17**(4): 170–8.

81. Van der Vleuten CPM. The assessment of professional competence: developments, research and practical implications. *Adv Health Sci Educ Theory Pract.* 1996; **1**(1): 41–67.

13

An International Review of the Recertification and Revalidation of Physicians

Progress toward Achieving Best Practices

W. Dale Dauphinee

THE PAST TWO DECADES HAVE SEEN MORE EFFORT, INNOVATIVE CHANGE, and documented progress in the fields of physician recertification or revalidation than at any time in the history of medicine. These changes have roots inside and outside of medicine. No stronger internal influences can be identified than widespread recognition of the ineffectiveness of classroom and other course-based lecturing and self-assessment based programs in continuing medical education[1,2] and the reality of quality of care disasters like the Royal Bristol Infirmary in the United Kingdom and similar events elsewhere.[3,4] Yet on careful examination of the quality of care and safety and the empirical education literatures, it is also clear that a shift in thinking about maintaining quality began long before these sentinel events or the focus on educational outcomes began. Reading either the *Quality Chasm* or *To Err Is Human* from the Institute of Medicine confirms the accumulated wisdom that holding a medical degree, a general license, or acquisition of a specialty certificate is insufficient evidence to ensure quality of care or patient safety.

Early formulations of ideas about recertification and continuous improvement came from within the profession and the certification boards.[5,6] For example, the American Board of Family Practice, now the American Board of Family Medicine, introduced time-limited certification in 1969.[7] In 1998, other initiatives were described when Bashook and Parboosingh[8] outlined the state of recertification and the maintenance of competence in North America. A year later, a series of articles on revalidation in the *British Medical Journal* focused on the United Kingdom, Canada, the United States, the Netherlands, and Australasia.[9-13] These articles outlined progress in the field but there were many challenges, as Norcini pointed out subsequently.[14] One was the relative lack of emphasis on the key element needed for any feedback loop in the assessment-feedback-learning cycle—the need for an educational or learning component. Now, in 2012, this chapter will focus on what has been learned in the last decade and will assess how the field is developing. The specific question is: have we reached the point of stating that there are clearly verifiable *best practices* that meet basic validity criteria due to their consequences for addressing the purposes of revalidation and recertification? But first, it is necessary to define terms, implied goals, and impacts expected from revalidation and recertification.

Terminology, Guiding Principles, and Concepts

Cunnington and Southgate[15] have noted that the key underlying concept—recertification, revalidation, re-licensure—has been that maintenance of competence of physicians in practice is intended to protect the public. Public protection is achieved by defining standards of care and by ensuring that physicians meet these practice standards, either individually or team-wise. Cunnington and Southgate[15] also point out that the common element is professional guidance about care standards, and the means to maintain those standards. The basic concepts implied in revalidation and recertification will be reviewed together but described separately, depending on the political and sociocultural context.

Crucial insights that frame this assessment have emerged in the educational and health services research literatures. Investigators questioned assumptions and principles that grounded continuing professional development (CPD), how physicians learn, and how doctors change their professional activities. Four significant shifts in educational thinking are directly related to revalidation and recertification practices.

1. Self-assessment and self-reflection were challenged as established principles, and their role in practice-based learning came in doubt. Reflective personal judgments are no longer promoted as an effective strategy in CPD. Eva and Regehr[16,17] have addressed key issues and evidence in a series of publications

from 2005 to 2008. Their syntheses have confirmed the importance of external feedback and support in the improvement cycle.

2. Deliberate practice needs focused peer or professional feedback to achieve optimal results. The writings of Anders Ericsson[18] have identified the need for afferent assessment feedback loops to be part of the improvement cycle, as will be noted repeatedly in this synthesis.

3. Peer feedback and review needs an underlying educational strategy to be optimally effective with physicians. Objective peer feedback or other professional guidance is needed for optimal change and results that stick. Illustrations include the CPD work of Sargeant and colleagues[19] and recertification studies sponsored by the American Board of Medical Specialties (ABMS).[20] More than peer feedback is needed for better patient outcomes. Peer support and interaction are key elements of the process.

4. Nothing can be argued about CPD results or validity without measurement of impact in actual practice that includes evidence of change in future practice performance or behaviors. The outcomes literature has shown that more activity or outputs are not necessarily better. Measurements of impact are needed.[21] An explanation of the shift in the validation process has been offered by Streiner and Norman[22] and also described by Clauser et al.'s[23] writing on validity and reliability in medical education assessment.

These findings and insights together suggest that the assumptions behind recertification or revalidation practices must include these key elements and must be part of the criteria for defining best practices for implementing revalidation, recertification, CPD, and continuous quality improvement (CQI) programs.

This chapter defines a *best practice* as one that, upon rigorous evaluation, demonstrates success, has an impact, and can be replicated.[24] Successful replication involves a cascade of activities that describe what works, or does not work, in a particular context. Evaluators must accumulate and apply knowledge about how and why *best practices* work in different situations, contexts, and cultural and environmental conditions. In keeping with the prior discussion of outcomes and impacts, the definition requires that impact analyses and an analysis of consequential validity should be included for a program to be considered a best practice. Otherwise, the fallacy of more is better operates. As witnessed by a recent discussion in the *New England Journal of Medicine* by grandfathered certificants,[25] and any look at the UK literature since the late 1990s, physicians care about costs without evidence of value to doctors or their patients.

The debate about the meaning of competence will be avoided by suggesting that the field of quality assurance and public policy has advanced to a more directly accountable framework. The intent in 2012 is to focus on the maintenance of clinical performance and its impact on patient care. This distinction is crucial to avoid the fallacy that educational outputs, such as competencies or their indicators, are useful to monitor the course of developing essential knowledge, skills, and clinical training. Educational outcomes are *not* viewed as proxies for clinical outcomes needed for public accountability in any health care system. This line of thinking, in the analysis of best practices, must also address inefficiency and making health care and education endeavors like recertification commercial products. It is not about units of continuing education sold, courses taken, or certification units achieved. This is a higher calling of standards than where the field was in 2000. The use of outcomes and consequences of current practices in CPD, for public benefit, will be discussed.

Finally, the chapter will examine other policies emerging in the health care environment. Will the impacts of other political or institutional policy shifts influence revalidation for licensure, certification, or recertification in the specialties? How will universally legislated quality of care policies play out, compared to those jurisdictions where they are recommended but not universally mandated? Will developments in institution-based quality of care and accreditation influence or dominate the field? Will expected cost-reduction strategies in health systems and institutions affect quality assurance and practice improvement?

Methodology

Inclusion Criteria: What?

Literature coverage included published peer-reviewed literature and gray literature consisting of reports by independent authors or internal documents that met the quality criteria and have been approved by the oversight board of an agency or organization. Reports or essays quoting existing literature that meet inclusion criteria are used for areas where reports exist in languages other than English.

Exclusion Criteria: Why Not?

Self-assessments are excluded because evidence shows they are unreliable performance measures.[26,27] Quantitative or qualitative analyses of any effect beyond chance or measurement error is expected to be included in program reports. The reasons are simple. To recommend a best practice, potential users should have solid evidence about how and why that conclusion was reached, that analyses were reliable and interpreted validly, and that the return on investment made in the program is reported. Return on investment includes potential benefits forgone from other means in lieu of the adopted approach (opportunity costs).[27]

Survey of Approaches in Use

Readers should appreciate what currently exists in medical revalidation or recertification programs in Europe, North America, and Australasia before considering best practices. The following table, adapted from Merkur et al.,[28] lists selected examples from Europe. The information does not imply best practices but, rather, states existing practices at the country level. For additional European programs, readers are referred to Merkur et al.'s 2008 paper for the World Health Organization.[29]

TABLE 13.1 Type and Features of Programs for Medical Revalidation by Country

Country	Time Frame (Years)	Type of Revalidation		Compulsory	Sanction or Reward	Primary Regulator
		CPD	Peer			
Austria	3	Yes	Yes	Yes	Legally required	Medical Chamber
Belgium	3	Yes	Yes	No	Fiscal Incentives	Ministry of Public Health
France	5	Yes	Yes	Yes	Lawsuit by regional MD councils	National Continuing Medical Education Council
Germany	5	Yes	Yes	Yes	Fiscal penalty and after 2 years, withdraw	Regional Chambers
Netherlands	5	Yes	Yes, specialties	Yes	Deregister	Central College of Specialists
Spain	–	Yes, 9/17 regions	–	No	Varies between regions	National Medical Association
United Kingdom	5	Yes	360-degree multisource feedback	Yes	Potential supervision	Department of Health
United States	Varies	Yes	Yes	Depends on age of certification	Decertify	Certifying Boards

(continued)

Country	Time Frame (Years)	Type of Revalidation		Compulsory	Sanction or Reward	Primary Regulator
		CPD	Peer			
Canada	5	Yes	Yes, with some 360-degree feedback	Only for certification	Decertify	National Colleges with some regulatory bodies
Australasia	Varies	Yes	Yes	Only for certification	Decertify	National Royal Colleges

As can be seen, practices vary. However, the pervasiveness of the move to revalidation, primarily using auditing of continuing medical education programs is clear. The following quotation from Merkur et al.[29] can summarize the overall conclusion:

> As this summary demonstrates, what is required of physicians and whether and how it is enforced vary significantly. This reflects the diversity of traditions, such as the concepts of the liberal professions, norms of the role of the state, the degree of devolution to regional bodies and the role of the payers, such as social insurance funds.

The question remains, what works in terms of demonstrating an impact on variations in care? In the case of compulsory programs with sanctions or penalties, there is a particular interest in following the consequences of these programs over time and determining the ultimate impacts.

Generic Models of Best Practices in Quality Assurance, Revalidation, and Recertification

A generic model of an improvement cycle is illustrated in Figure 13.1. The essential features are that it must be seen as a quality assurance process that uses the classical assessment cycle, described by many authors.

Revalidation or recertification models are much more complex than this simple model. The complexity of interactions and possible impacts of a national quality improvement model can be seen in an adaptation of Shaw's[30] model in Figure 13.2. The obvious difference is the number of stakeholders involved. This broader constituency will have an increasing impact in time.

In practice, most authors tend to classify revalidation and recertification

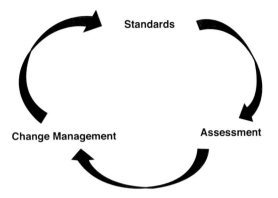

FIGURE 13.1 Improvement cycle

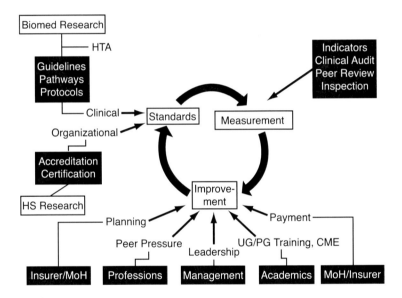

FIGURE 13.2 National continuous quality improvement system

processes by their requirements—independent of the stakeholders, incentives, or disincentives. Thus St. George et al.[31] classified current revalidation processes as either educational or assessment oriented. Creators of these programs are aware that both elements are needed for the ultimate goal—improvement—and that demonstration of an outcome must be part of the sequence. Further, promoters of educational programs should not focus on the numbers of educational units sold, as if units taken or sold were any indication of a successful change or outcome in clinical practice. Looking at the more interventionist models of revalidation in Table 13.1, there is a major distinction between the British model and the

American model that warrants attention. These models represent the extremes of revalidation or recertification as mandated by law, versus those mandated by professional agency-based regulatory programs. This points out that the structural intent of both approaches is to establish a program with features that are designed to benefit patients, other stakeholders, and the practicing profession by means of the improvement cycle.

From this initial examination of these two contrasting approaches, one question is immediately obvious. Is the central legal mandate necessary? In many areas of active change for the public, laws such as automobile drivers' permits or seat belt legislation are effective in reducing adverse outcomes. The UK model is a large-scale experiment in reaction to a set of accountability failures at many levels of their system.[32] However, a mandate alone does not necessarily produce immediate outcomes, like wearing a seatbelt or not, or downstream outcome indicators such as head injury or death. But in time, the program should show an impact via multiple indicators that would reassure the public by either identifying areas to be addressed in a classic CQI mode or demonstrating an effect. In keeping with that overall vision and its implied strategic goals, what evidence exists that would assure the public and other stakeholders that there are documented examples of best practices in recertification and revalidation?

Best Practices: Operational and Assessed for Impact

Existing recertification and revalidation programs that operate at either the general licensure or certification levels will be outlined. For a discussion of these differences, the readers are referred to either the chapter on Licensure and Certification in the *International Handbook of Research in Medical Education*[33] or the United States Agency for International Development's Quality Assurance Methodology refinement series by Rooney and van Ostenberg.[34]

At General Licensure and Certification Levels (Revalidation)

Only the United Kingdom is tackling the revalidation issue through both the licensure and certification processes. Government legislation has mandated the duties that both the General Medical Council (GMC) in the United Kingdom at the licensure level and the individual members of the Federation of Royal Colleges of Medicine in the United Kingdom, must administer for certification.[35] Figure 13.3 illustrates the model. The GMC and Royal Colleges are the points of action and their practicing members have no choice. Under a national

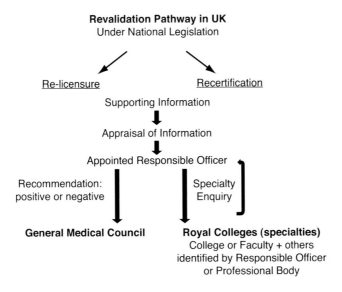

Revalidation Pathway in UK
Under National Legislation

Re-licensure   Recertification

Supporting Information

Appraisal of Information

Appointed Responsible Officer

Recommendation: Specialty
positive or negative   Enquiry

General Medical Council   **Royal Colleges (specialties)**
College or Faculty + others
identified by Responsible Officer
or Professional Body

FIGURE 13.3 Revalidation pathway in the United Kingdom

legislated mandate, all physicians must undergo mandatory revalidation every 5 years. This entails the general licensure route via the GMC or the certification route for specialists through their certificate-issuing Royal College. Each party and the specific regulatory or professional body are responsible for gathering the supporting data indicating that the physician has undergone the required assessment steps. That information and documentation is appraised by the GMC or Royal College. As part of the process, a responsible officer, as in the concept of a "trusted third party," is identified for each physician "candidate." In the case of the GMC route for general licensure, a recommendation is made about whether or not a physician has met the requirements. In the case of the route via one of the Royal Colleges, there will also be another step—a specialty enquiry to which the college or a faculty can add information. Thus the responsible officer and the implicated professional body can add information to the dossier. The whole package is then recycled back through the assessment or appraisal processes, and the final recommendation is made.

There are models in several countries that address revalidation at the general licensure level. The models are based on declarations with documented proof of attendance that operate via Continuing Medical Education credits.[29] The ability to enforce a true quality assurance model with assessment and feedback and an improvement arm as per Figure 13.1 does not exist, because there is no legal mandate in the certifying body or legislation to dictate the improvement cycle process. One exception was Canada, where a "monitor, offer feedback, and then enhance" model was promoted in the late 1990s.[12] In Canada, licensure is provincially based. As of early 2011, no provincial authority or territory has mandated the revalidation-enhancement model for all physicians in all cycles for general medical licensure.

Is the UK system grounded in best practices? The answer is the United Kingdom is moving in that direction but subsequent results will confirm its success or lack of success. To illustrate, the Royal College of Physicians of Edinburgh has described the standards building steps that each body must develop to create its College's framework.[36] The first step involves setting standards (generic and specialty-based criteria) that describe the features of good practice. The second step defines standards and criteria for the methods and the evidence to be used to demonstrate good practice. The third step develops and validates tools for the assessment of these standards. This is a huge undertaking. Because it is a legal process, the notion of evidence and natural justice versus opinion or offering conclusions without evidence will drive the process. As a necessary first step in evaluating an instrument based on its evaluation qualities, studies are being published as part of piloting and early validation. These studies are based on traditional measurement concepts of content or construct validity. They are too numerous to cite here and are often preliminary. Most have not yet finished addressing the generalization and extrapolation links in the Kane[37] validity argument chain or demonstrated outcome data aimed at a high level of adoption in practice, such as Kirkpatrick's level 4.[38] In 2012, most funding bodies and foundations expect a logic model of outcome-based documentation of an ultimate impact to declare successful adoption of change and improve a measureable outcome that is sustained.[39] The United Kingdom is not at the point where it can link the interpretation of their "actual results" against their intended use. This is the final and key step in Kane's validity argument chain. However, they are slowly and surely documenting the quality of their evaluation tools. Results are yet to come.

At Certification Level

In contrast to the UK model, the American model was not legislated centrally by the national parliament or other legislative body. It operates through the ABMS. After the American Board of Family Medicine placed a time limit on its certification diploma in 1969, the other 23 boards in the ABMS gradually joined the move to time-limited certification, using cycles of 7–10 years for all new diplomates.[5] The policy of recertification for the new diplomates was finally accepted by all ABMS specialty boards in 1999.[10] Benson,[5] a major leader and then head of the American Board of Internal Medicine, described the purposes of recertification as improving patient care, setting standards for the practice of internal medicine and its sub-specialties, promoting continuous learning, and reassuring all stakeholders that the new American Board of Internal Medicine diplomates would remain competent in practice. Thus recertification is mandated only for those who have volunteered to be certified, and recertification applies only for those certified after the date on which the recertification policy was adopted by their board. All other physicians who were certified beforehand are thus considered certified for life, unless they choose to be recertified. Currently, only 1% of those exempted have chosen recertification in one specialty.[25] However, during the time from the early adoption until the ABMS began to actually execute recertification, the nature of the processes and tools used varied greatly across member boards. Thus the American approach was iterative, compared with the United Kingdom's decreed approach. Weiss[40] has outlined the history of the implementation.

The next major step in the United States was the adoption of a competency-based model of certification. That step gave the first nationally agreed upon framework with national definitions of the categories of competency. A key actor was the Accreditation Council on Graduate Medical Education (ACGME), under the leadership of David Leach.[41] In 1999, the ABMS and the ACGME adopted the same competency framework for both certification and recertification.[42] This was a major step in pursuing a quality assurance program that was integrated across the entire educational lifetime of physicians. To outline the resulting framework and the needed process, Holmboe's[42] representation of the integrated ABMS and ACGME competency framework is illustrated in Figure 13.4.

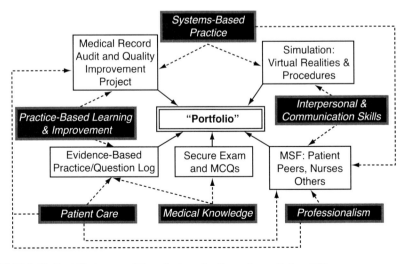

FIGURE 13.4 United States: multifaceted evaluation of practicing MD

The six competencies are represented in black and the white boxes represent the potential assessment processes. In this case, the suggested steps to meet the criteria are described and it will be noted that many of the potential tools overlap. There is a need to not only document activities and be assessed in actual practice but also to review the resulting data and information and make an assessment, not unlike the UK model. To illustrate, consider the six competencies (in black in Figure 13.4).

In 2000, the ABMS boards all agreed that they would move from a recertification model to a continuous professional development model, to be known as maintenance of certification (MOC). MOC included four major components to be phased in between 2004 and 2010. In this manner, a new cohort could enter the phase in each year, in the case of a board with a 7-year cycle, such that all diplomats would be covered before a new cycle began.[43] The four components are as follows:

- Part I—demonstration of professional standing
- Part II—participation in lifelong learning
- Part III—demonstration of cognitive expertise
- Part IV—demonstration of practice performance.

New standards for the MOC (Parts I–IV), which would serve as guiding principles and time frames for the 24 specialty boards, were adopted in 2009; highlights are summarized on the ABMS website.[43] This initiative was launched together with the ABMS Enhanced Public Trust Initiative for 2008–2011.

Prime examples of the programs and best practices components from among the boards using the ABMS model have evolved in an iterative manner. They will be highlighted in a subsequent section and their impact noted.

There are other frameworks to consider when planning a recertification or maintenance of performance program. The CanMEDS (Canadian Medical Education Directives for Specialists) physician competency framework of the Royal College of Physicians and Surgeons of Canada (RCPSC) is well known (see Figure 13.5).[44] It frames the RCPSC maintenance of competence strategy that differs from the ABMS maintenance of certification strategy. The CanMEDS framework originated from the Education of the Future Physicians of Ontario and was developed via a literature review and interviews of physicians and the public.[45] That framework was revised by the RCPSC with extensive consultation within the profession and public leaders. For the current National Assessment Strategy evolving in Canada, the two certifying bodies, the RCPSC, the College of Family Physicians of Canada, and the Medical Council of Canada, who run the national licensure qualification examinations, have all adopted the CanMEDS roles as an integrating framework.[46]

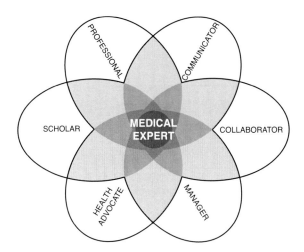

FIGURE 13.5 The CanMEDS (Canadian Medical Education Directives for Specialists) roles framework

The CanMEDS framework has not resulted in the move to recertification or revalidation per se. The element of knowledge re-examination, common in the ABMS strategy, is shunned in Canada. It is a widely studied framework.[47] As with all broad-based competency-based models, one of the challenges in applying the CanMEDS framework is the issue of varying the standards from the typically expected level of performance to new and very different responsibilities as physicians' activities in the different specialties and their field of practice change over time. This is particularly true for roles like manager or advocate, which are driven by changing levels of responsibility as physicians' careers mature. The same challenge exists for the ABMS competency-based schema.

Based on Merkur's survey and the initial overview of activities in the United Kingdom and North America, one should note that the development of any multifaceted process, such as recertification or revalidation, requires a set of long-term, iterative, strategic goals. Goals are essential if the steps are expected to demonstrate measureable impact and be replicable. Follow-up measurement of a program's impact takes many years. Even if legislated, legal due process, legal fairness challenges, the need for "evidence" and practice-based validity dictate that best practices still apply. The pathway to any revalidation or recertification program is a trajectory where many jurisdictions are moving up a developmental slope to achieve best practices. Figure 13.6 illustrates the pattern of development based on Merkur's survey and this review. The issue is not about making one-shot judgments of program quality. Instead, the idea is to locate and advance existing programs on this journey, a path where all parties will prosper and latecomers may benefit by shaping their future plans. This chart is not meant to be a forecast, because there are many other concurrent developments that affect quality at the system level and drive developments in other directions or at different rates. The challenges include institutional quality assurance programs in local jurisdictions, in existing health systems, cost-effectiveness initiatives, or legislated programs as in the United Kingdom.

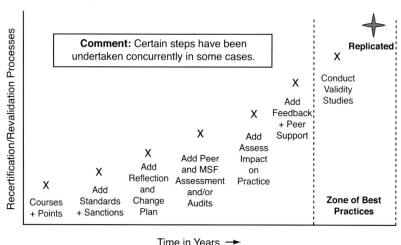

FIGURE 13.6 Long-term trajectory for best practices in recertification and revalidation

Institutional or System Level

The impact of recertification, maintenance of competence, or certification program on health care institutions is not as readily apparent. There is great interest among hospitals and other clinical facilities given their potential contribution to institutional accreditation and quality assurance programs. One of the consequences of the early MOC programs at the ABMS was that health care providers like health plans or hospitals systems used MOC status reports for re-credentialing and staff appointments, which provided an incentive for physicians to pursue MOC.[40] The new broad-scope, continuous accreditation model being implemented by the Joint Commission in the United States is also advancing concurrently.[48,49] The new focus on institutional accreditation in the United Kingdom and also among European clinics inside and outside hospitals (e.g., the International Organization for Standardization accreditation designation for health institutions) may affect revalidation and recertification.[50]

Thus, progress toward continuous documentation and analyses is becoming the new "norm." Downstream effects on clinical care outcomes are not yet known. However, almost any change is better than programs where physicians just tick off as meeting compliance with structural or educational process requirements.

Over a decade ago, Norcini argued that attribution—that is, linking patient outcomes to physician behavior—remains a difficult challenge for assessment of individuals at the in-patient level.[51] Fortunately, more insight is emerging from the patient safety literature at the level of teams.[52] Individually focused attribution around in-patient therapeutic safety issues and attention to system-based approaches for reducing medical errors and infection control is difficult unless done at the institutional level.[48] We do not yet know how individual accountability will be captured by recertification and revalidation. Accountability may be addressed at the institutional level as exemplified by the new Joint Commission approach in the United States or the new UK model at the National Health Service institutional and practice appraisal level.

Ambulatory Level

One-on-one physician-patient relationships and the resultant actions are clearer in the ambulatory setting in terms of attribution for accountability, recertification, or revalidation programs. This is especially the case for dyadic activities between the patient and the physician like prescribing.[53] As the cost of pharmaceuticals rises and institutional budgets are squeezed and lead to closer fiscal monitoring, it remains to be seen if this issue will become a point of interest in recertification or revalidation. This area will be watched closely given the growth of electronic medical records and the increased need for prescribing reconciliation. It is premature to assess their impact politically in terms of earlier adoption of MOC and patient outcomes.

Having reviewed the conceptual breakthroughs and opportunities around new methodologies, a key requirement defined in the purpose of this chapter remains to be addressed: best practices in revalidation and recertification. In summary, from this international overview, only two contenders have been identified for our predetermined definition of best practices: the United Kingdom and the ABMS and its boards in the United States. Elsewhere, the common practices are maintenance of competence programs based on learning strategies. Many programs offer selective options, where physicians can choose practice-based outcome assessments that approach, but do not yet meet, 2012 best practices criteria. Those situations will be examined more closely focusing on best practice "components" that exist at the time of writing.

If Not Best Practices Systems, then Practices Components: the United Kingdom and the American Board of Medical Specialties

The most dramatic changes since 2001 have occurred in the United Kingdom, thus its approach will be addressed first. The UK system is not yet tried and proven. The final phase has in fact been delayed for a least a year.[54] The reasons for delay, as one might expect, stem from problems with developing a completely new set of tools. New instrumentation is needed for virtually every aspect of the assessment toolbox. The new instruments must function for the variety of practice settings and specialties under the United Kingdom's legislated mandate. This is necessary to meet the definition of best practices. The importance of pilot testing to produce an adequate distribution of results over each scoring scale is needed to demonstrate discrimination. The validity of the scoring keys is also important. Matching of assessment content to practice context is tedious but should be done. Another set of problems concern the propriety of the practice outcome indicators used in the assessment and verifying their consistency. Pilot tests of these indicators to assure a high level of impact on the evidence hierarchy is essential.[38] That requires use of both diagnostic and impact-oriented score scales. A good example of this challenge is the use of multisource feedback. Developers must consider if the insight from 360-degree feedback from peers, coworkers, and patients has resulted in actual practice change by the doctor and not just intentions from surveys or declarations of "I plan to change." Did the physician change his or her practice and demonstrate an improved outcome?

To illustrate, in both the United Kingdom and the ABMS, recertification and revalidation programs are long-term developments. This was true for the processes created for the current certification assessments that exist today.[55] Development of measurement tools used in American certification was a decades-long journey.[40] The notion of deconstructing the broad-based competences and other expectations into measureable and observable events and then reconstructing them into new aggregates of clinical activity is just one step. The final steps involve showing that the anticipated results are reliable and demonstrating that interpretation of the outcome-based results are a consequence of the peer feedback and educational activities.

Consider the ABMS and the ACGME's six competencies for initial certification, recertification, or MOC and how they may be deconstructed and later reconstructed as observable events or measured behaviors. To start, one must break the competencies down and consider at what performance level and where the measurements and assessments will be made. Assessment planners must then reconstruct a new set of measurement indictors for each competency to reach assessment decisions and establish validity for interpretations of each indicator's results. Consider Stephen Miller's diagram for the deconstruct-reconstruct process.[*] In Figure 13.7, the outer circle labels the six competencies: (1) patient care, (2) interpersonal and communications skills, (3) professionalism, (4) medical knowledge, (5) systems-based practice, and (6) practiced-based learning and improvement. The second circle, moving inward, represents opportunities where the observations can be made.

The primary conceptual change over what was done in the previous decade is the idea of deconstructing the nature of practice into a series of activities or indicators of impact that frame the scope of expected and needed outcomes. This deconstruction is not without risks in an era where there is concern over oversimplifying the cultural, socioeconomic, and contextual factors often so important to addressing quality.[56] Thus the reconstruction of the world of real practice with measures and sampling frames becomes important if an assessment is to be representative of a medical specialty's practice profile. Interpretations given to assessment scores must be generalizable to that specialty area so they can be extrapolated to a physician's practice in terms of content and performance. These assessments must match the reality of the diplomate's practice situation and honor the scope of practice implied by the certificate. The congruence of "my practice" and the meaning of the certificate's standards is critical for the face validity of the credential. The third circle, inside, is the need to track these observations and document them so an appraisal can take place at regular and appropriate intervals.

A set of educational elements that are now widely recognized are often missing. Norcini[14] and Sargeant et al.[19] have identified the learning and enhancement components as the missing elements. The elements are implied, but in reconstructing and tracking measures, an educational strategy of learning and enhancement processes must be defined and planned. Note the central role of feedback and enhancement in Figure 13.7. Learning and enhancing approaches also need to be evaluated as part of the process of continuous improvement, especially for those who do poorly and have little insight into shortcomings.[57] The Canadian model of monitor, feedback, and enhance has been shown to be very useful in addressing physicians' underperformance in practice.[58] It may well be that many physicians only need a modest feedback or what can be called a

---

[*] Stephen Miller, personal communication with author, 2012.

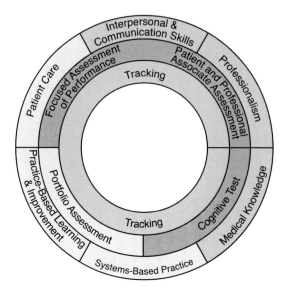

FIGURE 13.7 Deconstruct-reconstruct

"nudge" strategy for improvement.[59] But some critics in the United Kingdom are concerned about potential cohorts of physicians who cannot functionally learn without feedback and peer support and who need to undergo significant relearning.[60] This is a concern that suggests different tools are required to sort and classify learning and enhancement needs. The basic ABMS recertification model may work well for most physicians, but it can also be said that fallback strategies will be needed for outliers having atypical practice content and underperformance problems. Thus a continuous practice monitoring strategy is desirable and has been recommended long before the recertification deadline looms.[61]

Turning to the American scene, the ultimate test of the components of the various ABMS models is their application. With 24 boards and additional sub-specialties within some boards, portfolios of MOC programs, measurement tools, and results of the individual board programs need to be considered individually. The boards that have taken the iterative approach and developed new instruments and documented *practice impact* can be characterized as executing best practices. They include five of the largest boards.

1. The American Board of Internal Medicine[62,63]
2. The American Board of Surgery[64]
3. The American Board of Family Medicine[65]
4. The American Board of Emergency Medicine[66,67]
5. The American Board of Pediatrics.[68]

The characteristics for these sample programs are applicable to other ABMS boards, but space does not permit a board-by-board review. The key messages are the use of common operating criteria for MOC and a varied time course in meeting these standards, as in Figure 13.6. Most ABMS boards are closing in on the zone of best practices. Certainly, the American Board of Internal Medicine has been exemplary in is iterative and progressive documentation of the tools for its MOC program, including outcomes-based evaluations. The other ABMS boards are well within reach of the designation as using best practices. They are to be congratulated for their careful and transparent approaches. Significant questions remain for the future. What are the next steps in terms of the variation in practice context and content as many practitioner profiles become highly focused because of narrow clinical activities for reasons such as academic interests or "boutique-oriented care?" If the MOC format is sufficiently adaptable to deal with content variation, will the meaning of certification change compared with the original and wider content definition associated with the broadly based specialties? Or must the recertification model have a floor and a ceiling or left and right content variation limitations to validly address the so-called "national average" physician capability as implied by that specialty certificate?

Other Model Components to Consider: Canada and Australasia

Canada was a leader in the early days of the maintenance of competence movement. The initial action was in the certifying community with a focus on educational activities. That movement came from the two colleges, which, unlike the American boards, have to function in both certifying and educational advocacy roles. Interestingly, in Canada the pressure for a stronger feedback loop and enhancement began through the Federation of Medical Regulatory Authorities of Canada.[12] Arising from three national conferences, a monitor and enhance revalidation model was proposed in 1998–99 and included key monitor and enhancement (educational) elements. The model was focused at the practice level based on six strata of evidence, one of which clearly involved peer review and objective assessment of practice activities (Figure 13.8).

The maintenance of competence strategy existed through the certifying bodies. At the same time a strong movement around enhancement programs for underperforming physicians (both monitored and referred cases) was included and is underway in several jurisdictions, often with referral from smaller medical

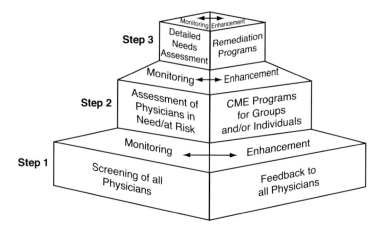

FIGURE 13.8 Monitoring and enhancement of physician performance

regulatory authorities (MRAs).[*] There has been an ongoing program of enhancement in most provinces but not directly involving the certifying colleges.[†] One
variation is Quebec where the MRA under their law functions as both licensing
and certifying body independent of the advocacy roles.

Other provinces have adopted office peer review and audit programs in
selected areas.[‡] Several MRAs have been active such as Quebec, Ontario,
Alberta, Manitoba, and Nova Scotia regarding recertification or revalidation.
The most active MRA over the past decade has been in Alberta, mainly using its
360-degree multisource feedback (MSF) program. The results are readily available in journals and online, thanks to the hard work of Lockyer and colleagues
at the University of Calgary who developed the program. Developed evaluation
instruments have been subjected to many validity studies. However the use of
traditional construct validity studies are not conventional in the performance
assessment world today.[55] Basically, the key validity issue remains: does the
360-degree MSF approach predict practice change and better practice outcomes?

Levinson, a former chair of the American Board of Internal Medicine, crafted
a challenging editorial in the *Canadian Medical Association Journal*. The editorial
suggested that Canada was not up to speed 10 years after a promising start by
promoting a basic CQI model of monitor and enhance.[69] The regulators and certifying bodies use instruments validated on the basis of measurement qualities in

---

[*]   B. Ward, personal communication with author regarding Annual Survey of Canadian Medical
    Regulatory Authorities, August 2010.
[†]   Ibid.
[‡]   Ibid.

discriminating between physicians on the MSF.[*] What is missing is an indication of improvement or documented change in practice behavior. The Calgary group has published the results of a 5-year follow-up study confirming the concern.[70] The study noted that the MSF program "was accompanied by very little formal opportunity to discuss results, set goals, and receive feedback within a short time frame." It suggests that upward changes in performance will be small or moderate. Without key impact indicators, evaluating self-assessment and self-reflection via a survey may fail for those who may need it most. Random verification checks could be imposed but may be insensitive for physicians who vary slightly from the norm. Thus work in Canada is in progress, ahead of the curve, but requires more study of effectiveness and impact confirmation about existing enhancement procedures through a modern validation process. Nonetheless, there are well-established referral programs for those who are reported as underperforming.[12,58,59]

In Canada, for the both the RCPSC and the College of Family Physicians of Canada, maintenance of competence programs remain educationally focused on required reflection associated with self-declared improvement. There are also categories for peer review and other forms of outcomes oriented in self-administered asssessment.[71] Re-examination processes are not used in Canada[69] despite the evidence from the United States about their predictive validity in assessing knowledge areas such as drug therapy.[72] The colleges follow-up with physicians who comply to offer an option of practice assessment. They also contact all members who do not comply. The programs apply to all certification holders, unless retired, and are accepted by most MRAs for their re-registration. Except for Alberta, no long- or even short-term outcome analyses have been published to indicate predictive validity of the processes or to confirm their impact on patient care.

In Australasia, the program is not established under one or two specialty colleges as in Canada. Like the United Kingdom, there is a Royal Colleges' collaborative or council that meets regularly. Again like Canada, the educational role of the colleges, as in the United States, and the independent certification role of the specialty boards are not separate functions. This offers an advantage of linking the recertification with educational or enhancement opportunities under one structure, their Royal College. The issue is that Canada and Australia and New Zealand are small in population compared with the United States so the relative cost burden of these quality assurance linkages is of concern. "Simpler" would likely be more cost-effective.

---

[*]   Ibid.

The currently proposed requirements for recognition of any recertification program in New Zealand have been set by its Medical Council.[73] These requirements are 50 hours of CPD that must include an annual learning plan made up of at least one clinical audit per year, measured against preset standards; a regular practice review, that follows uniform principles; peer review of at least 10 hours per year, such as peer MSF or review of charts; understanding and respect for cultural competence; and of course educational conferences and workshops.[74] The regular practice review acknowledges it is a formative process, that a 360-degree assessment must be included, and that external experts are a part of the process. They have also set out the requirements for records, and details about the system to manage poor performance for those parties offering such programs. If approved and once the impacts are assessed, it may well be a key model for smaller jurisdictions.

In Australia, the elephant in the room is the 2010 move to national medical registration by the federal government via the Medical Board of Australia, which in turn is under the Australian Health Practitioner Regulatory Authority.[75] That may change the scene significantly, and push matters toward the UK situation. The Productivity Commission in Australia has had a commitment to high-quality and safe outcomes. A title from an article in the *Australian Doctor* magazine said it clearly: "Testing times ahead," voicing concerns similar to those expressed earlier in this volume (*see* Chapter 10) about outcomes assessment in continuing education and training.[76] The current system is CPD based. There are options for practice audit and peer review, such as in the case of the Royal Australasian College of Physicians, which includes pediatricians.[77] It is carried out on the same model as the Royal College of Physicians and Surgeons of Canada. The Royal Australasian College of Surgeons offers variations of requirements that are flexible to accommodate variations in practice profiles, but fundamentally it is the same model as in Canada.[78] Outcome-based best practice components exist but are not essential requirements and have not undergone impact studies. There is a heavy emphasis on reflection and self-assessment without the educational or peer support enhancement options. The information manuals are available on line from specific Royal Colleges. In summary, the certifying bodies in Australia are moving cautiously, with outcome-oriented assessment options but little evidence of practice outcomes.[75,76] That may change as the methodologies and evidence of impact arise elsewhere. The federal government is standing by, watching.

An Assessment of the Recertification-Revalidation and its Impact?
• • • • • • • • • • • •

Internationally, the state of the science and politics of revalidation and recertification remains a work in progress. It would be easy to criticize, but establishing a process that actually changes practice and results is a Herculean task. The two models that most closely meet our preset criteria are the UK initiative and MOC in the United States. The UK model holds promise to have the greatest potential impact if the methodology can be established and proven effective. The reason for this is because the UK model reaches all physicians. In the United States, access to an MOC-like program is only available to holders of a certificate from an ABMS board (as do 80% of physicians), unless provided otherwise by the employers or via a health system. Even then, within that number, the grandfathered, older diplomats may be most at risk of underperforming due to advanced age. However, only 1% of grandfathered physicians with American Board of Internal Medicine certification have sought MOC status.

Does the American model have a flexibility advantage since it is not legally driven? It really depends on the political philosophy of the country and the public's expectations. In the end, like certification itself, health care institutions and public pressure help close compliance gaps. Otherwise, for the public, the phrase "let the buyer beware!" is very fitting. Improvement is needed to close the enhancement gap in the United States. With the separation of certification from education and advocacy, organizations such as the American College of Physicians or the American College of Surgeons offer enhancement linkages that continue to evolve.

Some of the same enhancement issues exist in the United Kingdom but the Colleges who must be involved, and the availability of the National Health Services clinical support teams, including reappraisal services and revalidation support teams, offer excellent potential. Despite outcries, the existing support services can identify and deal with those at very high risk of offering poor care or who are incompetent. Loopholes will close given the new accountability oversight for the GMC, the Royal Colleges, the National Health Service assessment services, and the Council of Healthcare Regulatory Excellence.

The educational approach prevails in other jurisdictions. This is true in Europe even though there are sanctions available. But are the sticks aligned with improved outcomes? That remains to be seen. Canada is in a state of evolution and the stimulus to drive the process toward true best practices may come from the MRAs or even from the outcome lessons of recertification and revalidation processes being developed in the United States and the United Kingdom. Professional structures in Canada are closely aligned to those in the United States and it may be less costly to let the bigger American bodies pay the price for progress. If that happens, the MRAs in Canada will undoubtedly push that agenda, given the large number of public members on MRA boards with voting privileges.

Other countries of interest, with shared specialty Royal Colleges, are Australia and New Zealand. Given their decentralized and separate specialty colleges, with smaller resources, progress may have other parents. The nature of New Zealand's quality misfortunes in the 1980s and 1990s resulted in a different culture in the public's mind and in the MRA community, where the governance is more shared but still a physician-led self-regulation.[74] The Australian federal government is pushing for greater accountability. A national registration body, the Medical Board of Australia, will place standards on the state-based regulators including verification and assessment of recency for each physician's current credentials.[75] This response arose from their recent Bristol equivalent, the Patel affair,[4] where state processes were casual and did not observe best practices of primary source verification of credentials. The mood will likely continue for greater performance accountability. The Australians may also be greatly influenced by the progress and resulting impacts of MOC in the United States along with the revalidation progress in the United Kingdom.

The lessons learned since 2000 are clear. We have cited principles and publications since 1999 that are particularly important for success and impact for any organization considering how to respond to revalidation or recertification demands. First, ensure that real outcomes are measured for evidence of impact. Processes are expected and provide the feedback loop information. Systems should monitor constantly and respond appropriately rather than focus on a great rush a few months before a review deadline. Learning is most effective near the time of error or omission. Feedback is needed but must include peer support. The plan must also include developing enhancement strategies for high-risk groups because physicians functioning at the margin or worse are a concern. Whatever the shortfall in performance, structures and processes for guided learning strategies and improvement must be readily available.

Concluding Comments
• •

A look back in 2020 will be certain of only one thing: given international fiscal constraints and the impact of the internet as an informal equalizer of public opinion, accountability will not lessen. The impact of information technology expansion and the increasing penetration of electronic health record and institu- tional- and health system-based quality assurance programs are already underway. Access to data will not be the problem. The crucial issue is whether the evid- ence needed to predict improvement in the quality of care and thus inform the outcome debates has been validated and applied appropriately to the physician's practice context, especially if the practice is very specialized. If a physician works within an expected range of practice content, commensurate with the intent of the certification diploma, a true MOC will be appropriate. This is a challenge for all systems. The concurrent involvement trajectory of the public and other stakeholders[79] including insurers, health plan providers,[80,81] and combinations of public-private partnerships will be upward. The reader is invited to review Figure 13.2 to recall the scope of quality improvement movement. The CQI scope is not focused solely on hospitals and physicians. Corrigan[79] has chal- lenged the professions in the United States that other initiatives may overtake the profession-led CQI field.

Will there be additional examples of improved and valid methodologies and impact studies available by 2020? Will the UK top-down response to the events of the 1990s via a legislated route prove effective and cost-effective and yield the impact anticipated? Will the American bottom-up, profession-led MOC model demonstrate similar, better, or worse results? Economic and cultural con- siderations will influence those outcomes and strategies. Perhaps a European country, Canada, or Australasia will step up and outperform the UK or American approaches by promoting deeper penetration of programs to reach high-risk physicians and thus impact their patient populations. Whatever the result, the profession must continue to assume part of the responsibility for improvement solutions, working with partners like health care institutions, or anticipate being mandated by law or by their health care institutions, which in turn will also be under greater scrutiny for the foreseeable future.

References

1. Davis DA. Does CME work? An analysis of the effect of educational activities on physician performance or health care outcomes. *Int J Psychiatry Med.* 1998; **28**: 21–39.
2. Davis DA, Mazmanian PE, Fordis M, et al. Accuracy of physician self-assessment compared with observed measures of competence: a systematic review. *JAMA.* 2006; **296**(9): 1094–102.

3. Bristol Royal Infirmary Inquiry. *Learning from Bristol: the report of the public inquiry into children's heart surgery at the Bristol Royal Infirmary 1984–1995*. London: The Stationery Office; 2001.

4. Burton B. Queensland report on deaths recommends sweeping changes. *BMJ*. 2005; **331**(7508): 70.

5. Benson JA Jr. Certification and recertification: one approach to professional accountability. *Ann Intern Med*. 1991; **114**(3): 238–42.

6. Berwick DM. Continuous improvement as an ideal in health care. *N Engl J Med*. 1989; **320**(1): 53–6.

7. Graham R. Family medicine has a second chance to make a good first impression. *J Am Board Fam Med*. 2010; **23**(Suppl. 1): S46–8.

8. Bashook PG, Parboosingh J. Continuing medical education: recertification and the maintenance of competence. *BMJ*. 1998; **316**(7130): 545–9.

9. Southgate L, Pringle M. Revalidation in the United Kingdom: general principles based on experience in general practice. *BMJ*. 1999; **319**(7218): 1180–3.

10. Norcini JJ. Recertification in the United States. *BMJ*. 1999; **319**(7218): 1183–5.

11. Newble D, Paget N, McLaren B. Revalidation in Australia and New Zealand: approach of the Royal Australasian College of Physicians. *BMJ*. 1999; **319**(7218): 1185–8.

12. Dauphinee WD. Revalidation of doctors in Canada. *BMJ*. 1999; **319**(7218): 1188–90.

13. Swinkels JA. Reregistration of medical specialists in the Netherlands. *BMJ*. 1999; **319**(7218): 1191–2.

14. Norcini JJ. Where next with revalidation? *BMJ*. 2005; **330**(7506): 1458–9.

15. Cunnington J, Southgate L. Relicensure, recertification and practice-based education. In: Norman GR, van der Vleuten CPM, Newble DI, editors. *International Handbook of Research in Medical Education*. Dordrecht, the Netherlands: Kluwer Academic Publishers; 2002. pp. 883–912.

16. Eva KW, Regehr G. Self-assessment in the health professions: a reformulation and research agenda. *Acad Med*. 2005; **80**(Suppl. 10): S46–54.

17. Eva KW, Regehr G. I'll never play professional football and other fallacies of self-assessment. *J Contin Educ Health Prof*. 2008; **28**(1): 14–15.

18. Ericsson KA. Deliberate practice and the acquisition and maintenance of expert performance in medicine and related domains. *Acad Med*. 2004; **79**(Suppl. 10): S70–81.

19. Sargeant J, Mann K, van der Vleuten CPM, et al. "Directed" self-assessment: practice and feedback within a social context. *J Contin Educ Health Prof*. 2008; **28**(1): 47–54.

20. Hawkins RE, Weiss KB. Building the evidence base in support of the American Board of Medical Specialties maintenance of certification program. *Acad Med*. 2011; **86**(1): 6–7.

21. Perrin B. *Moving from Outputs to Outcomes: practical advice from governments around the world*. IBM Center for The Business of Government; 2006. Available at:

http://siteresources.worldbank.org/CDFINTRANET/Resources/PerrinReport.pdf (accessed February 8, 2011).

22. Streiner DL, Norman GR. *Health Measurement Scales*. Oxford: Oxford University Press; 2008.

23. Clauser BE, Margolis MJ, Swanson DB. Issues in validity and reliability for assessments in medical education. In: Holmboe ES, Hawkins RE, editors. *Practical Guide to the Evaluation of Clinical Competence*. Philadelphia, PA: Mosby Elsevier; 2008. pp. 10–23.

24. Bogan CE, English MJ. *Benchmarking for Best Practices: winning through innovative adaptation*. New York: McGraw-Hill; 1994.

25. Levinson W, King TE Jr., Goldman L, et al. Clinical decisions: American Board of Internal Medicine maintenance of certification program. *N Engl J Med*. 2010; **362**(10): 948–52.

26. Grol R, Wensing M, Eccles M, editors. *Improving Patient Care: the implementation of change in clinical practice*. Maarssen, the Netherlands: Elsevier; 2004.

27. Maynard A, Bloor K. Optimizing the medical workforce by improving efficiency and physician training. In: *Paper Prepared for the International Medical Workforce Collaborative*. New York, NY; 2010. pp. 1–9. Available at: http://rcpsc.medical.org/publicpolicy/IMWC12/2010-IMWC12/imwc2010_Canada_Maynard_section.pdf (accessed October 16, 2012).

28. Merkur S, Mossialos E, Long M, et al. Physician revalidation in Europe. *Clin Med*. 2008; **8**(4): 371–6.

29. Merkur S, Mladovsky P, Mossialos E, et al. *Do Lifelong Learning and Revalidation Ensure that Physicians are Fit to Practice? Policy brief*. Copenhagen: World Health Organization Regional Office for Europe; 2008.

30. Shaw C. World Bank Health Reform in Kazakhstan: connecting national quality assurance components. In: *Presentation on Behalf of the Canadian Society for International Health before the Ministry of Public Health and World Bank Officials December 10, 2010*. Astana, Kazakhstan; 2010.

31. St. George I, Kaigas T, McAvoy P. Assessing the competence of practicing physicians in New Zealand, Canada, and the United Kingdom: progress and problems. *Fam Med*. 2004; **36**(3): 172–7.

32. Department of Health, Workforce Directorate. *Medical Revalidation: principles and next steps; the report of the Chief Medical Officer for England's Working Group*. London: Department of Health; 2008. Available at: www.dh.gov.uk/prod_consum_dh/groups/dh_digitalassets/@dh/@en/documents/digitalasset/dh_086431.pdf (accessed March 18, 2011).

33. Dauphinee WD. Licensure and certification. In: Norman GR, van der Vleuten CPM, Newble DI, editors. *International Handbook of Research in Medical Education*. Dordrecht, the Netherlands: Kluwer Academic Publishers; 2002. pp. 835–82.

34. Rooney AL, van Ostenberg PR. *Licensure, Accreditation, and Certification: approaches to Health Services Quality*. Quality Assurance Methodology Refinement Series. USAID Quality Assurance Project/URC; 1999. pp. 1–38. Available at: www.urc-chs.com/resource?ResourceID=30 (accessed June 15, 2011).

35. Royal College of Physicians, London. *Revalidation: how it works*. Available at: http://old.rcplondon.ac.uk/Professional-Issues/revalidation/Pages/Structures-and-Processes.aspx (accessed February 9, 2011).

36. Royal College of Physicians of Edinburgh. *Standards, Evidence and Tools*. Available at: www.rcpe.ac.uk/revalidation/standards.php (accessed February 21, 2011).

37. Kane M. An argument based approach to validation. *Psychol Bull*. 1992; **112**: 527–35.

38. Smidt A, Balandin S, Sigafoos J, et al. The Kirkpatrick model: a useful tool for evaluating training outcomes. *J Intellect Dev Disabil*. 2009; **34**(3): 266–74.

39. W. K. Kellogg Foundation. *Logic Model Development Guide: using logic models to bring together planning, evaluation and action*. Battle Creek, MI: W. K. Kellogg Foundation; 2004.

40. Weiss KB. Future of board certification in a new era of public accountability. *J Am Board Fam Med*. 2010; **23**(Suppl. 2): S32–9.

41. Leach DC. A model for GME: shifting from process to outcomes; a progress report from the Accreditation Council for Graduate Medical Education. *Med Educ*. 2004; **38**(1): 12–14.

42. Holmboe ES. Assessment of the practicing physician: challenges and opportunities. *J Cont Educ Health Prof*. 2008; 28(S1): S4–10.

43. American Board of Medical Specialties. *Standards for ABMS MOC© (Parts 1–4) Program: approved March 16, 2009*. Evanston, IL: American Board of Medical Specialties; 2009. Available at: www.abms.org/News_and_Events/Media_Newsroom/pdf/Standards_for_ABMS_MOC_Approved_3_16_09.pdf (accessed June 15, 2011).

44. Frank J, editor. *The CanMEDS 2005 Physician Competency Framework: better standards, better physicians, better care*. Ottawa, CA: Royal College of Physicians and Surgeons of Canada; 2005.

45. Neufeld VR, Maudsley RF, Turnbull JM, et al. Educating future physicians for Ontario. *Acad Med*. 1998; **73**(11): 1138–48.

46. Medical Council of Canada. *NAC Program Overview*. Available at: www.mcc.ca/en/NAC/NAC_Program_overview.shtml (accessed March 17, 2011).

47. Davis D, Ringsted C. Accreditation of undergraduate and graduate medical education: how do the standards contribute to quality? *Adv Health Sci Educ Theory Pract*. 2006; **11**(3): 305–13.

48. Chassin MR, Loeb JM, Schmaltz SP, et al. Accountability measures: using measurement to promote quality improvement. *N Engl J Med*. 2010; **363**(7): 683–8.

49. The Joint Commission. *Improving America's Hospitals: The Joint Commission's annual report on quality and safety*. Oakbrook Terrace, IL: The Joint Commission; 2010. Available at: www.joint commission.org/annualreport.aspx (accessed June 15, 2011).

50. Shaw C, Bruneau C, Kutryba B, et al. Towards hospital standardization in Europe. *Inter J Qual Health Care*. 2010; **22**(4): 244–9.

51. Norcini JJ. Psychometric issues in the use of practice performance assessment for physician evaluation. In: Mancall EI, Bashook PG, editors. *Evaluating Residents for Board Certification*. Evanston, IL: American Board of Medical Specialties; 1999. pp. 95–101.

52. Baker DP, Day R, Salas E. Teamwork as an essential component of high-reliability organizations. *Health Serv Res.* 2006; **41**(4 Pt. 2): 1576–98.

53. Tamblyn R, Abrahamowicz M, Dauphinee D, et al. Influence of physicians' management and communication ability on patients' persistence with antihypertensive medication. *Arch Intern Med.* 2010; **170**(12): 1064–72.

54. Royal College of Physicians of Edinburgh. *Revalidation: The Key Proposals. Revalidation date set for 2012: results of GMC consultation and RCPE comment.* Available at: www.rcpe.ac.uk/revalidation/revalidation-date-set-for-2012.php (accessed February 21, 2011).

55. Dauphinee WD. Self regulation must be made to work. *BMJ.* 2005; **330**(7504): 1385–7.

56. Holmboe ES, Arnold GK, Weng W, et al. Current yardsticks may be inadequate for measuring improvements from the medical home. *Health Aff (Millwood).* 2010; **29**(5): 859–66.

57. Regehr G, Mylopoulos M. Maintaining competence in the field: learning about practice, through practice, in practice. *J Contin Educ Health Prof.* 2008; **28**(Suppl. 1): S19–23.

58. Goulet F, Gagnon R, Gingras ME. Influence of remedial professional development programs for poorly performing physicians. *J Contin Educ Health Prof.* 2007; **27**(1): 42–8.

59. Norton PG, Ginsburg LS, Dunn E, et al. Educational interventions to improve practice of nonspecialty physicians who are identified in need of peer review. *J Contin Educ Health Prof.* 2004; **24**(4): 244–52.

60. Dyer C. GMC's revalidation plans don't tackle poorly performing doctors, MPs say. *BMJ.* 2011; **342**: d872.

61. Dauphinee WD, Case S, Fabb W, et al. Standard setting for recertification. In: Newble DI, Wakeford R, Jolly B, editors. *The Certification and Recertification of Doctors: issues in the assessment of competence.* Cambridge: Cambridge University Press; 1994. pp. 201–15.

62. Levinson W, Holmboe E. Maintenance of certification in internal medicine. *Arch Intern Med.* 2011; **171**(2): 174–6.

63. Holmboe ES, Lynn L, Duffy FD. Improving the quality of care via maintenance of certification and the web. *Perspect Biol Med.* 2008; **51**(1): 71–83.

64. The American Board of Surgery. *Maintenance of Certification (MOC): overview.* Available at: http://home.absurgery.org/default.jsp?exam-moc (accessed March 18, 2011).

65. Bazemore AW, Xierali IM, Petterson SM, et al. American Board of Family Medicines (ABFM) maintenance of certification: variations in self-assessment modules uptake within the 2006 cohort. *J Am Board Fam Med.* 2010; **23**(1): 49–50.

66. American Board of Emergency Medicine. *Emergency Medicine Continuous Certification Overview.* Available at: www.abem.org/public/portal/alias_Rainbow/lang_en-US/tabID_3422/DesktopDefault.aspx (accessed September 28, 2012).

67. American Board of Emergency Medicine. *Maintenance of Certification: Part IV. Performance in practice.* Available at: https://www.theabfm.org/moc/part4.aspx (accessed March 18, 2011).

68. Miles PV. Maintenance of Certification: the role of the American Board of Pediatrics in improving children's health care. *Pediatr Clin North Am.* 2009; **56**(4): 987–94.

69. Levinson W. Revalidation of physicians in Canada: are we passing the test? *CMAJ.* 2008; **179**(10): 979–80.

70. Violato C, Lockyer JM, Fidler H. Changes in performance: a 5-year longitudinal study of participants in a multi-source feedback programme. *Med Educ.* 2008; **42**(10): 1007–13.

71. Gutkin C. Mandatory continuing professional development. *Can Fam Physician.* 2007; **53**(8): 1396.

72. Holmboe ES, Meechan TP, Tate JP, et al. Association between maintenance of certification examination scores and quality of care for Medicare beneficiaries. *Arch Intern Med.* 2008; **168**(13): 1396–403.

73. Medical Council of New Zealand. *Consultation on Strengthening Recertification Requirements for Doctors Registered in a General Scope of Practice* [consultation paper]. Wellington: Medical Council of New Zealand; 2010.

74. Medical Council of New Zealand. *Recertification and Continuing Professional Development.* Available at: www.mcnz.org.nz/assets/News-and-Publications/Booklets/Continuing-Professional-Development.pdf (accessed October 16, 2012).

75. Medical Board of Australia. *Types of Medical Registration.* Available at: www.medical board.gov.au/Registration/Types.aspx (accessed March 22, 2011).

76. Mazmanian PE, Feldman M, Berens TE, et al. Evaluating outcomes in continuing education and training. In: McGaghie WC, editor. *International Best Practices for Evaluation in the Health Professions.* London: Radcliffe Publishing; 2013. pp. 199–227.

77. The Royal Australasian College of Physicians (RACP). *Continuing Professional Development. Guide to MyCPD.* RACP; 2008. Available at: www.racp.edu.au/page/educational-and-professional-development/continuing-professional-development (accessed June 15, 2011).

78. The Royal Australasian College of Surgeons. *A Guide by The Royal Australasian College of Surgeons. Continuing Professional Development Program Information Manual 2010–2012.* The Royal Australasian College of Surgeons; 2009. Available at: www.surgeons.org/media/310989/CPD_Info_Manual_2010-2012.pdf (accessed June 15, 2011).

79. Corrigan JM. The specialty board movement at the crossroads: reaction to the paper by Keven B. Weiss, MD. *J Am Board Fam Med.* 2010; **23**(Suppl. 2): S40–1.

80. Asch SM, McGlynn EA, Hogan MA, et al. Comparison of quality of care for patients in veterans health administration and patients in a national sample. *Ann Intern Med.* 2004; **141**(12): 938–45.

81. Shelley M, Judkins K; for National Health Service Revalidation Support Team. *Assuring the Quality of Medical Appraisal for Revalidation.* National Health Service; 2009. Available at: www.revalidationsupport.nhs.uk/CubeCore/.uploads/pdfs/links/Assuring_the_Quality_of_Medical_Appraisal_for_Revalidation.pdf (accessed June 15, 2011).

14

Evaluation of Health Professions Leadership and Management and Programs that Teach these Competencies

Henry de Holanda Campos, Stacey Friedman,
Page S. Morahan, Francisco Eduardo de Campos,
and Ana Estela Haddad

WE FRAME THIS CHAPTER WITH APPROACHES TO EVALUATE LEADERSHIP and management in different situations where health and education are linked closely. We address two interrelated aspects for leadership and management in health professions in the twenty-first century: (1) leadership and management competencies needed for individuals in the health professions and (2) approaches to evaluate leadership and management development programs designed to inculcate the necessary competencies.

There is a general call to further develop leadership and management skills in the health professions. An important first step to improving these skills in individuals and organizations is a needs assessment to identify key competencies expected among health professionals in a given context. Skill development programs can then be designed to address these needs with program evaluation being used to determine program effectiveness and needed improvements. Leadership can also be developed as a social process because people engage to reach common directions and accomplishments. Evaluation of leadership and management attributes in any of these initiatives is an important strategy to incorporate these elements in the health care professional profile of the twenty-first century.

Two specific examples are used to describe these processes. The first addresses a proposal for evaluation of leadership and management in educational initiatives developed in Brazil. This is a component of the country's long-term commitment to invest in its primary care-based national health system with the intent to deliver care that is universal, equitable, and holistic. Second, strategies for program evaluation of leadership and management development initiatives are described within the scope of two institutions devoted to leadership and academic career development in health professions education: (1) the Foundation for Advancement of International Medical Education and Research (FAIMER) Institute, with its Regional Institute fellowships, and (2) the Executive Leadership in Academic Medicine (ELAM) program for women faculty in medicine, dentistry, and public health.

Leadership and Management Competency Gap in Health Care
•••••••••••••••

There is consensus that health care professionals and biomedical scientists—clinical practitioners such as physicians and nurses, and faculty in health professions schools—lack knowledge and skills in the leadership and management disciplines.[1] Moreover, health care professionals and academic organizations do not value leadership and management as being equivalent to disciplines such as biochemistry or neurosurgery.[2]

Many publications have appeared describing competencies in leadership and management required in health care. Competencies have been identified by personal reflections of experienced health care leaders.[3] Investigations of leadership effectiveness across a broad group of individuals and perspectives from a broad group of health care leaders and leadership researchers are available.[4-6] The Center for Creative Leadership's recent study is the most comprehensive documentation about the current leadership gap. The center measured leadership effectiveness among nearly 35 000 health care leaders and managers in the United States compared with its well-researched list of 16 leadership competencies and five "derailment factors."[4] The five competencies that health care organizations viewed as most important for success were (1) leading employees, (2) resourcefulness, (3) straightforwardness and composure, (4) change management, and (5) participative management. Unfortunately, some of these important competencies were those rated as least skilled—leading employees, change management, and participative management (*see* Table 14.1). Alignment of importance and skill level only occurred with the resourcefulness and straight-forwardness and composure competencies.

TABLE 14.1 Leadership and Management Competencies in Health Care[4]

Leadership Skills Ranked Most Important for Organizational Success (Top 5)	Ranking in Skills in Competency (Out of 16, Where 1 = Most Skilled and 16 = Least Skilled)
1. Leading employees	15
2. Resourcefulness	4
3. Straightforwardness and composure	6
4. Change management	10
5. Participative management	11

Collaborative, participatory, and team leadership are terms being used to encompass many of the aforementioned specific competencies that public health, education, and health care leaders need to develop.[3,4,7–9] Souba[3] emphasizes the need for coordinated health care, entrepreneurial teamwork, commitment to doing shared work and creating solutions together, mutual respect for the other's worldview, and transparency. Others have emphasized similar competencies for *interdisciplinary collaborative leadership* required for biomedical research that interfaces laboratory and patient-oriented research, population-based research, and community-based participatory research.[10,11] *Relationship-centered care* is another term used to emphasize the importance of relationships in leading and managing health care organizations and systems—whether between health care providers and patients, between faculty and students, between faculty and staff, or between health care professionals themselves.[12–14]

Increasing Interest in Leadership and Management Development in Health Care

There is increasing interest in providing formal leadership and management development for health professionals and scientists due to the gap in required competencies. Souba[3] concluded that, "leadership development becomes the single most important organizational competency for ensuring long-term sustainable success."

Approaches to leadership and management development for health professionals and scientists have included internal leadership development programs;[15–17] external leadership development programs focused on clinical health care leadership such as physician executive programs that are offered by business colleges and associations;[18] external leadership development programs focused on public health and health delivery;[19,20] or on leadership in academic health centers;[15,21-27] and formal degree programs offering master's degrees in disciplines such as business, health administration, public health, and health professions education.[28] It is interesting to note that 27% of US medical school deans appointed between 1980 and 2006 have such formal degrees in addition to their primary MD or PhD degree.[29]

Evaluation of Leadership and Management during Health System Reform

Reform of the Brazilian health system toward universal access and primary care presents an opportunity to evaluate leadership in a new context. Citizen mobilization and the primary care emphasis[30] are profound changes that allow evaluation of leadership using more shared and relational approaches, what has been termed "organized complexity."[30,31]

Another important aspect is the integration of the Brazilian health and education sectors.[32] It is necessary to move from traditional health education to participatory and engaging learning strategies to shift the focus of the system to primary care and family health teams.[33] A multilayer educational program was established to prepare students to benefit from community-based education[34-36] and "better prepare them for their roles as professionals who can meet the demands and challenges of health care delivery in the 21st century."[37] This combination sets the stage for social accountability of educational institutions,[38,39] and reinforces the understanding that the "real movement of leadership development occurs more effectively in the context of the work itself."[40]

Collaboration between the Brazilian Ministries of Health and Education and the active engagement of the Secretariat of Labor Management and Health Education, created in 2003, led to the progressive construction (2003–10) of a pathway of educational initiatives harbored within the unique Brazilian health system (*see* Table 14.2).[34,41-44]

There are opportunities for management and leadership development to forge new ways of learning in educational initiatives like the ones developed in Brazil.[45-47] This is an objective of twenty-first-century health professions education.[48] The approach to evaluate leadership and management attributes in this situation, as proposed by Day,[40] should consider leadership a complex interaction between individuals and their social and organizational environments. For example, assessing dimensions of the validated *Team Climate Inventory*[49] offers opportunities to evaluate team accomplishments, functionality, effectiveness, and capacity to innovate (*see* Table 14.3).[50]

TABLE 14.2 Educational Programs for the Health Professions Jointly Developed by the Brazilian Ministries of Health and Education[34]

Educational Program	Scope	Focus/Objective
Pro-Saúde	354 schools	Support to curriculum reforms through grants
PET-Saúde	461 tutorial groups 543 schools 17 057 students	Tutorial education and interdisciplinary team-based community work and research project—Fellowship granted program
PET-Vigilância	122 tutorial groups	Similar to PET-Saúde: focus on epidemiological surveillance
Pró-Residência	60 programs 1255 new placements	Development of medical residency programs in underserved medical specialties through granted program with tutoring and recipient institutions
Especialização em Saúde da Família	22 400 students enrolled	Graduate diploma course in Family Health; blended learning; physicians, dentists and nurses members of family health teams
Telehealth Brazil	1150 Tele-health points Universities telemedicine network Portfolio of diversified courses Educational repertoire	Second opinion to remote family health teams; open university for the health system; permanent education for health system workers

TABLE 14.3 Leadership Dimensions of the Team Climate Inventory[49]

Dimensions	Elements
Vision	Idea of valued outcome; clarity; shared vision; commitment to the group; reachable outcomes
Participative Safety (two components: team participation and team safety)	Reinforced involvement in decision making; shared information; group trust and support; safe environment; new ideas; local approach to problem solution
Task Orientation (two components: climate for excellence and constructive controversy)	Quality of task performance: commitment to excellence Support for adoption of improvements to established policies, procedures, and methods; relation to shared vision or outcome; individual and team accountability; reflection upon work method and team performance; intra-team advice; feedback and cooperation; mutual monitoring; appraisal of performance and ideas; clear outcome criteria; exploration of opposing opinions; constructive controversy
Support for Innovation	"The expectation, approval and practical support of attempts to introduce new and improved ways of doing things in the work environment."[51]

Directing evaluation to team performance is also aligned with present trends and recommendations to include interdisciplinary team work as one of the main competences of health professionals.[3,4,7-9,12-14] Evaluation of leadership and management using the team approach can be embedded in an overall program evaluation strategy as described in the following section.

General Approaches to Evaluation of Leadership and Management Development Programs

Each organization or government system needs to tailor its leadership and management development programs based on the findings of an organizational needs assessment. Needs assessments should take into account organizational strategy (i.e., what approach to leadership development is needed to support the strategy) and organizational gaps in key leadership competencies identified by internal and external information sources.

This needs assessment is the first step in an ongoing relationship between *program evaluation*, *program planning and improvement*, and *organizational effectiveness*. There are many ways that program evaluation can be used to support individual and organizational leadership and management development including:

- informing program and policy decisions (e.g., program planning)
- generating knowledge (e.g., lessons learned, evidence-based practice)
- assessing program benefits
- program improvement
- measuring effectiveness
- obtaining needed resources
- celebrating successes.

An important component to achieve any of these uses is involvement of stakeholders (i.e., end users of the evaluation findings) in the evaluation process, including evaluation planning.[52,53] Participatory program evaluation seeks to involve stakeholders deeply in the evaluation process[54] and a variety of specific approaches of this type can be used. For example, *appreciative inquiry* can be applied to evaluation, using in-depth appreciative interviews around the desired outcomes of the program.[55,56] The process discovers what has worked best in a program to achieve its outcomes and builds on program successes going forward. Appreciative inquiry may be particularly helpful in situations where there is, for any number of reasons, resistance or lack of trust about evaluation. Appreciative inquiry is also useful where there is a desire to build evaluation capacity or a community of practice.

Assessment of leadership and management competencies forms a foundation of what will be measured for each stage of the evaluation. Examples include the competencies that need to be improved among individuals, and other competencies the program or intervention is designed to improve (e.g., teamwork). However, program outcomes and thus evaluation is not restricted to assessment of competencies. There are other areas for consideration pertaining to changes from *application* of competencies such as systems level outcomes involving change at organizational and community levels.

The following describes practical approaches to development of an evaluation plan that includes and extends beyond assessment of competencies. In each case, it is critical to determine as soon as possible in the design of the program:

1. Who are the major stakeholders for the evaluation? To whom is the program accountable? Who will use the evaluation findings and how will they use them?

2. What is the purpose of the evaluation? (e.g., needs assessment, formative evaluation, summative evaluation, or some combination).

3. What research methods will result in data that will be useful, believable, credible, and valid to the primary intended users of the evaluation? Are the methods practical, cost-effective, and ethical?

An important message is that no single program evaluation approach is best. The appropriate approach depends on the type of program and organizational context.[57] As researchers, we often equate rigorous program evaluation with experimental design with randomized, double-blinded control groups as the gold standard. This is often not appropriate or feasible for educational or social change programs. It is useful to have multiple data sources, including multiple stakeholder perspectives (not only participant perspectives) and both quantitative and qualitative measures.[58,59]

Models and Approaches for Development of a Program Evaluation Plan
••••••••••••••••••••

Logic Model

The many varieties of logic models are program-planning tools that also support program evaluation planning. Most models include program resources, activities, outputs, and outcomes (short-term, intermediate, and long-term) and may also include other aspects related to program context. Development of a logic model enables identification of indicators, data sources, and methods of data collection. The process is designed to create clarity and avoid vagueness about program processes, outcomes, and their measurement.[60]

EvaluLEAD

This newer framework for conceptualizing leadership development programs and their program evaluation was developed by the Kellogg Foundation for community leadership development programs. The process emphasizes the need for two forms of inquiry, collecting both evidential (quantitative) and evocative (qualitative) data. It also organizes program results and data collection methods into a nine-cell grid, with individual, organization, and society/community domains on the vertical axis, and episodic, developmental and transformative types of results on the horizontal axis.[60,61]

Leadership Development Investment Matrix

This evaluation approach is similar to EvaluLEAD and adds program evaluation to development of policy and practice fields.[62,63] The research leading to this framework investigated top leadership programs in the United States and resulted in a 25-cell matrix combining goals of development effort (five levels: individual, team, organization, network, and systems capacity) with the system targeted (five levels: individuals, teams, organizations, communities, and fields of policy and practice). By using the matrix, designers of leadership development or other educational interventions can focus on the unique matrix cell for which their program is intended and design their program and evaluation more specifically.

All three of these program evaluation frameworks often include the approach developed by Kirkpatrick[64] 50 years ago to encompass all levels of program outcomes (rather than solely participants' knowledge/skills).

Kirkpatrick's Four Levels of Assessment

This approach is still a mainstay for evaluation of education effectiveness. Phillips[65] added an additional fifth level to measure institutional impact, as shown in Table 14.4.

TABLE 14.4 Description of Kirkpatrick's[64] and Phillips's[65] Level of Assessment of Effectiveness of Educational Training

Level	Description	Potential Data Source
1	*Participant Reaction:* participant satisfaction	End of program or session survey of participants regarding their satisfaction, ratings of facilitator knowledge/skills, participant intent to use learning
2	*Knowledge and Skill Acquisition or Attitude Change by Participants:* has learning taken place	Pre- and post-assessment self-report, knowledge test instruments, focus groups
3	*Behavior Change:* have participants transferred learning to their job	Surveys, workplace observations, 360-degree assessment, focus groups, interviews with supervisors, data from former participants Some of the methods described in Level 2 can also be useful to measure this dimension
4	*Outcomes/Results:* has the educational intervention made a difference to the organization	Numbers of successful faculty (with "successful" needing to be operationally defined by stakeholders), 360-degree assessment, organizational measures of effectiveness (scorecard)
5	*Return on Investment* (noted to be the most difficult to measure)	Self-report descriptions of changes, coupled with asking what percentage of the change the participants attribute to the educational program, and how confident the participant is in that number. These two percentages can be multiplied to obtain a relatively realistic score of the change impact of the educational intervention. For example, if participants say that they obtained a grant because of the program, and they attribute 80% to the program (e.g., mentoring), and they have 50% confidence that it was the mentoring that made the change, then the change impact is $0.8 \times 0.5 = 0.4 \times$ the grant award dollar amount. Financial impact (e.g., grant awards), comparing this with the money invested in the program (time of mentor, time of mentee, program administration, etc.). Cost of turnover analysis could also be performed and compared with the cost of the intervention program.

There are a variety of pre- and post-assessments that are useful for level 2. These include *pre- and post-tests of participants' knowledge, attitude and skills*: multiple choice questions, essay questions, simulation and other hands-on exercises, and so forth; *pre- and post-survey of participants' perceived (self-report) knowledge, skills and attitudes*, as shown by self-report. It is often helpful to delay the post-survey for several months, to avoid a "halo effect" that may surround the program participants. This is a retrospective pre- and post-survey of participants' perceived (self-reported) knowledge, skills and attitudes. This approach can be helpful in situations where a pre-survey may be inflated, where participants may not know the extent of what they do not know about a topic. The approach is also useful when it is difficult to obtain follow-up information from participants because these surveys are administered at the end of the program. Data from any of these self-report instruments can be triangulated with data from focus groups, interviews with supervisors, and 360-degree assessments.

Examples of Leadership Development Program Evaluations in Health Care: FAIMER and ELAM Fellowships

The following summarizes approaches we have used in evaluating two programs for health professions faculty—the 10 years of experience with the Foundation for Advancement of International Medical Education and Research (FAIMER) Institute and Regional Institute fellowships for international health professions educators[66–68] and 15 years of experience with the Executive Leadership in Academic Medicine (ELAM) program for women faculty in medicine, dentistry, and public health.[22,69,70] Table 14.5 shows brief examples of outcomes and measures, based on evaluation of the FAIMER and ELAM fellowships for health professions educators, cast in the EvaluLEAD framework.

TABLE 14.5 Examples of Outcomes and Measures used in the FAIMER and ELAM Leadership Development Programs, in Context of the EvaluLEAD Model[62]

Impact	Level: Individual	Level: Organizational	Level: Region
Type: Episodic	Increased knowledge and skills in education and leadership Project implementation achieved	Increase in schools participating in fellowship, or with multiple fellows Fellow projects sustained and generalized to other components of school School convenes stakeholders around educational improvement themes (e.g., regional meetings and workshops)	Fellows and their schools conduct pilot projects to improve health in community or region Fellows and their schools convene meetings regarding education related to improving health of community or region

Impact	Level: Individual	Level: Organizational	Level: Region
	Measure example: ELAM—pre- and post-survey (1 year after program completion)	*Measure example*: ELAM and FAIMER—fellowship application data	*Measure example*: FAIMER—tracking convening of meetings or workshops
Type: Developmental	Project expansion Active in and/or expanded community of practice Academic promotion and/or administrative appointment based on educational leadership in health	Medical education unit started Increased number of women tenured or women in leadership positions Institutionalization of fellow project	Collaborations between fellows' schools and community to implement new health projects Fellows influence government policy on health and education through leadership positions and scholarly writing Increase in fellowship graduates in leadership positions in national organizations
	Measure example: FAIMER—project progress reports ELAM—social network analysis	*Measure example*: FAIMER—professional development portfolio data on institutionalization of FAIMER project (sustained, enlarged, policy/procedure change) ELAM—career tracking by positions across the United States	*Measure example*: FAIMER—tracking collaborative presentations and publications
Type: Transformative	National/international leadership role in medical education and/or health organizations	Curriculum aligned with regional health needs (e.g., common regional diseases, rural clinical rotations, integrating community physicians into leadership roles) Revised appointments and promotions criteria to broaden the definition of scholarship	National policy mandates health professions schools address regional health issues National societies of health professions education and journals established Number, education and retention of health professionals meets regional health needs
	Measure example: ELAM—comparative longitudinal study of ELAM program participants compared with two other groups	*Measure example*: ELAM and FAIMER—interview or survey of medical and dental school deans	*Measure example*: FAIMER—tracking national mandates that involve FAIMER Institutes

Future: Need for Research in Health Care Leadership and Management

A compelling need for profound changes in the organization and delivery of health care is paving the road for a more universal conceptual framework of health systems. Universal access and a primary care orientation are distinctive guiding features of the health systems framework.[71–73] The imperative to strengthen the health workforce globally and the simultaneous need to redesign health care systems are clearly dependent on the development of health professionals "that can personify the new health systems' core values."[74] Leadership development and effective teamwork play a pivotal role in meeting these challenges. They also are the agenda for this chapter.[75,76]

Leadership and management are closely related to organizational context and can be developed in structured programs and relationships created through personal interchange. It is noteworthy that evaluation of leadership and management and research development in this field will reinforce valuing these attributes among health professionals.

Continued research in leadership development and evaluation will provide a more consistent use of evidence-based applications.[77] The health professions and their education are well suited for new research investigations in this fast-paced field. Leadership and management are transitioning to a more holistic view, encompassing approaches based on positive psychology, leadership distributed and shared throughout organizations, and on leadership in clusters.[78] Such new understanding of leadership and management allows not only for the intended actions but also for emergent properties of social order. It also encompasses not just the immediate but also the wider historical, political, and cultural context of social practices.[78]

References

1. Souba WW. The new leader: new demands in a changing, turbulent environment. *J Am Coll Surg.* 2003; **197**(1): 79–87.
2. Gilmore TN. *Dilemmas of Physicians in Administrative Roles: dealing with the managerial other within.* Paper delivered at International Society for the Psychoanalytic Study of Organizations Symposium, Jun 20–22, 2002; Melbourne, Australia. Available at: www.cfar.com/Documents/physadmin.pdf (accessed April 22, 2011).
3. Souba WW. New ways of understanding and accomplishing leadership in academic medicine. *J Surg Res.* 2004; **117**(2): 177–186.

4. Patterson TE, Champion H, Browning H, et al.; for Center for Creative Leadership. *Addressing the Leadership Gap in Healthcare: what's needed when it comes to leader talent?* Greensboro, NC: Center for Creative Leadership; 2010. Available at: www.ccl.org/leadership/pdf/research/addressingleadershipGapHealthcare.pdf (accessed April 22, 2011).

5. Martin A, Willburn P, Morrow P, et al.; for Center for Creative Leadership. *What's Next? The 2007 Changing Nature of Leadership Survey.* Greensboro, NC: Center for Creative Leadership. Available at: www.ccl.org/leadership/pdf/research/WhatsNext.pdf (accessed April 28, 2011).

6. Mouradian WE, Huebner CE. Future directions in leadership training of MCH professionals: cross-cutting MCH leadership competencies. *Matern Child Health J.* 2007; **11**(3): 211–18.

7. www.collaborative-leaders.org

8. Rubin H. *Collaborative Leadership: developing effective partnerships for communities and schools.* Thousand Oaks, CA: Corwin Press; 2009.

9. Archer D, Cameron A. *Collaborative Leadership: how to succeed in an interconnected world.* Burlington, MA: Butterworth Heinemann; 2008.

10. Bonham AC, Rich EC, Davis DA, et al. Putting evidence to work: an expanded research agenda for academic medicine in the era of health care reform. *Acad Med.* 2010; **85**(10): 1551–3.

11. Stokols D, Hall KL, Taylor BK, et al. The science of team science: overview of the field and introduction to the supplement. *Am J Prev Med.* 2008; **35**(Suppl. 2): S77–89.

12. Caring Matters. *Defining Relationship-Centered Care.* Available at: www.caringmatters.com/html/DefiningRCC.htm (accessed June 1, 2011).

13. Suchman AL. A new theoretical foundation for relationship-centered care: complex responsive processes of relating. *J Gen Intern Med.* 2006; **21**(Suppl. 1): S40–4.

14. Safran DG, Miller W, Beckman H. Organizational dimensions of relationship-centered care: theory, evidence, and practice. *J Gen Intern Med.* 2006; **21**(Suppl. 1): S9–15.

15. McDade SA, Richman RC, Jackson GB, et al. Effects of participation in the Executive Leadership in Academic Medicine (ELAM) program on women faculty's perceived leadership capabilities. *Acad Med.* 2004; **79**(4): 302–9.

16. Morahan PS, Diserens DF, Richman RC, et al. Women health scientists from developing countries: a pilot effort for meeting their career and leadership aspirations and needs. *AWIS.* 2006; Summer: 5–10.

17. Kuo AK, Thyne SM, Chen HC, et al. An innovative residency program designed to develop leaders to improve the health of children. *Acad Med.* 2010; **85**(10): 1603–8.

18. www.acpe.org

19. Miller DL, Umble KE, Frederick SL, et al. Linking learning methods to outcomes in public health leadership development. *Leadersh Health Serv (Bradf Engl).* 2007; **20**(2): 97–123.

20. www.msh.org

21. Morahan PS, Kasperbauer D, McDade SA, et al. Training future leaders of academic

medicine: internal programs at three academic health centers. *Acad Med.* 1998; **73**(11): 1159–68.

22. Morahan PS, Gleason KA, Richman RC, et al. Advancing women faculty to senior leadership in U.S. academic health centers: fifteen years of history in the making. *J Women High Educ.* 2010; **3**(1): 137–62.

23. Burdick WP, Morahan PS, Norcini JJ. Slowing the brain drain: FAIMER education programs. *Med Teach.* 2006; **28**(7): 631–4.

24. Burdick WP, Morahan PS, Norcini JJ. Capacity building in medical education and health outcomes in developing countries: the missing link. *Educ Health (Abingdon).* 2007; **20**(3): 65.

25. Norcini J, Burdick W, Morahan P. The FAIMER Institute: creating international networks of medical educators. *Med Teach.* 2005; **27**(3): 214–18.

26. Gruppen LD, Frohna AZ, Anderson RM, et al. Faculty development for educational leadership and scholarship. *Acad Med.* 2003; **78**(2): 137–41.

27. Steinert Y, Nasmith L, McLeod PJ, et al. A teaching scholars program to develop leaders in medical education. *Acad Med.* 2003; **78**(2): 142–9.

28. Cusimano MD, David MA. A compendium of higher education opportunities in health professions education. *Acad Med.* 1998; **73**(12): 1255–9.

29. White FS. The Relationship Between Gender and Career Progression Variables and Service Factors for Deans of U.S. Medical Schools from 1980–2006 [dissertation]. Washington, DC: The George Washington University; 2009.

30. Cornwall A, Shankland A. Engaging citizens: lessons from Brazil's national health system. *Soc Sci Med.* 2008; **66**(10): 2173–84.

31. Garajedaghi J. *Systems Thinking: managing chaos and complexity.* Boston, MA: Butterworth Heinemann; 1999.

32. World Health Organization (WHO). *Transformative Scale Up of Medical, Nursing and Midwifery Education: an effort to increase the numbers of health professionals and to strengthen their impact on population health.* Geneva: WHO; 2011.

33. Man KV. Theoretical perspectives in medical education: past experience and future possibilities. *Med Educ.* 2011; **45**(1): 60–8.

34. Ministry of Health, Secretariat of Management of Labor and Education in Health, Department of Management of Education in Health (MS-SGTES-DEGES). *Relatório de Gestão. 2010.* Brasília, Brazil: MS-SGTES-DEGES; 2011.

35. Kristina TN, Majoor GD, van der Vleuten CP. Comparison of outcomes of a community-based education programme executed with and without active community involvement. *Med Educ.* 2006; **40**(8): 798–806.

36. Nair M, Webster P. Education for health professions in the emerging market economies: a literature review. *Med Educ.* 2010; **44**(9): 856–63.

37. Gwee MC. Medical and health care professional education in the 21st century: institutional, national and global perspectives. *Med Educ.* 2011; **45**(1): 25–8.

38. Woollard RF. Caring for a common future: medical schools' social accountability. *Med Educ.* 2006; **40**(4): 301–13.

39. Boelen C, Woollard B. Social accountability and accreditation: a new frontier for educational institutions. *Med Educ.* 2009; **43**(9): 887–94.

40. Day DV. Leadership development: a review in context. *Leadership Quart.* 2001; **11**(4): 581–613.

41. Ministry of Education, Secretariat of Higher Education (MEC-SESu); Ministry of Health, Secretariat of Public Policy (MS-SPP). *Programa de Incentivo a Mudanças Curriculares nos Cursos de Medicina. Uma nova escola médica para um novo sistema de saúde* (PROMED). Brasília, Brazil: MEC-SESu, MS-SPP; 2002.

42. De Souza PA, Zeferino AM, Ros MA. Changes in medicine course curricula in Brazil encouraged by the Program for the Promotion of Medical School Curricula (PROMED). *BMC Med Educ.* 2008; **8**: 54.

43. Castro Lobo MS, Lins MP, da Silva AC, et al. Assessment of teaching: health care integration and performance in university hospitals [article in English, Portuguese]. *Rev Saude Publica.* 2010; **44**(4): 581–90.

44. Haddad AE, Morita MC, Pierantoni CR, et al. Formación de profesionales de salud en Brasil: un análisis en el período de 1991 a 2008 [Undergraduate programs for health professionals in Brazil: an analysis from 1991 to 2008]. *Rev Saude Publica.* 2010; **44**(3): 383–91.

45. Millican J, Bourner T. Student-community engagement and the changing role and context of higher education. *Educ Train.* 2011; **53**(2–3): 89–99.

46. Mennin S. Self-organisation, integration and curriculum in the complex world of medical education. *Med Educ.* 2010; **44**(1): 20–30.

47. Goldstein AO, Calleson D, Bearman R, et al. Teaching advanced leadership skills in community service (ALSCS) to medical students. *Acad Med.* 2009; **84**(6): 754–64.

48. Burch VC. Medical education in the 21st century: what would Flexner ask? *Med Educ.* 2011; **45**(1): 22–4.

49. Anderson NR, West MA. Measuring climate for work group innovation: development and validation of the team climate inventory. *J Organ Behav.* 1998; **19**(3): 235–58.

50. West MA, Borrill CS, Dawson JF, et al. Leadership clarity and team innovation in health care. *Leadership Quart.* 2003; **14**: 393–410.

51. West MA. The social psychology of innovation in groups. In: West MA, Farr JL, editors. *Psychological and Organizational Strategies.* Chichester, UK: Wiley; 1990. pp. 4–36.

52. Preskill H, Jones N. *A Practical Guide for Engaging Stakeholders in Developing Evaluation Questions.* Princeton, NJ: Robert Wood Johnson Foundation; 2009. Available at: www.rwjf.org/pr/product.jsp?id=49951 (accessed April 28, 2011).

53. Patton M. *Utilization-Focused Evaluation.* 4th ed. Thousand Oaks, CA: Sage Publications; 2008.

54. Cousins JB, Whitmore E. Framing participatory evaluation. *New Dir for Eval.* 1998; (80): 5–23.

55. Coghlan AT, Preskill H, Tzavaras Catsambas T. An overview of appreciative inquiry evaluation. *New Dir for Eval.* 2003; (100): 5–22.

56. Mohr BJ, Smith E, Watkins JM. Appreciative inquiry and learning assessment: an embedded evaluation process in a transnational pharmaceutical company. *OD Pract.* 2000; **32**(1): 36–52.

57. Hannum KM, Martineau JW, Reinelt C, editors. *The Handbook of Leadership Development Evaluation*. San Francisco, CA: Jossey-Bass; 2007.

58. Reinelt C, Russon C. Evaluating the outcomes and impacts of leadership development programs: selected findings and lessons learned from a scan of 55 programs. In: Cherrey C, Gardine JJ, Huber N, editors. *Building Leadership Bridges*. Baltimore, MD: International Leadership Association; 2003. pp. 119–36.

59. Goldie J. AMEE Guide no. 29: Evaluating educational programmes. *Med Teach.* 2006; **28**(3): 210–24.

60. *W.K. Kellogg Foundation Logic Model Development Guide*. Battle Creek, MI: WK Kellogg Foundation; 2006. Available at: www.wkkf.org/knowledge-center/resources/2006/02/WK-Kellogg-Foundation-Logic-Model-Development-Guide.aspx (accessed October 23, 2012).

61. Hatry HP. *Measuring Program Outcomes: a practical approach*. 10th printing. Alexandria, VA: United Way Sales Services; 1996.

62. Grove JT, Kibel BM, Haas T. *EvalULEAD: a guide for shaping and evaluating leadership development programs*. Sustainable Leadership Initiative, The Public Health Institute; 2005. Available at: www.wkkf.org/knowledge-center/resources/2005/05/EVALULEAD-A-Guide-For-Shaping-And-Evaluating-Leadership-Development-Programs.aspx (accessed October 23, 2012).

63. McGonagill G, Pruyn PW. *Leadership Development in the U.S.: principles and patterns of best practice*. Bertelsmann Stiftung Leadership Series. Berlin: Bertlesmann Siftung; 2010.

64. Kirkpatrick DL. *Evaluating Training Programs*. San Francisco, CA: Berrett-Koehler; 1959.

65. Phillips JJ. *Handbook of Training Evaluation and Measurement Methods*. Houston, TX: Gulf Publishing; 1997.

66. www.faimer.org

67. Burdick WP, Diserens D, Friedman SR, et al. Measuring the effects of an international health professions faculty development fellowship: the FAIMER Institute. *Med Teach.* 2010; **32**(5): 214–21.

68. Burdick WP, Friedman SR, Diserens D. Faculty development projects for international health professions educators: vehicles for institutional change? *Med Teach.* 2012; **34**(1): 38–44.

69. Drexel University College of Medicine. *Executive Leadership in Academic Medicine*. Available at: www.drexelmed.edu/elam (accessed June 2, 2011).

70. Dannels SA, Yamagata H, McDade SA, et al. Evaluating a leadership program: a comparative, longitudinal study to assess the impact of the Executive Leadership in Academic Medicine (ELAM) program for women. *Acad Med.* 2008; **83**(5): 488–95.

71. Institute of Medicine. A new health system for the 21st century. In: *Crossing the Quality Chasm: a new health system for the 21st century*. Washington, DC: National Academy Press; 2001. pp. 23–38.

72. World Health Organization (WHO). Executive summary to *The World Health Report 2010: Health Systems Financing; the path to universal coverage*. Geneva: WHO; 2010.

73. World Health Organization (WHO). Executive summary to *The World Health Report 2008: Primary Health Care (Now More Than Ever)*. Geneva: WHO; 2008.

74. Institute of Medicine. Building organizational support for change. In: *Crossing the Quality Chasm: a new health system for the 21st century*. Washington, DC: National Academy Press; 2001. pp. 111–44.

75. World Health Organization (WHO). Executive summary to *The World Health Report 2006: Working Together for Health*. Geneva: WHO; 2006.

76. Reich MR, Takemi K. G8 and strengthening of health systems: follow-up to the Tokyo summit. *Lancet*. 2009; **373**(9662): 508–15.

77. Avolio BJ, Walumbwa FO, Weber TJ. Leadership: current theories, research, and future directions. *Annu Rev Psychol*. 2009; **60**: 421–49.

78. Sydow J, Lerch F, Huxham C, et al. A silent cry for leadership: organizing for leading (in) clusters. *Leadership Quart*. 2011; **22**: 328–43.

15

Evaluation for Program and School Accreditation

Barbara Barzansky, Dan Hunt, and Nick Busing

ACCREDITATION HAS BEEN DEFINED AS "RECOGNITION OF AN EDUCA-
tional institution or program that is awarded based on achieving standards or
criteria established by an agency or association."[1] This statement raises a number
of questions about how to implement accreditation. Some of the questions are
policy related. They include the following:

- What is the authority of the group that sets the accreditation standards (e.g.,
  governmental or professional)?
- What is the structure and composition of the group(s) that make the accreditation decision?
- What is the benefit to programs or institutions received by being
  accredited?

However, because accreditation is a type of program evaluation, there are a
number of questions that are directly relevant to evaluators.

- What are the accreditation implications for the set of standards (quantitative
  or qualitative) that are used?
- How can stakeholders be assured that the standards used in accreditation are
  relevant to program quality and outcomes (i.e., validity)?
- How are accreditation standards applied in a uniform (i.e., reliable) manner
  to make accreditation decisions?
- How can the accreditation process unify the need for a summative judgment
  about accreditation with formative goals of program improvement?

These evaluation questions have been answered in different ways by higher education accreditation systems that exist in more than 70 countries.[2] This chapter addresses various approaches to program accreditation used by different accreditation bodies. The chapter also suggests ideas for accreditation "best practices." Several examples are presented based on methods used by the Liaison Committee on Medical Education (LCME)—the accrediting body for educational programs leading to the MD degree in the United States and Canada—and the Committee on the Accreditation of Canadian Medical Schools (CACMS, the LCME's partner in Canadian medical school accreditation). These accrediting bodies use a process that combines institutional self-assessment and peer review that is similar to many accrediting bodies around the world. The process usually includes several steps that occur on a regular review cycle.

1. Institutions collect prespecified information (e.g., class size, teaching and laboratory space, curriculum content, financial resources), conduct an internal review of this information in the context of predefined accreditation standards, and identify areas of strength and weaknesses. This is the self-assessment phase.

2. An individual or group external to the institution visits and, using the information collected by the institution along with on-site data collection (e.g., interviews with faculty and students), makes an independent judgment about compliance with accreditation standards. The evaluator(s) develop a report of findings and conclusions for the accrediting body.

3. The accrediting body makes a decision about the accreditation status of the program or institution and any follow-up that is required about areas of non-compliance with standards. Steps 2 and 3 represent the peer-review phase.

While many accreditation systems use this process, there are specific differences among them that are important to evaluators. These differences come from variations in the following elements.

Accreditation Standards

Accreditation actions must be based in predefined standards; that is, no area outside the standards may be used to make decisions about the accreditation status of an institution. This requires that standards, individually and in aggregate, have certain characteristics. The standards must:
- be clear and understandable

- be linked to appropriate data elements so that compliance can be determined
- cover all areas of importance to all stakeholder groups.

Accreditation bodies differ in the nature and the number of their standards. Each of these has implications for the accreditation process.

Nature of Standards

Quantitative standards specify the components that must exist for educational program compliance. Examples include requirements for specific departments to be present in the institution; the minimum number of faculty within departments, including required faculty-student ratios; specific courses to be included in the curriculum, often with required hours or credits; and teaching space that must be available.[3] For example, in the early twentieth century in the United States, the Association of American Medical Colleges specified the number of hours for each subject in the medical curriculum, based on 4000 total hours of instruction, for medical school recognition.[4]

In contrast, qualitative standards only specify that a condition must be met. However, they do not prescribe the means by which compliance should be reached. To illustrate this point, LCME/CACMS accreditation standard FA-2 related to the adequacy of faculty states:

> A medical education program must have a sufficient number of faculty members in the subjects basic to medicine and in the clinical disciplines to meet the needs and missions of the program.[5]

Such a standard leaves the requirements for compliance open to interpretation. In this approach, a decision about compliance with this standard will be made taking into account institutional characteristics. These may include the presence of an in-depth biomedical or other research program, a robust patient care enterprise, the structure of the medical education program (lecture-based, small-group based), and the educational programs for other learners (e.g., physiotherapists). Each of these features would affect the total number and the types of faculty needed.

If a standard is stated in general (qualitative) terms, accrediting bodies can provide explanatory language to clarify the compliance expectations. For example, the annotation to standard FA-2 states:

> In determining the number of faculty needed for the medical education

program, the program should consider the other responsibilities that its faculty may have in other academic programs and in patient care activities required to conduct meaningful clinical teaching across the continuum of medical education.[5]

This language is not prescriptive yet it provides direction to institutions and serves as a guide for the data elements that will be used to judge compliance. Accrediting bodies with qualitative standards have to decide how detailed they choose to be in describing their compliance expectations. For example, institutional flexibility is diminished if expectations are stated only as numerical benchmarks.

Each approach to accreditation standards has strengths and weaknesses. Quantitative standards are easy to understand and permit uniform evaluation and decision-making across institutions. However, quantitative standards limit variation, institutional flexibility, and may not be based on a definition of organizational effectiveness.[3] By contrast, qualitative standards permit variation among institutions but require more specification of the required data to be collected and the meaning of and boundaries for compliance.

Number of Standards

Accreditation bodies vary widely in the number of their standards. For example, the LCME/CACMS have 129 individual standards while the Commission on Osteopathic College Accreditation, which accredits colleges of osteopathic medicine in the United States, has eight standards, each with a number of subsections.[6] Despite the difference in absolute numbers, the standards of these accrediting bodies cover many of the same areas. Accrediting bodies define compliance as individual concepts or as concept clusters. These definitions are shaped by ways that accreditation bodies set compliance rules.

Validity of Standards and Reliability of their Application

The purpose of accreditation is to assure stakeholder groups including current and prospective students, the public, regulatory bodies, and others about the quality of an educational institution.[7] The terms "valid" and "reliable" are not used in the rigorous sense typical of evaluation discourse. Instead, they are meant to remind us that there needs to be:

- transparency in the standard-setting process and belief by stakeholder groups that standards are appropriate (valid) measures of quality
- application of the standards in a consistent (reliable) manner across institutions and within institutions over time.

Setting and Evaluating Accreditation Standards

In the LCME/CACMS process, standards may originate from any source, including professional and student groups or the LCME/CACMS itself. Proposed standards are judged sequentially through (a) the accrediting body itself; (b) the sponsoring organizations of the LCME/CACMS (the Association of American Medical Colleges and the Council on Medical Education of the American Medical Association in the US and the Association of Faculties of Medicine of Canada and the Canadian Medical Association in Canada); and (c) the public, including the medical education community, through a public hearing.

This process, which may take a year or more, allows broad input from stakeholders related to new standards. This allows stakeholders to provide evidence that supports or refutes the importance of the standard change. If there is significant disagreement with a proposed standard change, it is sent back through the process for review and revision. This is the predominant approach used for gaining agreement on the "validity" of new standards.

Once a new standard has been approved, it is assigned an effective date and posted on the LCME's website. Such transparency in the accreditation system, including using predefined standards and publicizing them to stakeholders, has been cited as an important element in accreditation.[2,8]

Review of existing LCME/CACMS standards takes place on a regular 5-year cycle. Representatives from relevant stakeholder groups are sent standards related to a specific area (for example, the educational program, medical students) and asked to rate each of the standards about its clarity and importance. These reviews allow a contemporary look at standards and provide a systematic process and timeline for standard revision.

Applying Standards

In addition to broad dissemination of standards, several things need to be in place for standards to be applied consistently across institutions.

Identifying Relevant Data Elements

For quantitative standards, the types of data needed are specified in the standard. The confirmation that the specified data element(s) exist at the institution (e.g., predetermined faculty-to-student ratio, presence of a course with a set number of credit hours) indicates that there is compliance with that standard.

For qualitative standards, there is a need for a prospective definition of information that will be used to judge compliance because this may not be obvious from the language of the standard. For example, for the LCME accreditation standard on faculty (FA-2) noted earlier, schools are asked to provide:

- the number of faculty by department and faculty rank
- the number of courses taught by each department to a variety of learners
- the percentage of salaries that are covered for course directors and others with leadership responsibilities in medical education to fulfill these responsibilities
- a description of the extent to which research and clinical service missions of the medical school have impacted the ability to fulfill the faculty's educational responsibilities.[9]

Such specification allows all institutions to submit the same categories of information but also allows reviewers to judge compliance in the context of institutional characteristics.

The decision about what information to collect for a qualitative standard should be driven by expert opinion. The decision must be filtered through those who use qualitative data in compliance decisions related to a standard and the accreditation status of an institution or program. This means that those who visit institutions as reviewers, as well as members of accrediting bodies, should provide feedback about the utility of the information available for use in determining compliance with each standard. As with the accreditation standards themselves, the information that will be used to determine compliance with each accreditation standard should be shared openly.[2] That is, standards and the questions asked about each standard as part of the accreditation review should be posted for institutions or programs to use not only as they prepare for their formal accreditation review but also for ongoing self-assessment.

Preparing Evaluators to Determine Compliance with Standards

In addition to defining accreditation standards and specifying data elements to be collected for each standard, selection and training of on-site evaluators is critical to bring as much consistency as possible to the accreditation process. On-site evaluators need not be content experts in the field of the institution or program being evaluated for accreditation systems with strictly quantitative standards. In this case, they must be able to identify and record the presence of actuarial data and summarize the results of data collection in a report for the accrediting body. If the standards have been well written and the data elements specified clearly, there will be little variation among institutions or programs in what to look for and little judgment required of the on-site evaluator except to state if information related to a specific standard was "found" or "not-found."

By contrast, qualitative standards often are associated with variability among institutions or programs. In this case, the on-site evaluators must be able to apply the accreditation standards to an institution with a specific set of characteristics. For example, how many faculty and of what types are needed in a community-based versus a research-intensive medical school or in medical schools with a lecture-based versus a problem-based curriculum? The on-site evaluators must be able to interpret standards and make judgments for a particular set of circumstances.

One strategy is to select some evaluators from an institution or program with characteristics similar to those of the institution or program undergoing evaluation. The assumption is that peer-reviewers from similar institutions will have a better understanding of the meaning of compliance in those circumstances. But similar does not mean identical. Care is needed to assure that visitors are not prescriptive and use their own institution as an ideal standard.

Another good strategy is to use data from multiple sources to judge compliance with a standard. The data sources include written descriptions provided by the institution, interviews with representatives from different groups within the institution (i.e., faculty, administrators, students), and review of documentation from external sources. Together these give a "three-dimensional" picture that allows an informed judgment about compliance with a given standard.

Another way to enhance transparency and support consistency is to share with institutions the accreditation standards that are cited most commonly. Practices that allow institutions to be judged in compliance can also be shared.

Training of evaluators to understand the meaning and application of standards is an important element to support consistency across institutions. This can be done in many ways, including in-person workshops, online modules, and written materials. However, training cannot cover all circumstances. Mechanisms need to be created to look across institutions to assure that standards are being applied fairly and consistently. This is the province of the accrediting body.

Accreditation Action

Accreditation is a single summative judgment. Accrediting bodies need to turn the findings about compliance with individual accreditation standards into an accreditation decision. Accreditation bodies do not usually state publicly the formula they use to decide if an institution satisfies requirements; that is, they do not explicitly tie loss of accreditation or the imposition of another type of adverse action (e.g., putting the institution or program on probation) to noncompliance with a specific number of standards. They may, however, set guidelines for themselves, which they may share in the interests of transparency. The LCME/CACMS, for example, has stated that the adverse action of probation may be taken for longstanding noncompliance with one or more standards or current patterns of noncompliance that "seriously jeopardize the quality of the educational program."[10]

In addition to being consistent with the guidelines they have set related to granting of accreditation or the imposition of an adverse action, accreditation bodies must act consistently across institutions with similar findings of noncompliance. This can be more straightforward for accrediting bodies that use quantitative standards, since two institutions cited for noncompliance with the same standard will have the same deficit (e.g., the deficit of a required course).

Dual Goals of Accreditation

The primary goal of accreditation is to attest that an institution or program has met standards. This is typically a decision that is made public, with the institution's accreditation status posted or otherwise disseminated to stakeholders. However, accreditation often has the secondary goal of program improvement. This adds another dimension to the process.

Issues for Accreditors and Institutions

The following are issues that evaluators should take into account when considering their role in program improvement. There is no one way that accrediting bodies currently address these dichotomies and each side has positive and negative aspects.

Site Visitor as Evaluator Versus Consultant

The role of the site visitor is to collect information and to report findings related to compliance with accreditation standards. Especially when site visitors are content experts from similar programs or institutions, there is a temptation to share what the visitor's own institution is doing related to a specific area. This could create a role tension, which may be difficult to manage. The LCME/CACMS considers the role of the site visitor to be restricted solely to information gathering. This is because the LCME/CACMS has the final authority to make the decision about compliance with accreditation standards, so the "consultation" about how to improve provided by the site visitor may be misleading. However, others argue that the site visitor, as a peer, may be able to provide useful information. Accrediting bodies should set guidelines about whether and to what extent consultation during survey visits is permitted and include such guidelines in policy as well as visitor training.

Confidentiality versus Transparency of Accreditation Findings

Accrediting bodies also differ on whether their detailed findings about an institution or program's compliance with accreditation standards are made public, as opposed to revealing just the institution's accreditation status. In addition, institutions themselves may or may not make public the results of their accreditation reviews.

Transparency by accrediting bodies provides information to stakeholders about educational program quality but also potentially inhibits candor in accreditor's appraisal of institutions. Transparency by the institution motivates and informs its members to correct identified deficiencies. The downside is that transparency might damage institutional reputation to outsiders.

Strategies to Support Program Improvement

After these issues have been addressed in the policies and processes of accreditors, several steps would support their role in program improvement, outlined as follows.

Follow-Up after Accreditation Reviews

After an accreditation review, accrediting bodies must define the follow-up that is required to assure that compliance has been achieved with all accreditation standards. This may be done through written reports from the program or institution or by on-site inspections. This follow-up continues until full compliance has been achieved with all accreditation standards.

Clear Description of the Areas Needing Correction

Accrediting bodies typically provide institutions with a list of areas where improvement is needed. These include areas of noncompliance with accreditation standards and specific data elements or information that will be used to monitor compliance. Noncompliance problems should be clear so that institutions know what changes must be made and the timeframe for their completion.

Ongoing Follow-Up Outside the Regular Accreditation Cycle

The LCME/CACMS conduct a full review of medical school every 8 years. Other accrediting bodies use a different cycle. Some collect data on an interim basis to check for ongoing compliance with accreditation standards, even if the institution or program was not out of compliance in its last full review. This low-stakes review allows problem areas to be identified and corrected early.

Information about Good Practices

While it is problematic for accrediting bodies to recognize a single way ("best practice") to achieve compliance with qualitative standards, it is useful to identify a range of acceptable approaches. These could be derived from recent surveys and shared by the accrediting body or some other group. Care is needed, however, to reserve the judgment that adopting one of these approaches will ensure compliance. Institutional characteristics and circumstances need to be taken into account.

Consultation about the Meaning and Interpretation of Standards

While an accrediting body may choose to not have its evaluators provide consultation, the staff of the accrediting body may be able to fill this role. Staff are typically knowledgeable about what constitutes compliance since they have the "institutional memory" about the actions taken by the accrediting body over time. They typically do not participate in deliberations of the accrediting body and vote on accreditation actions, so they do not have a conflict of interest as consultants.

Summary: Elements to Consider in Developing Best Practices
• • • • • • • • • • • • • • • • • • •

Accreditation is a form of applied program evaluation that has not been formally grounded in any single program evaluation model. Study of both the process of accreditation of health professions education programs and accreditation outcomes is limited, and is mainly descriptive in nature. A model of education program accreditation has emerged over time that is widely used throughout the world. Although there is significant consistency in the overall approach to accreditation in the United States and internationally, there are important variations, such as the nature of standards, the roles of evaluators, and the transparency of accreditation findings.

There is at least anecdotal consensus that a good accreditation system should include the following general elements.

Trustworthiness

An accreditation system must appear trustworthy to the relevant constituencies, including the institutions to be accredited, their applicants and students, and other stakeholders.[2] What makes an accreditation system trustworthy has not been specified or studied, except by inference, but likely includes features such as (a) an absence of conflict of interest and fairness in decision making and (b) the perceived relevance and appropriateness of accreditation standards and practices.

Competence

Accreditation systems must function efficiently and effectively, in such things as (a) selecting and training appropriate on-site reviewers, (b) developing and implementing policies and practices, (c) keeping appropriate records related to accreditation actions, and (d) managing reviews.

Transparency

Accrediting bodies should make the standards, processes, and policies of an accreditation system widely available and open to comment.

Outcome Orientation

Accrediting bodies should evaluate their policies, procedures, and standards to assure that they are, as well as can be determined, consistent with generally accepted practices. Working to determine if accreditation makes a difference in the quality of health professions' graduates is an important task for all accrediting bodies.

In summary, accreditation has an important place in the educational system for health professionals around the world. For example, in the United States, graduation from an accredited medical school provides access to postgraduate training and to licensure to practice. Through engaging in high-quality evaluation, accreditation as a process must work to ensure that it meets this responsibility.

References

1. Blauch LE. The meaning of accreditation. In: Blauch LE, editor. *Accreditation in Higher Education*. Washington, DC: Department of Health, Education, and Welfare; 1959. pp. 3–8.
2. Karle H. Global standards and accreditation in medical education: a view from the WFME. *Acad Med*. 2006; **81**(Suppl. 12): S43–8.
3. Norcini JJ, Banda SS. Increasing the quality and capacity of education: the challenge for the 21st century. *Med Educ*. 2011; **45**(1): 81–6.
4. Darley W. AAMC milestones in raising the standards of medical education. *J Med Educ*. 1965; **40**: 321–8.
5. *Functions and Structure of a Medical School*. May 2011 edition. Available at: www. lcme.org/functions2011may.pdf (accessed October 18, 2012).
6. Commission on Osteopathic College Accreditation. *Accreditation of Colleges of Osteopathic Medicine: COM Accreditation Standards and Procedures* (July 2012). Available at: www.osteopathic.org/inside-aoa/accreditation/predoctoral%20accreditation/Documents/COM-accreditation-standards-Effective-7-1-2012.pdf (accessed October 18, 2012).
7. Simpson I, Lockyer T, Walters T. Accreditation of medical training in Australia and New Zealand. *Med J Malaysia*. 2005; **60**(Suppl D): S20–3.
8. Van Zanten M, Parkins LM, Karle H, et al. Accreditation of undergraduate medical education in the Caribbean: report on the Caribbean accreditation authority for education in medicine and other health professions. *Acad Med*. 2009; **84**(6): 771–5.
9. Liaison Committee on Medical Education. *Medical Education Database*, 2012–2013. Available at: www.lcme.org/database12_13.htm#database (accessed October 18, 2012).
10. LCME *Rules of Procedure*, April 2012. Available at: www.lcme.org/rules_of_procedure.pdf (accessed October 18, 2012).

16

Looking to the Future

S. Barry Issenberg and William C. McGaghie

THIS CHAPTER CONCLUDES THE PRESENTATION OF *INTERNATIONAL Best Practices for Evaluation in the Health Professions*. The fifteen preceding chapters set forth "cutting edge" ideas about health professions education by thought leaders from around the world. In this coda we focus on three specific aims to round out the discussion about evaluation best practices. The first aim is to reveal and discuss a growing awareness that traditional methods of clinical education and evaluation in the health professions are becoming obsolete. The second aim is to propose a new unifying educational framework for health professions individuals and teams that incorporates the science of mastery learning and deliberate practice, to better prepare health professionals for patient care responsibilities. A key feature of this framework is reliance on rigorous learner measurement and reliable outcome evaluation. The third specific aim is to advance a roadmap for best practices research in health professions education that goes beyond *educational science* featuring mastery learning with deliberate practice, to include *translational science* and *implementation science* and the implications these developments have on health sciences evaluation.

Obsolete Clinical Education

The first aim of this chapter is to raise awareness that many current methods of clinical education and evaluation in the health professions are growing obsolete. Today's clinical education of physicians, nurses, and many other health professionals is grounded in nineteenth-century thinking about the acquisition of clinical competence, as pointed out in Sir William Osler's quote in Chapter 1 of this book, concerning ideas about the hospital as a college expressed in 1903. Osler[1] also stated in that essay, "In what may be called the *natural method of teaching* the student begins with the patient, continues with the patient, and ends his studies with the patient" (emphasis added).

Osler's *natural method of teaching*, echoed by his Johns Hopkins surgeon colleague William Halsted,[2] endorses the idea that the clinical curriculum is embodied in patients. In practice, this view holds that longitudinal clinical exposure and experience with many patients is sufficient for physicians in training to become competent doctors. The belief is that there is no real need for structured exercises, skills practice, objective evaluation with feedback, and guided reflection for young physicians to master their craft. Thus the traditional Osler clinical curriculum is passive on educational grounds, based solely on patients seen over time, with faculty performance evaluations of learners given subjectively using clinical criteria. The Osler clinical curriculum tradition has dominated twentieth-century medical education and still persists in the early twenty-first century.

The problem with Osler's *natural method of teaching* based on longitudinal clinical education is that it does not work very well, especially in comparison with contemporary educational approaches. We know this because rigorous evaluations of clinical skills among postgraduate residents during clinical medical education produce consistent, disturbing results. For example, research by Mangione et al.[3] and Mangione and Nieman[4] shows that postgraduate primary care trainees in family medicine and internal medicine performed poorly on objective measures of cardiac auscultation. Year of resident training did not affect results because senior residents performed the same as first-year residents. Cardiology fellows performed slightly better than residents (22% correct) on these basic skills. Six hundred fifty-six residents and cardiology fellows in both studies were no better than medical students at evaluating heart sounds correctly. The poor performance of primary care residents and cardiology fellows on cardiac auscultation has been replicated in another large study evaluating primary care residents' proficiency at pulmonary auscultation.[5] Many other studies that evaluate educational outcomes of traditional clinical education in medicine reveal similar, weak results. To illustrate, a 3-year study involving objective evaluations of 126 pediatric residents showed these trainees failed to meet faculty expectations about acquisition of such basic clinical skills as physical examination, history taking, laboratory use, and telephone management.[6] Clinical skill and knowledge deficits among new residents whose undergraduate medical education was grounded chiefly in the traditional natural method of teaching have been documented in studies performed at the University of Michigan[7] and at Northwestern University.[8] The skill and knowledge deficits include such basic competencies as critical laboratory values, cross-cultural communication, evidence-based medicine, radiographic image interpretation, aseptic technique, advanced cardiac life support, and cardiac auscultation. Clinical skill and knowledge deficits were widespread among new residents at both institutions. United States Medical Licensing Examination scores, and the prestige of residents' undergraduate medical schools, had no effect on their readiness for supervised patient care measured objectively. A study of anesthesiology residents learning epidural anesthesia demonstrated a strong correlation between increased clinical experience and manual skills measured by a checklist and a global rating scale. However, clinical experience was not associated with improvement in aseptic technique while performing epidural anesthesia. The investigators state:

> The most significant conclusion of the study is that in contrast to the teaching of manual skills, our didactic and practical teaching of the aseptic principles as they should be applied to epidural anesthesia was, as our results clearly demonstrate, insufficient.[9]

A recent study by Bell et al.[10] documented the operative experience of residents in US general surgery programs. Surgery program directors graded 300 operative procedures A, B, or C using these criteria:

> A—graduating general surgery residents should be competent to perform the procedure independently; B—graduating residents should be familiar with the procedure, but not necessarily competent to perform it; and C—graduating residents neither need to be familiar with nor competent to perform the procedure.

The actual operative experience of all residents completing general surgery training in June 2005 was reviewed and compared with the three procedural criteria.

The study results are enlightening and address Osler's natural method of teaching directly. Bell et al.[10] report:

> One hundred twenty-one of the 300 operations were considered A level procedures by a majority of program directors (PDs). Graduating 2005 US residents (n = 1022) performed only 18 of the 121 A procedures, an average of more than 10 times during residency; 83 of 121 procedures were performed on average less

than 5 times and 31 procedures less than once. For 63 of the 121 procedures, the mode (most commonly reported) experience level was 0. In addition, there was significant variation between residents in operative experience for specific procedures.

The investigators conclude:

Methods will have to be developed to allow surgeons to reach a basic level of competence in procedures which they are likely to experience only rarely during residency. Even for more commonly performed procedures, the numbers of repetitions are not very robust, stressing the need to determine objectively whether residents are actually achieving basic competency in these operations.[10]

The consistent finding from these and other studies is that clinical experience alone does not guarantee the acquisition of clinical competence. Osler's natural method of teaching, grounded solely in longitudinal clinical experience without curriculum objectives and management, learner supervision, rigorous assessment with feedback, learner performance expectations, and educational milestones, yields poor results.

Alternative approaches to traditional clinical education are beginning to gain traction in medicine and other health professions. Simulation-based education (SBE), in particular, is gaining popularity throughout the health professions because a growing body of empirical evidence shows it produces strong, sustained results in terms of clinical skill acquisition among individuals and teams.[11,12]

The power and utility of SBE is reinforced by new knowledge from comparative effectiveness research.[13] A recent meta-analytic study of clinical medical education involved a comparison of SBE with deliberate practice (DP)[14,15] versus traditional clinical education toward skill acquisition goals. The meta-analysis combined data from 14 eligible research studies involving 633 learners: 389 internal medicine, surgical, and emergency medicine residents; 226 medical students; 18 internal medicine fellows. The SBE studies address a wide variety of competencies and skills, including advanced cardiac life support, laparoscopic surgical techniques, central venous catheter insertion, cardiac auscultation, and thoracentesis. Measured outcomes in these studies include procedural skill acquisition, medical problem recognition, clinical decision making, communication skills, teamwork, and team leadership. The results show that all comparisons, without exception, favored SBE with DP versus traditional clinical education.[13]

The overall results translate to a Cohen's *d* coefficient of ~2.00, a "large" effect.[16] The evidence clearly shows that traditional clinical education, compared with SBE with DP, has *never* been a better option for learner skill acquisition.

Studies are now underway to extend the SBE model to other clinical competencies, including physician-patient communication and code status discussions about end-of-life issues with patients and their families.[17] Such "soft" clinical skills are no less important than "hands on" procedures such as intubation and suturing as markers of clinical competence.

These studies are clear indicators that Osler's nineteenth-century natural method of teaching, now referred to as the "apprenticeship" or "see one, do one, teach one" approach to clinical education in the health professions, has outlived its usefulness. The traditional model of learning through clinical encounters and accumulation of clinical experience alone is insufficient to reach expert status in a given field or for a specific clinical skill. Change is needed in health professions education to better prepare a more competent health professions workforce and to better serve patient safety goals.

The many flaws in the traditional approach to clinical education in medicine and other health professions demonstrate a need for a new, evidence-based educational framework. The time has come to create, implement, deliver, manage, and evaluate programs of clinical education in the health professions that produce measureable, competency-based outcomes among learners.

A New Educational Framework

The second specific aim of this chapter is to propose a new unifying educational science framework for training clinical health professionals as individuals and teams. The new framework has two prominent features: (1) *mastery learning*[18,19] and (2) opportunities for *deliberate practice*.[14,15] Rigorous learner measurement and reliable outcome evaluation are foundation features of this framework. The new educational framework also relies heavily on new learning technologies covered in Chapter 3 of this volume on "Technology-Enabled Assessment of Health Professions Education." The premise is that clinical competence can be achieved by all health professions learners—nurses, physicians, physiotherapists, pharmacists, and many others in their own way—with little or no outcome variation. This is a radical departure from traditional health professions education. Traditional clinical education endorses the idea that learning outcomes are expressed as individual differences among persons and teams distributed on a

Gaussian normal curve. The new framework expects high and uniform competence from everyone.[18,19]

Mastery Learning

Mastery learning begins with educational engineering. The key question is, "How shall we design an educational environment that produces maximum learning outcomes among all trainees?" The answer is to create a set of educational conditions, a curriculum, and an assessment plan that facilitates high achievement among all learners.

Mastery learning is a stringent form of competency-based education.[18] Mastery learning requires that learners acquire essential knowledge, skill, and professionalism attributes, measured rigorously and compared with fixed achievement standards, without regard to the time needed to reach the outcome. Mastery indicates a much higher level of performance than competence alone. In mastery learning, educational *results* are uniform, with little or no variation, while educational *time* can vary among trainees.

As expressed elsewhere,[19]

> mastery learning has the following seven complementary features:
> 1. Baseline, or diagnostic testing;
> 2. Clear learning objectives, sequenced as units in increasing difficulty;
> 3. Engagement in educational activities (e.g., skills practice, data interpretation, reading) focused on reaching the objectives;
> 4. A set minimum passing standard (e.g., test score) for each educational unit;
> 5. Formative testing to gauge unit completion at a preset minimum passing standard for mastery;
> 6. Advancement to the next educational unit given measured achievement at or above the mastery standard;
> 7. Continued practice or study on an educational unit until the mastery standard is reached.
>
> The goal in mastery learning is to ensure that all learners accomplish all educational outcomes with little or no variation in outcome. The amount of time needed to reach mastery standards for a unit's educational objectives varies among the learners.[19]

Mastery learning in health professions education is advanced by reliance on new learning technologies, as described in Chapter 3 of this volume. Given learning objectives, educational resources, and skillful teaching faculty, learners may use, for example, simulation technology that varies in fidelity to practice and acquire key clinical competencies. Simulation technology has been used successfully to help learners master a variety of clinical skills, including advanced cardiac life support,[20] central venous catheter (CVC) insertion,[21] thoracentesis,[22] and ventilator patient management.[23] Mastery learning with or without new educational technologies calls for a structured and sequenced curriculum, skillful faculty instructors, flexible scheduling, a focus on skill acquisition, a noncompensatory policy (i.e., one cannot "make up for" poor performance on one unit with superior performance on another unit), and is driven by rigorous measurement that yields reliable data.

Rigorous measurement that produces reliable data is essential in mastery learning for two reasons. First, reliable data are a source of trustworthy information to give learners feedback about their progress toward mastery goals. Second, reliable data serve as a database for research and program evaluation. Such measurement qualifies as "dynamic testing"[24,25] because it is instructive and elicits responses. "[Dynamic] testing involves learning at the time of the test, rather than just static testing of what has been learned before."[24] As implied by Boulet and McKinley in Chapter 2 of this volume, dynamic testing is an example of formative assessment—assessment *for* learning, not just assessment *of* learning.

An example of mastery learning in medical education is seen in a recent study by Barsuk and colleagues[26] of internal medicine (IM) residents' acquisition of lumbar puncture (LP) skills in a mastery learning curriculum compared with neurology residents' LP skill acquisition using traditional clinical education. Figure 16.1 shows that IM residents express wide variation in LP skills at baseline testing using an LP simulator. However, after a minimum 3-hour education session featuring deliberate practice and feedback, all IM residents met or exceeded a mastery standard for LP skills. By contrast, only a handful of the traditionally trained neurology residents met the passing standard measured on the LP simulator, even though they had much more LP clinical experience. The research report concludes, "Few [traditionally trained] neurology residents were competent to perform a simulated LP *despite clinical experience with the procedure*"[26] (emphasis added). An editorial that accompanied publication of the LP research comments:

> The Barsuk et al. study is clearly a wake-up call for all of us who were trained in the era of "see one, do one, teach one"—the so-called "apprenticeship" model of clinical training. The old training methods are no longer enough to ensure the best education, and thus the best care for patients.[27]

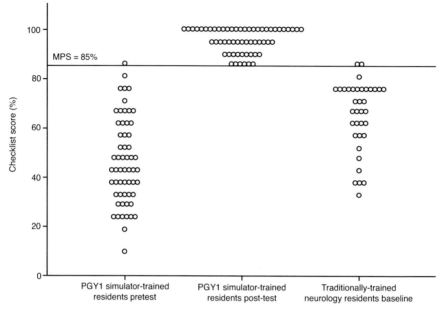

Clinical skills examination (checklist) pre- and final posttest performance of 58 first-year simulator-trained internal medicine residents and baseline performance of 36 traditionally trained neurology residents. Three internal medicine residents failed to meet the minimum passing score (MPS) at initial post-testing. PGY = postgraduate year.

FIGURE 16.1 Clinical skills examination (checklist) performance

Source: Barsuk J, Cohen E, Caprio T, et al. Simulation-based education with mastery learning improves residents' lumbar puncture skills. *Neurology.* 2012; **79**(2): 132–7. Reprinted with permission of Wolters Kluwer Health.

Deliberate Practice

The utility of DP as a mechanism for skill and knowledge acquisition in the health professions is now well established. Briefly,

> Deliberate practice is an educational variable associated with delivery of strong and consistent educational treatments as part of the mastery learning model. Although demanding of learners, deliberate practice is grounded in information processing and behavioral theories of skill acquisition and maintenance.[19]

The theoretical foundations and early empirical research on deliberate practice have been pioneered by learning psychologist K. Anders Ericsson (Ericsson,[14,15] Ericsson et al.,[28] Ericsson and Charness[29]).

Deliberate practice has at least 10 components that match features of the mastery learning model.[19]

1. Highly motivated learners with good concentration;
2. Engagement with a well-defined learning objective or task; at an
3. Appropriate level of difficulty; with
4. Focused, repetitive practice; that leads to
5. Rigorous, precise measurements; that yield
6. Informative *feedback* from educational sources (e.g., simulators, teachers); and where
7. Trainees also monitor their learning experiences and correct strategies, errors, and levels of understanding, engage in more DP; and continue with
8. *Evaluation* to reach a mastery standard; and then
9. Advance to another task or unit.
10. The goal of DP is constant improvement, not just maintenance of the status quo.

The power and utility of DP for knowledge and skill acquisition and mainten-ance have been demonstrated in a variety of professions and skilled endeavors, including competitive sports, chess, musical performance, medicine, acting, and other domains.[15] DP and mastery learning are complementary ideas, which when enacted together in a health professions education curriculum, can produce extraordinary learning results.[20–23,26] This new evidence-based educational frame-work is beginning to replace the "apprenticeship," "see one, do one, teach one" approach to clinical education that has defined knowledge and skill acquisition in the health professions for more than a century.

Research Roadmap

The third specific aim of this chapter is to advance a roadmap for best practices research in health professions education and evaluation that addresses five fac-ets: (1) research opportunities, (2) research methods, (3) *translational science*, (4) *implementation science*, and (5) scholarship by individuals and teams. This aim amplifies the *educational science* theme of the previous section with its emphasis on mastery learning and deliberate practice.

Research Opportunities

A 2008 essay identified 10 research opportunities in simulation-based med-ical education (SBME) using deliberate practice that still warrant attention throughout the health professions.[30] These 10 research opportunities, with brief annotation, are as follows.

1. *Wither randomized trials? Mastery learning!* Randomized trials are no longer needed to evaluate the effectiveness of health professions curricula featuring mastery learning and deliberate practice. Strong evidence shows that these educational interventions work, especially when used with new education and evaluation technologies. Instead, research opportunities reside in engineering mastery learning environments that increase and maintain acquisition of skill, knowledge, and professionalism and to evaluate results rigorously.

2. *Stretch the endpoint!* Several schemes have been proposed to classify health professions education research outcomes. One typology identifies educational outcomes measured in the classroom or laboratory (T1), compared to downstream educational results measured as better patient care practices (T2), and improved health outcomes for individuals and the public (T3).[31] More translational research is needed to reinforce recent studies that show T1 educational outcomes transfer to T2 and T3 results.[32]

3. *Study DP quality.* DP can have many variations, and research is needed to isolate the conditions, intensity, duration, feedback features, and other moderator variables that make DP effective. We assume, but lack empirical evidence, that DP is a powerful variable for all forms of skill and knowledge acquisition, among all health professions, at all levels of training and experience.

4. *Research design features.* Strong research designs with rigorous measures and large sample sizes (i.e., individuals, teams) are needed for both comparative and correlational quantitative studies. This work should embrace established principles of health professions education research design to produce informative, robust results.[33]

5. *Measurement development.* A great need exists to develop and refine new measures of the complex human behaviors that account for clinical competence in the health professions. Future research in health professions education can only advance with the availability of rigorous measures that yield reliable data that permit valid judgments about the progress or competence of learners.

6. *Affective educational outcomes.* Most health professions education programs produce strong affective results among individuals and teams, but the outcomes are rarely measured. Trainee morale, self-efficacy, team spirit, team cohesiveness, mutual trust, and other outcome variables are all metrics of

educational program effectiveness and of professional practice in clinics and wards. More research on affective outcomes in health professions education is warranted.

7. *Clinical skill maintenance.* Past research shows that professional skills can decay rapidly without frequent practice or use.[34] More recent studies provide mixed retention results, with one reporting maintenance of acquired advanced cardiac life support clinical skills over time,[35] while another shows uneven CVC skill decay among clinical learners.[36] These studies warrant replication with fresh data sets about other clinical skills to determine if their findings are generalizable.

8. *Faculty development.* Research on new and better approaches to prepare faculty for new, more active, clinical teaching roles is needed to move beyond the dated "apprenticeship" model of clinical education. This is a key message of the 2007 Colloquium on Educational Technology sponsored by the Association of American Medical Colleges.[37] Issenberg[38] has amplified this faculty development theme by arguing that clinical education "best practice" is a multiplicative product of (a) new educational technologies, (b) teachers prepared to use the technologies to maximum educational advantage, and (c) curriculum integration. Studies of faculty development training models are needed to prepare clinical teachers for new roles and competencies.

9. *UTOST model.* Behavioral science research scholars point out that our investigations are usually grounded in the five-component UTOST model, often without investigator awareness: **U**nit (individual or team) + **T**reatment (e.g., SBME with DP) + **O**bservations (measurements) + **S**etting (laboratory, clinic) + **T**ime (occasions).[39] Each of these components can vary in many ways. Science advances when the variations are implemented systematically, in controlled settings, allowing rigorous studies that can be replicated elsewhere. Kenneth Hammond has pronounced a scientific moral imperative:

> "Every method . . . implies a methodology, expressed or not; every methodology implies a theory, expressed or not. If one chooses not to examine the methodological base of his or her work, then one chooses not to examine the theoretical context of that work, and thus becomes an unwitting technician at the mercy of implicit theories."[40]

Research methods must be studied, selected, and used judiciously.

10. *Team science.* Modern science is rarely done by solitary scholars working alone. Team science is normative today and is the source of scholarly

productivity and impact. A distillation of team science research suggests there are 10 attributes of productive academic teams: (i) shared goals— common mission and vision; (ii) functional diversity; (iii) clear leadership that may change or rotate; (iv) shared mental models and language; (v) high standards, recognition, and credit; (vi) sustained hard work and commitment; (vii) physical proximity; (viii) minimize status differences *within* the team; (ix) maximize status *of* the team; (x) shared activities that breed trust.[41–43] Formulating and operating research teams based on these principles, and evaluating academic team outcomes rigorously, will advance the research agenda.

Research Methods

The research methods used by investigators in health professions education in scientific studies should be matched to the focused question being addressed. Comparative questions (e.g., "Is instructional method A better than method B?") call for randomized trials and cohort studies. Research questions about associations (e.g., "Do Medical College Admission Test scores predict clinical performance?") are addressed in correlational studies. There is no one best research approach. Selection of research methods should be informed by theory and practical matters, used judiciously, as stated earlier.[33] Research in health professions education is governed chiefly by three traditions: (1) quantitative, (2) qualitative, and (3) mixed methods.

Quantitative research in health professions education has been the dominant model for more than 6 decades. This scholarship is grounded in structured prospective and retrospective research designs, quantitative measurement, concern for data reliability, attention to valid inferences, and attempts to generalize findings from local studies to wider populations.[39,40,44,45] This empirical research is inspired by a research tradition throughout the world that values objectivity, parsimony, and intellectual detachment. There are many examples of quantitative research in health professions education that have informed both theory and practice. Much of this work is summarized in the 2002 *International Handbook of Research in Medical Education*,[46] edited by G. R. Norman, C. P. M. van der Vleuten, and D. I. Newble.

Health professions education qualitative research, by contrast, uses a different investigative model. Qualitative research relies on words rather than numbers, is inductive more than deductive, and frequently engages the researcher as a participant and an observer in the research enterprise. Qualitative research is no less rigorous than quantitative research but employs different rules of evidence.[47]

Classic examples of qualitative research in health professions education include *Boys in White: Student Culture in Medical School*,[48] an exposition of student culture in medical school at the University of Kansas in the 1950s, *Getting Rid of Patients: Contradictions in the Socialization of Physicians*,[49] and *Forgive and Remember: Managing Medical Failure*,[50] a coming-of-age study about surgeons in training. A new example of qualitative health professions research is a study about the problems and obstacles that diabetes patients encounter when they try to self-manage their disease.[51] Côté and Turgeon[52] offer a set of 12 guidelines for methodological appraisal of qualitative research journal articles in medicine and medical education.

Mixed-methods research combines the strongest features of the quantitative and qualitative traditions in the same study. Mixed-methods research allows investigators to study health professions education questions with the rigor embedded in systematic research design, reliable measurement, and quantitative data analysis, together with the rich and thick descriptions that qualitative research employs. A recent illustration of mixed-methods research in health professions education is a report by Dixon-Woods and colleagues[53] that sought to identify the reasons why the Michigan Project, which aimed to reduce catheter related bloodstream infections in medical intensive care units, was so successful. Earlier quantitative research demonstrated significant statewide reductions in medical intensive care unit infection rates due to aggressive clinical interventions focused on care processes addressing patient safety.[54,55] The mixed-methods study amplified the quantitative research by revealing that clinical staff education, hospital rivalries, and social pressures also contributed to infection rate reductions.[53] Methodological best practices for the conduct of mixed-methods research in health professions education have been published by Cresswell and colleagues[56] and by Lopez-Fernandez and Molina-Azorin.[57]

Translational Science

Translational science (TS) is usually defined as biomedical or biomedical engineering research designed to accelerate movement of results from the laboratory bench to the patient bedside. The biomedical translational science model has recently been extended to medical and health professions education, especially education programs that use simulation technology coupled with mastery learning and deliberate practice.[31]

A long and rich research legacy shows that under the right conditions, simulation-based medical education (SBME) is a powerful intervention to increase medical learner competence. SBME translational science demonstrates that results achieved in the educational laboratory (T1) transfer to improved downstream patient care practices (T2) and improved patient and public health (T3).[32]

Translational education outcomes in the health professions cannot be achieved from single, isolated studies. Instead, TS results in health professions education derive from educational and health services research *programs* that are thematic, sustained, and cumulative. Such translational education research programs must be carefully designed and executed to capture and *measure* downstream results.

An example of an SBME TS research program is seen in the work of a team led by Northwestern University hospitalist physician Jeffrey Barsuk. This thematic, sustained, and cumulative research program has addressed training internal medicine residents in CVC insertion in the medical simulation laboratory, later studying the effects of this training on downstream results. The research program has reported that acquisition of CVC insertion skills by medical residents to mastery standards in the simulation laboratory (T1)[21] translates to improved patient care practices (i.e., fewer needle passes, arterial punctures, needle adjustments, higher success rates (T2)[58]) and improved patient outcomes (T3) (i.e., 85% reduction in medical intensive care unit catheter-related infection rate) because of the educational intervention.[59]

Other examples of downstream translational outcomes resulting from the SBME mastery learning educational intervention include CVC skill and knowledge retention over time;[36] unexpected, yet welcome, collateral effects that document systemic educational improvement among subsequent internal medicine residents, due to rigorous training of prior resident cohorts;[60] the need to increase the mastery learning minimum passing standard, due to the systemic improvement in trainee quality;[61] and cost-effectiveness expressed as a 7 : 1 rate of return on financial investment from the SBME CVC mastery learning program.[62]

The Barsuk team's ability to demonstrate such impressive translational science results is a consequence of careful research planning, hard work, and frequent attention to the importance of team science. Educational research groups across the health professions should emulate the thematic, sustained, and cumulative research program carried out by the Barsuk team.

Implementation Science

Implementation science, as discussed in Chapter 1, addresses the science of education and health care delivery. Implementation science studies, and aims to break down barriers to efficient and effective health professions education and the provision of health care.[63,64]

An example of an implementation science question in health professions education is, "Why has the mastery learning concept taken so long to be adopted in undergraduate and postgraduate education programs?" John Carroll[65] established the intellectual foundation for mastery learning in 1963, 5 decades ago. Subsequent incarnations of the idea have been reported in the behavioral sciences.[66,67] A monograph published by the World Health Organization in 1978, 35 years ago, devoted a chapter to mastery learning.[18] We suspect that educational inertia grounded in Osler's natural method of teaching, now known as the "apprenticeship model" of clinical education, is chiefly responsible. We anticipate broad adoption of the mastery learning model in health professions education as habitual modes of clinical education give way to evidence-based competency models.

Individual and Team Scholarship

Evaluation best practices in the health professions will be identified, refined, disseminated worldwide, and adapted to local conditions as a result of scholarship and publication by individuals, and increasingly, by teams. Scholarship in health professions is not just a responsibility of the academic professoriate. Scholarly ideas and products are also needed from scientists and clinicians in professions including nursing, pharmacy, physiotherapy, dentistry, medicine, and many others, as they care for patients and educate the next generation of health professionals. Scholarship should not be seen as an exclusive, "ivory tower" activity.

We encourage health professions education colleagues to design research and evaluation programs that are grounded in theory, address and test best practices with rigor, and insist on strong evidence for learner evaluation and policy formation. Teamwork and interprofessional collaboration is often the most efficient and productive approach to achieving scholarly goals. The "bottom line," however, is the importance of reporting individual and team scholarship as presentations at meetings, journal articles, book chapters, and monographs. Advancement of the health professions education field depends on thematic, sustained, and cumulative scholarship from its members.

References
• • • • • • • • • • • • • • •

1. Osler W. The hospital as a college [1903]. In: Osler W, editor. *Aequanimitas.* Philadelphia, PA: P. Blakiston's Son & Co.; 1932. pp. 313–25.

2. Halsted WS. The training of the surgeon. *Bull Johns Hopkins Hosp.* 1904; **15**: 267–75.

3. Mangione S, Nieman LZ, Gracely E, et al. The teaching and practice of cardiac auscultation during internal medicine and cardiology training. *Ann Intern Med.* 1993; **119**(1): 47–54.

4. Mangione S, Nieman LZ. Cardiac auscultatory skills of internal medicine and family practice trainees: a comparison of diagnostic proficiency. *JAMA.* 1997; **278**(9): 717–22.

5. Mangione S, Nieman LZ. Pulmonary auscultatory skills during training in internal medicine and family practice. *Am J Respir Crit Care Med.* 1999; **159**(4 Pt. 1): 1119–24.

6. Joorabchi B, Devries JM. Evaluation of clinical competence: the gap between expectation and performance. *Pediatrics.* 1996; **97**(2): 179–84.

7. Lypson ML, Frohna JG, Gruppen LD, et al. Assessing residents' competencies at baseline: identifying the gaps. *Acad Med.* 2004; **79**(6): 564–70.

8. Cohen ER, Barsuk JH, Moazed F, et al. Making July safer: mastery learning of clinical skills during intern bootcamp. *Acad Med.* 2013; **88**: in press.

9. Friedman Z, Siddiqui N, Katznelson R, et al. Experience is not enough: repeated breaches in epidural anesthesia aseptic technique by novice operators despite improved skill. *Anesthesiology.* 2008; **108**(5): 914–20.

10. Bell RH Jr., Biester TW, Tabuenca A, et al. Operative experience of residents in US general surgery programs: a gap between expectation and experience. *Ann Surg.* 2009; **249**(5): 719–24.

11. Issenberg SB, McGaghie WC, Petrusa ER, et al. Features and uses of high-fidelity medical simulations that lead to effective learning: a BEME systematic review. *Med Teach.* 2005; **27**(1): 10–28.

12. McGaghie WC, Issenberg SB, Petrusa ER, et al. A critical review of simulation-based medical education research: 2003–2009. *Med Educ.* 2010; **44**(1): 50–63.

13. McGaghie WC, Issenberg SB, Cohen ER, et al. Does simulation-based medical education with deliberate practice yield better results than traditional clinical education? A meta-analytic comparative review of the evidence. *Acad Med.* 2011; **86**(6): 706–11.

14. Ericsson KA. Deliberate practice and the acquisition and maintenance of expert performance in medicine and related domains. *Acad Med.* 2004; **79**(Suppl. 10): S70–81.

15. Ericsson KA. Enhancing the development of professional performance: implications from the study of deliberate practice. In: Ericsson KA, editor. *Development of Professional Expertise: toward measurement of expert performance and design of optimal learning environments.* New York, NY: Cambridge University Press; 2009. pp. 405–31.

16. Cohen J. *Statistical Power Analysis for the Behavioral Sciences*. 2nd ed. Hillsdale, NJ: Erlbaum; 1988.

17. Szmuilowicz E, Neeley KJ, Sharma RK, et al. Improving residents' code status discussion skills: a randomized trial. *J Palliat Med.* 2012; **15**(7): 768–74.

18. McGaghie WC, Miller GE, Sajid A, et al. *Competency-Based Curriculum Development in Medical Education*. Public Health Paper No. 68. Geneva: World Health Organization; 1978.

19. McGaghie WC, Siddall VJ, Mazmanian PE, et al.; for American College of Chest Physicians Health and Science Policy Committee. Lessons for continuing medical education from simulation research in undergraduate and graduate medical education: effectiveness of continuing medical education; American College of Chest Physicians Evidence-Based Educational Guidelines. *CHEST.* 2009; **135**(Suppl. 3): S62–8.

20. Wayne DB, Butter J, Siddall VJ, et al. Mastery learning of advanced cardiac life support skills by internal medicine residents using simulation technology and deliberate practice. *J Gen Intern Med.* 2006; **21**(3): 251–6.

21. Barsuk JH, McGaghie WC, Cohen ER, et al. Use of simulation-based mastery learning to improve the quality of central venous catheter placement in a medical intensive care unit. *J Hosp Med.* 2009; **4**(7): 397–403.

22. Wayne DB, Barsuk JH, O'Leary KJ, et al. Mastery learning of thoracentesis skills by internal medicine residents using simulation technology and deliberate practice. *J Hosp Med.* 2008; **3**(1): 48–54.

23. Schroedl CJ, Corbridge TC, Cohen ER, et al. Use of simulation-based education to improve resident learning and patient care in the medical intensive care unit: a randomized trial. *J Crit Care.* 2012; **27**(2): 219e7–13.

24. Grigorenko EL, Sternberg RJ. Dynamic testing. *Psychol Bull.* 1998; **124**: 75–111.

25. Sternberg RJ, Grigorenko EL. *Dynamic Testing: the nature and measurement of learning potential*. New York, NY: Cambridge University Press; 2002.

26. Barsuk JH, Cohen ER, Caprio T, et al. Simulation-based education with mastery learning improves residents' lumbar puncture skills. *Neurology.* 2012; **79**(2): 132–7.

27. Nathan BR, Kincaid O. Does experience doing lumbar punctures result in expertise? A medical maxim bites the dust. *Neurology.* 2012; **79**(2): 115–16.

28. Ericsson KA, Krampe RT, Tesch-Römer C. The role of deliberate practice in the acquisition of expert performance. *Psychol Rev.* 1993; **100**(3): 363–406.

29. Ericsson KA, Charness N. Expert performance: its structure and acquisition. *Am Psychol.* 1994; **49**(8): 725–47.

30. McGaghie WC. Research opportunities in simulation-based medical education using deliberate practice. *Acad Emerg Med.* 2008; **15**(11): 995–1001.

31. McGaghie WC. Medical education research as translational science. *Sci Transl Med.* 2010; **2**(19): 19cm8.

32. McGaghie WC, Draycott TJ, Dunn WF, et al. Evaluating the impact of simulation on translational patient outcomes. *Simul Healthc.* 2011; 6 Suppl.: S42–7.

33. McGaghie WC, Pugh CM, Wayne DB. Fundamentals of educational research using clinical simulation. In: Kyle RR, Murray WB, editors. *Clinical Simulation:*

operations, engineering, and management. Burlington, MA: Academic Press; 2008. pp. 517–26.

34. Arthur W Jr., Bennett W Jr., Stanush PL, et al. Factors that influence skill decay and retention: a quantitative review and analysis. *Hum Perform.* 1998; **11**(1): 57–101.

35. Wayne DB, Siddall VJ, Butter J, et al. A longitudinal study of internal medicine residents' retention of advanced cardiac life support skills. *Acad Med.* 2006; **81**(Suppl. 10): S9–12.

36. Barsuk JH, Cohen ER, McGaghie WC, et al. Long-term retention of central venous catheter insertion skills after simulation-based mastery learning. *Acad Med.* 2010; **85**(Suppl. 10): S9–12.

37. Association of American Medical Colleges Institute for Improving Medical Education. *Effective Use of Educational Technology in Medical Education: Colloquium on Educational Technology; Recommendations and Guidelines for Medical Educators.* Washington, DC: Association of American Medical Colleges; 2007.

38. Issenberg SB. The scope of simulation-based healthcare education. *Simul Healthc.* 2006; **1**(4): 203–8.

39. Shadish WR, Cook TD, Campbell DT. *Experimental and Quasi-Experimental Designs for Generalized Causal Inference.* Boston, MA: Houghton Mifflin; 2002.

40. Hammond KR. Introduction to Brunswikian theory and methods. In: Hammond KR, Wascoe NE, editors. *Realizations of Brunswik's Representative Design.* New Directions for Methodology of Social and Behavioral Science, No. 3. San Francisco, CA: Jossey-Bass; 1980. pp. 1–11.

41. Hong L, Page SE. Groups of diverse problem solvers can outperform groups of high-ability problem solvers. *Proc Nat Acad Sci USA.* 2004; **101**(46): 16385–9.

42. Wuchty S, Jones BF, Uzzi B. The increasing dominance of teams in production of knowledge. *Science.* 2007; **316**(5827): 1036–9.

43. Bennett LM, Gadlin H. Collaboration and team science: from theory to practice. *J Investig Med.* 2012; **60**(5): 768–75.

44. Maxwell SE, Delaney HD. *Designing Experiments and Analyzing Data.* 2nd ed. Mahwah, NJ: Lawrence Erlbaum Associates; 2004.

45. Regehr G. The experimental tradition. In: Norman GR, van der Vleuten CPM, Newble DI, editors. *International Handbook of Research in Medical Education.* Dordrecht, the Netherlands: Kluwer Academic Publishers; 2002. pp. 5–44.

46. Norman GR, van der Vleuten CPM, Newble DI, editors. *International Handbook of Research in Medical Education.* Dordrecht, the Netherlands: Kluwer Academic Publishers; 2002.

47. Harris IB. Qualitative methods. In: Norman GR, van der Vleuten CPM, Newble DI, editors. *International Handbook of Research in Medical Education.* Dordrecht, the Netherlands: Kluwer Academic Publishers; 2002. pp. 45–95.

48. Becker HS, Geer B, Hughes EC, et al. *Boys in White: student culture in medical school.* Chicago, IL: University of Chicago Press; 1961.

49. Mizrahi T. *Getting Rid of Patients: contradictions in the socialization of physicians.* New Brunswick, NJ: Rutgers University Press; 1986.

50. Bosk CL. *Forgive and Remember: managing medical failure.* Chicago, IL: University of Chicago Press; 2003.
51. Hinder S, Greenhalgh T. "This does my head in." Ethnographic study of self-management by people with diabetes. *BMC Health Serv Res.* 2012; **12**: 83.
52. Côté L, Turgeon J. Appraising qualitative research articles in medicine and medical education. *Med Teacher.* 2005; **27**(1): 71–5.
53. Dixon-Woods M, Bosk CL, Aveling EL, et al. Explaining Michigan: developing an ex post theory of a quality improvement program. *Milbank Q.* 2011; **89**(2): 167–205.
54. Pronovost PJ, Needham D, Berenholtz S, et al. An intervention to decrease catheter-related bloodstream infections in the ICU. *N Engl J Med.* 2006; **355**(26): 2725–32.
55. Pronovost PJ, Goeschel CA, Colantuoni E, et al. Sustaining reductions in catheter related bloodstream infections in Michigan intensive care units: observational study. *BMJ.* 2010; **340**: c309.
56. Cresswell JW, Klassen AC, Plano Clark VL, et al. *Best Practices for Mixed Methods Research in the Health Sciences.* Bethesda, MD: Office of Behavioral and Social Sciences Research, National Institutes of Health; 2011.
57. Lopez-Fernandez O, Molina-Azorin JF. The use of mixed methods research in the field of behavioural sciences. *Qual Quant.* 2011; **45**(6): 1459–72.
58. Barsuk JH, McGaghie WC, Cohen ER, et al. Simulation-based mastery learning reduces complications during central venous catheter insertion in a medical intensive care unit. *Crit Care Med.* 2009; **37**(10): 2697–701.
59. Barsuk JH, Cohen ER, Feinglass J, et al. Use of simulation-based education to reduce catheter-related bloodstream infections. *Arch Intern Med.* 2009; **169**(15): 1420–3.
60. Barsuk JH, Cohen ER, Feinglass J, et al. Unexpected collateral effects of simulation-based medical education. *Acad Med.* 2011; **86**(12): 1513–17.
61. Cohen ER, Barsuk JH, McGaghie WC, et al. Raising the bar: reassessing standards for procedural competence. *Teach Learn Med.* 2013; **25**: in press.
62. Cohen ER, Feinglass J, Barsuk JH, et al. Cost savings from reduced catheter-related bloodstream infection after simulation-based education for residents in a medical intensive care unit. *Simul Healthc.* 2010; **5**(2): 98–102.
63. Implementation Science. *About Implementation Science: aims & scope.* Available at: www.implementationscience.com/about (accessed June 28, 2012).
64. Bonham AC, Solomon MZ. Moving comparative effectiveness research into practice: implementation science and the role of academic medicine. *Health Aff (Millwood).* 2010; **29**(10): 1901–5.
65. Carroll JB. A model of school learning. *Teach Coll Rec.* 1963; **64**(8): 723–33.
66. Keller FS. "Good-bye, teacher . . ." *J Appl Beh Anal.* 1968; **1**(1): 79–89.
67. Bloom BS. Time and learning. *Am Psychol.* 1974; **29**(9): 682–8.

Index

References in **bold** denote tables and figures.